Cranio-Maxillofacial Surgery - Orthognathic and Orthodontic Techniques

Edited by Farid Bourzgui

Published in London, United Kingdom

Cranio-Maxillofacial Surgery - Orthognathic and Orthodontic Techniques
http://dx.doi.org/10.5772/intechopen.1005992
Edited by Farid Bourzgui

Contributors
Cynthia Minerva Gonzalez-Cantu, Devin Su, Fadia Awadalkreem, Farid Bourzgui, Farid El Quars, Gloria Francesca Pia Bennici, Haifa Kamal, Hossam Barghash, Joan Birbe, Melissa Fernanda Ochoa Cortez, Moncef Boutissante, Orazio Bennici, Ruchi Pathak Kaul, Soukaina Sahim, Sushma Sagar, Yanko Castro-Govea, Zineb Safi-Eddine

First published in London, United Kingdom, 2025 by IntechOpen
IntechOpen is the global imprint of INTECHOPEN LIMITED, registered in England and Wales, registration number: 11086078, 167-169 Great Portland Street, London, W1W 5PF, United Kingdom

For EU product safety concerns: IN TECH d.o.o., Prolaz Marije Krucifikse Kozulić 3, 51000 Rijeka, Croatia, info@intechopen.com or visit our website at intechopen.com.

British Library Cataloguing-in-Publication Data
A catalogue record for this book is available from the British Library

Cranio-Maxillofacial Surgery - Orthognathic and Orthodontic Techniques
Edited by Farid Bourzgui
p. cm.
Print ISBN 978-1-83634-893-1
Online ISBN 978-1-83634-892-4
eBook (PDF) ISBN 978-1-83634-894-8

Meet the editor

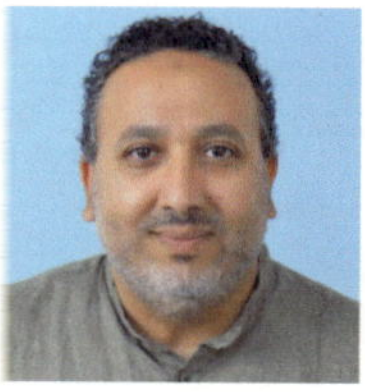

Prof. Farid Bourzgui obtained his DMD and his DNSO option in Orthodontics at the Dental School, University Hassan II of Casablanca, Morocco, in 1995 and 2000, respectively. Currently, Prof. Bourzgui is a Professor of Orthodontics in the Dental School at Hassan II University of Casablanca, Morocco. In addition to his educational qualifications, Prof. Bourzgui has served as the Head of the Orthodontics and Dentofacial Orthopedics Department from 2013 to 2020 and as a member of the Council of the Casablanca Dental School. He is the author of numerous articles and scientific chapters, as well as the editor of several books.

Contents

Preface

The cranio-maxillofacial region is a crucial anatomical area, constituting the cephalic extremity, which includes many noble elements of the human body. This area is anatomically, physiologically, and pathophysiologically complex and is also the site of numerous medical and surgical disciplines. These particularities gave rise to the idea for this book, which will enable readers to benefit from the shared skills and experiences in the vast field of cranio-maxillofacial surgery.

This book, therefore, presents an opportunity for a wide range of researchers and clinicians to update and establish the state of knowledge by contributing a small stone to this great edifice of understanding, expertise, and clinical practice in the field of maxillofacial surgery.

To this end, the book is divided into three sections. The first section, entitled "Background and Overview", outlines the theoretical framework of the subject by recalling the history of orthognathic surgery and reviewing the surgical techniques and procedures. The second one, entitled "Techniques and Procedures", reviews the details of surgical techniques and procedures. The last one, entitled "Artificial Intelligence and Workflow", is where the authors focus on the future vision of our practice by assessing the place of artificial intelligence, workflow, three-dimensional imaging, and digital printing in our daily practice.

This book is intended for all practitioners working on the cephalic extremity, medical and dental students and residents, as well as anyone else interested in the subject.

Before closing this preface, I'd like to thank all the authors and everyone else who has made this book possible, enabling it to be shared in an easily and openly accessible way.

Farid Bourzgui
Dental School,
University of Hassan II Casablanca,
Casablanca, Morocco

Section 1

Background and Overview

Chapter 1

History of Orthognathic Surgery and Its Interdisciplinarity with Orthodontics

Farid Bourzgui, Zineb Safi-Eddine and Farid El Quars

Abstract

Orthognathic surgery, a key subfield within cranio-maxillofacial surgery, plays a crucial role in the treatment of skeletal deformities of the jaws and face, offering significant improvements in both function and facial aesthetics, as well as enhancing patients' overall quality of life. The historical foundations of orthognathic surgery trace back to René Le Fort's classification of midface fracture patterns in the early twentieth century, which laid the groundwork for modern osteotomy techniques. Subsequent contributions from surgeons such as Hugo Obwegeser, who introduced the bilateral sagittal split osteotomy, marked transformative milestones in elective jaw surgery. Over the past century, orthognathic surgery has advanced considerably, fueled by enhanced surgical techniques and increased interdisciplinary collaboration. A major milestone in this progress was the integration of orthodontics, which marked a pivotal shift in the approach to treating patients. It has highlighted the critical role of precise occlusion in the achievement of optimal surgical outcomes. Thus, the aim of this review is to provide an overview of the history of orthognathic surgery and to explore its interdisciplinarity with orthodontics.

Keywords: orthognathic surgery, orthodontics, history, maxillar osteotomies, mandibular osteotomies, genioplasty

1. Introduction

Dentofacial anomalies, characterized by irregularities in the maxillary and mandibular regions, can significantly impact both aesthetics and functionality, often arising from a combination of genetic and environmental factors [1]. While orthodontics alone can address minor discrepancies, severe deformities typically require surgical intervention to achieve effective correction.

In such cases, orthognathic surgery becomes essential, targeting maxillomandibular dysmorphologies to resolve occlusal disorders and improve facial harmony, thereby meeting both functional and aesthetic objectives. This approach includes a range of surgical techniques tailored to individual patient needs, with commonly performed procedures.

It was *Simon P. Hullihen* who first performed orthognathic surgery in 1847 [2]. Then the history of this procedure got deeply intertwined with advancements in the management of facial trauma, beginning with *René Le Fort's* pioneering work on midface fracture patterns, which later formed the basis for elective osteotomies developed by visionaries like *Wassermund, Trauner, Paul Tessier, Hugo Obwegeser, and William Bell*, to name a few [3].

The development of orthognathic surgery is often recounted through the innovative techniques introduced by its pioneers. The field has been further transformed by contemporary technological advancements like digital imaging and virtual surgical planning, which give surgeons a better understanding of three-dimensional jaw movements and increase their ability to precisely navigate complex anatomy. However, this field extends far beyond a simple collection of surgical methods. Breakthroughs in the broader craniofacial treatment domain have significantly improved both treatment planning and the evaluation of outcomes, making surgical interventions more reliable and successful.

Therefore, the aim of this chapter is to examine the historical development of orthognathic surgery, focusing on the major turning points that have led to the establishment of the current concepts of this discipline, culminating to the codification of the collaboration between orthodontics and orthognathic surgery. This chapter also focuses on the future directions of this collaboration.

2. Maxillary osteotomies/osteotomy

2.1 The Le Fort I-type maxillary osteotomy

The nomenclature for the Le Fort fractures and corresponding osteotomies owes its origin to *René Le Fort's* 1901 experiments on cadaveric skulls, which identified natural planes of maxillary and facial fractures and led to the identification of consistent fracture patterns in the maxilla and midface (**Figure 1**) [5]. These fractures, classified as Le Fort I, II, and III, revolutionized orthognathic surgery (**Figure 2**) [6]. Surgeons soon began using these naturally occurring fracture planes to guide surgical interventions, allowing for the controlled mobilization of the maxilla in therapeutic procedures such as osteotomies [4].

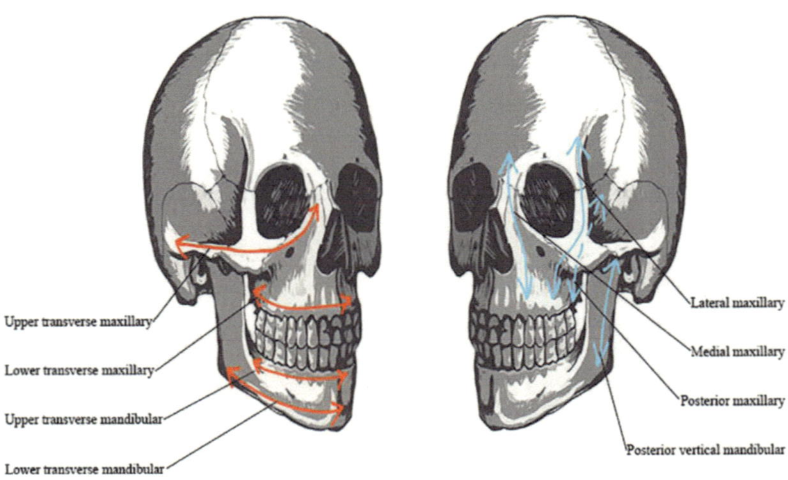

Figure 1.
Vertical and transverse buttress systems [4].

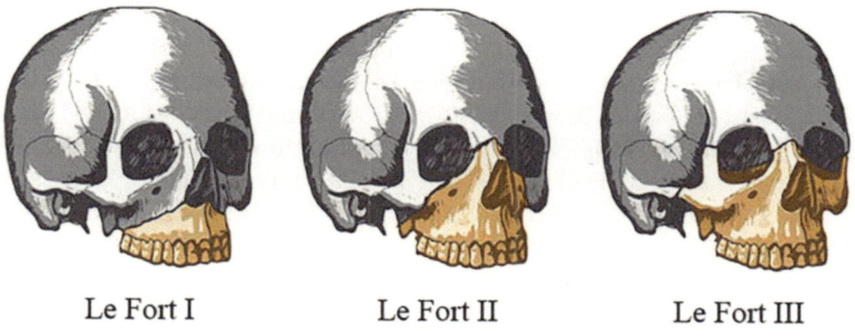

Figure 2.
Le Fort fracture patterns [4].

The Le Fort I osteotomy, a cornerstone in craniofacial surgery, has its roots deeply embedded in the nineteenth century, with its development shaped by numerous surgeons over the decades (**Figure 3**).

The initial conceptual framework for the procedure was laid by *Bernhard Rudolf Konrad von Langenbeck* (1810–1887) in 1859 [7]. *Von Langenbeck's* technique, detailed in 1861, demonstrated the potential for horizontally cutting through the maxilla from the sphenopalatine foramen forward, facilitating surgical access for polyp removal. In 1861, he demonstrated a technique termed "osteo-plastic resection of the maxilla" and described it as the potential for horizontally cutting through the maxilla from the sphenopalatine foramen forward, facilitating surgical access for polyp removal. This horizontal osteotomy of the upper jaw at the level later identified as the Le Fort I fracture line enabled temporary mobilization and inferior displacement of the upper jaw, pedicled on its soft tissue attachments, which would subsequently heal in its original position.

At the time, these procedures were referred to as "osteo-plastic" or "temporary" resections, as prior surgeries for nasopharyngeal tumors typically involved the complete removal of the maxilla [7, 8]. The hemimaxilla was transversely cut above the level of the dental roots and then downfractured to provide access to the posterior nasopharynx. The innovative aspect of the European technique was that

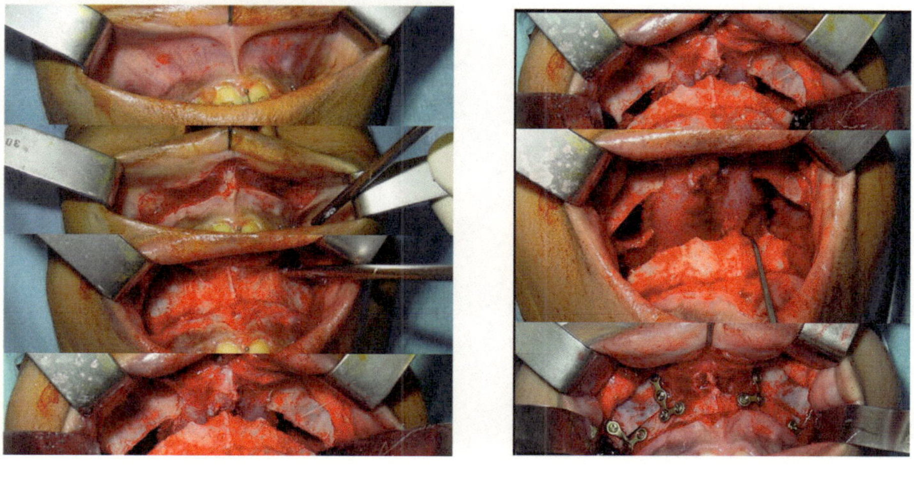

Figure 3.
Clinical illustrations of a Le Fort I osteotomy (original creations).

the hemimaxilla was repositioned, secured with wire, and allowed to heal. *Cheever* advanced the technique by extending the hemimaxillary osteotomy into a bilateral procedure, which came to be known as Cheever's double operation [8].

In 1870, *David Williams Cheever* (1831–1915) authored a report for the *First Medical and Surgical Report of the Boston City Hospital*, in which he described what is now recognized as the Le Fort I osteotomy [9]. This report predates Le Fort's own publications on experimental facial fracture lines by 31 years. Cheever also included a quote from Langenbeck, who stated that the osteoplastic resection of both jaws up to that time had never been performed in Germany or in Europe [8, 9]. The maxilla was then divided horizontally and tilted inferiorly [10].

In 1893, *Lanz* provided an account of a technique developed earlier by Kocher, involving a midline incision of the upper lip to expose the maxilla. He extended von Langenbeck's 1859 method by dividing the maxilla sagittally and expanding it along the midline, which allowed for access to the pituitary fossa. Lanz's diagram from 1893 (**Figure 4**) described the procedure as a two-section Le Fort I osteotomy. He also quoted von Dieffenbach, who remarked on the challenging nature of maxillary resection, emphasizing the need for a skilled surgeon capable of controlling bleeding [10].

According to Drommer [10], and by the turn of the century, several reports of reasonably large series on the temporary mobilization of the maxilla appeared, including those by Winkler (1903), Hertle (1905), Payer (1904), Borchardt (1908), Vorschiitz (1908), Kocher (1909) in Ref. [10].

Loewe conducted extensive experimental work on the temporary osteotomy of the maxilla. In his "Surgery of the Nose" (1905), he presented a historical summary of the methods up to that point, discussed technical difficulties such as bleeding, and introduced wire fixation [10].

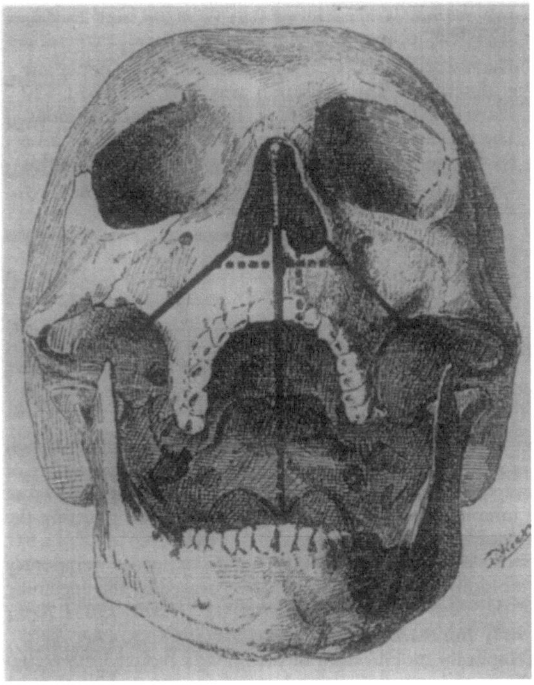

Figure 4.
Osteoplastic section of both halves of the maxilla (Kocher's method) (Lanz, 1893) [10].

Wassmund recognized the necessity of correcting midface deformities with a total maxillary osteotomy [11] and described the first LeFort I osteotomy for the correction of dentofacial deformities in 1921 [11] using orthopedic traction instead of intraoperative mobilization [12]. He carried out the first such procedure, which involved dividing the maxilla using a Guerin's transverse fracture with a chisel, without cutting the pterygoid plates. The maxilla was displaced after 14 days using intermaxillary elastic bands [10, 12]. For displacement, he used elastic bands; however, relapse resulted from the absence of bone grafting.

In 1934, Georg Axhausen from Kiel, Germany, was the first to describe an osteotomy that involved intraoperative mobilization of the maxilla to correct an open bite [13]. He performed a Le Fort I osteotomy along with an additional vertical osteotomy to advance a malunited maxillary fracture. He published three articles describing osteotomies of the maxilla for the correction of its position after trauma (1934) [13] and in cases due to other etiological factors resulting in anomalies of the maxilla (1936 and 1939) (**Figure 5**) [14, 15].

A crucial moment came in 1942 when Schuchardt described a two-stage Le Fort I osteotomy involving pterygomaxillary separation. He separated the pterygomaxillary junction, allowing anterior repositioning, and utilized external traction with weights for postoperative maxillary advancement, addressing issues of vascular supply preservation [16].

Subsequent recommendations by Moore and Ward in 1949 emphasized horizontal transection of the pterygoid plates for improved outcomes [17]. The 1950s marked a transition toward modern techniques. In 1954, Gillies and Rowe described a maxillary osteotomy in a cleft patient, which included maxillary advancement and the use of autogenous bone grafts [18]. However, they also had to set back the mandible, resulting in a "flattened" profile, indicating that the desired maxillary advancement was not fully achieved. Gillies and Rowe later presented additional cases involving cleft patients [18, 19]. Most of the techniques described involved partial mobilization of the maxilla, followed by the application of some form of external orthopedic force to reposition it. However, these methods were associated with significant relapse rates [19].

By the 1960s, Hans-Peter Obwegeser revolutionized the Le Fort I osteotomy. His studies on the complete mobilization of the maxilla, including pterygomaxillary disjunction, allowed for precise repositioning without tissue resistance [20–25].

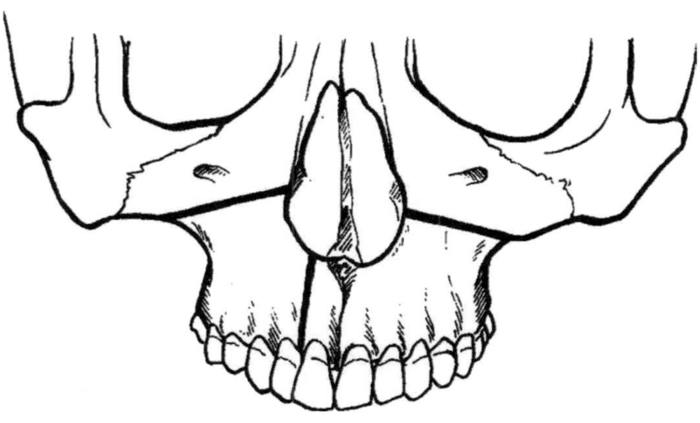

Figure 5.
Le Fort I osteotomy with an additional vertical bone cut for the correction of a malunited fracture (this technique was first described by Axhausen in 1934) [2].

Obwegeser introduced interposed bone grafts between the pterygoid plates and maxillary tuberosities, significantly enhancing stability and reducing relapse rates. Long-term follow-up studies, such as those by de Hailer, corroborated the effectiveness of Obwegeser's refinements, establishing the Le Fort I osteotomy as a foundational technique in maxillofacial surgery (**Figure 6**).

As for revascularization, from the late 1960s, studies conducted by William H. Bell significantly advanced the understanding of the biological foundations of maxillary (and mandibular) surgery and its techniques [26–33]. His work demonstrated that the maxilla could be sectioned at the Le Fort I level and even further segmented and repositioned, with only temporary ischemic effects and minimal impact on revascularization and bone healing. Through microangiography and histological analysis, it was shown that the vascular supply to the anterior maxillary segment remained intact when a soft tissue pedicle was preserved. This confirmed the biological importance of maintaining a viable labial/buccal or palatal pedicle to ensure blood flow to the osteotomized segment. In contrast, non-pedicled segments were found to undergo necrosis within 1 week. Bell's research also demonstrated that as long as vascularity was preserved during the osteotomy, bone union occurred within 6 weeks, and the dental pulp's vascularity was maintained, provided the osteotomies were performed at a sufficient distance from the root apices. His findings showed that the descending palatine arteries could be sacrificed without disrupting the blood supply, supporting the feasibility of osseous healing following a complete maxillary osteotomy. This work laid the biological foundation for performing a complete down-fracture of the maxilla [19].

2.2 The Le Fort II-type maxillary osteotomy

The Le Fort II-type osteotomy is one of the less frequently performed midfacial procedures, typically indicated for patients with severe nasomaxillary retrusion. While the exact individual who first performed the Le Fort II-type advancement osteotomy remains unclear, both Tessier and Obwegeser contributed to its development. In 1973, Henderson and Jackson formally described the procedure [19].

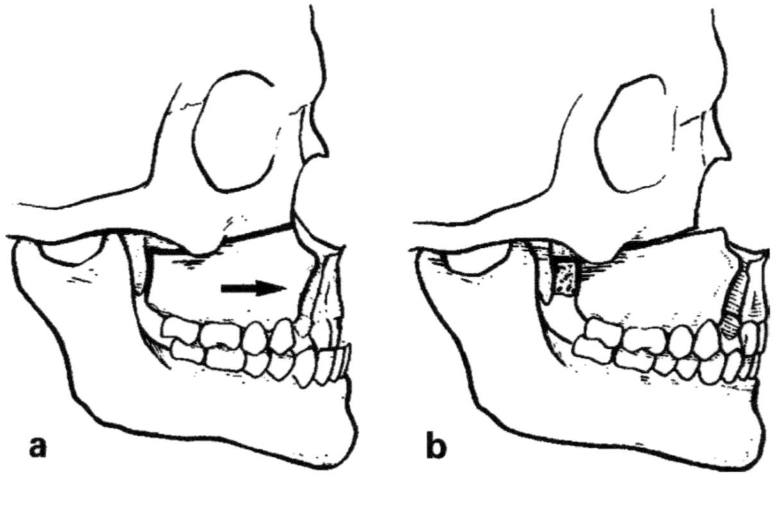

Figure 6.
Total maxillary advancement by a Le Fort I osteotomy in a cleft palate patient as published by Obwegeser in 1969 [2].

2.3 The Le Fort III-type maxillary osteotomy

Concerning Le Fort III, in 1943, Sir Harold Gillies in London performed the first radical advancement of a recessed face in an adult woman with Crouzon syndrome [34]. However, he never repeated the operation and discouraged other surgeons from attempting it, considering it too risky [34, 35].

In the 1960s, Paul Tessier and Gérard Guiot broke the barrier between the face and the cranium, allowing for combined operations around the orbits and forehead. This collaboration opened the door for close cooperation between plastic surgeons and neurosurgeons, especially for treating major malformations such as hypertelorism and significant facial retrusion [35].

In 1967, Paul Tessier published his techniques for mobilizing the middle third of the facial skeleton (Le Fort III-type osteotomy) and for dislocating the orbital curve to correct hypertelorism [36, 37]. He began to approach Gérard Guiot, a neurosurgeon at the Hospital Foch in Paris, where they both worked, with the idea of an intracranial approach to treat facial clefts with hypertelorism [34]. In response to Tessier's inquiry about the possibility of approaching the midface and the interorbital region through an intracranial frontal approach, Guiot famously replied, "Pourquoi pas?" ("Why not?"). This answer shattered the barrier between plastic surgery and neurosurgery [19, 34]. This moment marked the beginning of their groundbreaking collaboration. By the late 1960s, Tessier and Guiot started performing the combined approach, first cautiously with a frontal osteotomy, dissection of the anterior cranial base, and sacrificing the olfactory nerves: A dermal graft was placed to reinforce the dura, and the hypertelorism correction was done after several months. Later, it became possible to preserve the olfactory nerves in most cases, eliminating the need for this preliminary step [37].

In 1983, the International Society of Craniofacial Surgery was founded, with Paul Tessier as its first president. The organization's logo incorporated the words "Pourquoi pas?" in tribute to the collaboration between Tessier and Guiot [38].

3. Mandibular osteotomies

Simon P. Hullihen published a significant case report in 1849 in the *American Journal of Dental Science*, titled *"Case of Elongation of the Underjaw and Distortion of the Face and Neck, Caused by a Burn, Successfully Treated,"* which marked the first documented instance of true orthognathic surgery [3, 39]. He detailed the case of a 20-year-old woman who sought treatment for severe facial deformities resulting from a burn she sustained 15 years earlier. The burn caused significant scarring, pulling her head forward, restricting jaw movement, and leading to marked prognathism, with her chin nearly touching her sternum and her jaw projecting over an inch beyond her upper jaw. Hullihen devised a three-phase surgical plan:

1. Correcting the skeletal deformity of the mandible,

2. Resection of the large scar tissue on the right side of the face and neck, and

3. Correction of the lower lip defect.

He performed a wedge resection of the mandible bilaterally, similar to what would later be described as an anterior subapical osteotomy by Köle in 1959 [3]. Using a

V-shaped saw, Hullihen removed elongated bone portions and the first bicuspid on the left side, then performed a horizontal osteotomy of the upper mandible. Hullihen's pioneering procedure is even more impressive considering it was performed intraorally, employed the concept of immobilizing the osteotomized segments with an intraoral occlusal splint, and was carried out without the use of general anesthesia or antibiotics. Tragically, Hullihen's career was cut short at the age of 47 when he contracted typhoid pneumonia (**Figures** 7 and **8**). His obituary in Wheeling stated, "amongst American surgeons he had no superior, probably no equal. In dentistry, he was not equaled in America" [19].

Another attempt to address mandibular prognathism did not occur for nearly 50 years [19]. In 1898, James Whipple reported a case involving a patient whom he had followed for several years [40]. Whipple noted that the lower jaw exhibited significant prognathism, with a space appearing between the first and second bicuspids. Whipple referred the patient to Edward H. Angle (1855–1930), a pioneer of modern orthodontics, in 1896. Angle suggested a "double resection of the lower maxilla" to correct the severe protrusion [41]. However, the patient opted against surgery [40].

In 1897, Vilray Papin Blair (1871–1955) performed the first "double resection of the mandible" on the same patient [40]. This procedure involved a bilateral ostectomy of the mandibular body *via* an extraoral approach, with parallel cuts in the premolar regions and removal of the osteotomized blocks. Copper wire interosseous ligatures were used to secure the bony segments. Four months later, Whipple fabricated gold crowns for the posterior teeth to improve the occlusion. Whipple's publication of

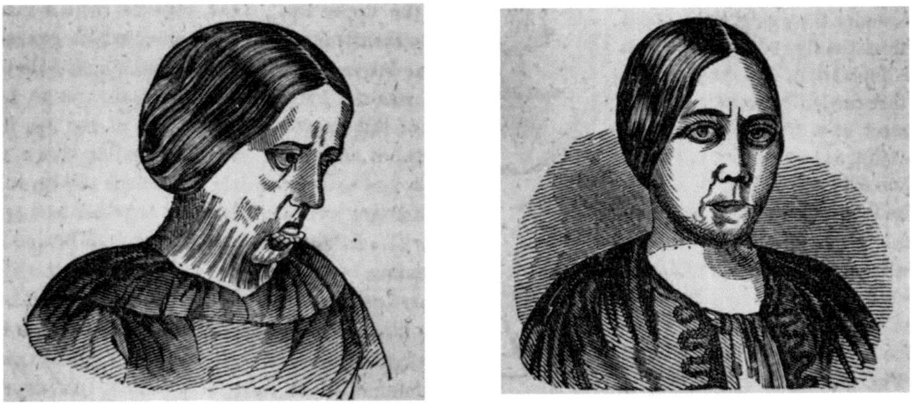

Figure 7.
Preoperative and postoperative appearance (from Hullihen SP: Case of elongation of the underjaw and distortion of the face and neck, caused by a burn, successfully treated. Am J Dent Sci 9:157, 1849) *[39]*.

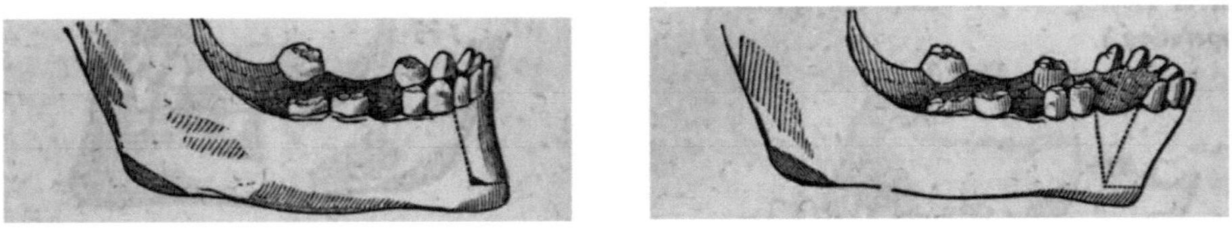

Figure 8.
A wedge ostectomy and setback of the anterior mandible via *an intraoral approach* (from Hullihen SP: Case of elongation of the underjaw and distortion of the face and neck, caused by a burn, successfully treated. Am J Dent Sci 9:157, 1849) *[39]*.

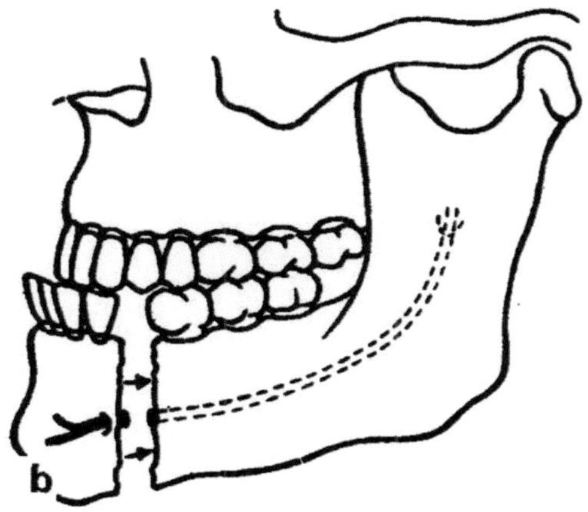

Figure 9.
Ostectomy of the mandibular body as performed by Blair in 1897 in the so-called "St Louis operation" [2].

Blair's procedure, which was written without Blair's direct involvement as he was out of the country, marked a significant step in the advancement of orthognathic surgery (**Figure 9**) [40].

Blair was also the first to recognize the importance of collaboration between orthodontists and surgeons, as highlighted in his 1907 article [42]. During World War I, he served as chief consultant to the American military forces. After the war, he and Robert Ivy established military hospital centers for treating facial and jaw injuries. This marked the end of the early period of orthognathic surgery in the U.S., with the specialty not being revisited for many years (**Figure 10**).

Rodrigues Ottolengui (1861–1937) criticized Angle's use of a splint in mandibular osteotomy procedures, suggesting instead a single template splint to guide postoperative occlusion, a concept ahead of its time and similar to modern surgical wafer splints [43]. He acknowledged Angle's efforts to advance the procedure for future collaboration between surgeons and orthodontists (**Figure 11**).

Mandibular orthognathic surgery in the nineteenth century saw limited progress in Europe, with key exceptions: In 1897, Paul Berger in Lyon described the first bilateral condylectomy to correct mandibular prognathism, [44] a technique later practiced by other French surgeons like Mathieu Jaboulay and Léon Bérard [2]. This approach involved removing the condyles *via* a preauricular incision. His work marked a significant advancement in orthognathic surgery, though Robert Henry Ivy (1881–1974) later pointed out that the procedure often resulted in suboptimal dental occlusion [45]. Berger and Mikulicz (head of the surgery department of the University of Breslau (now Wroclaw, Poland)) are credited with being the first to wear a surgical mask during operations to reduce the risk of infection [46]. It is important to note that earlier, the first documented condylar resection was performed by George Murray Humphry (1820–1896) in 1856 at Addenbrooke's Hospital in Cambridge, treating a young woman with condylar hyperplasia. His successful extraoral resection corrected the asymmetry and improved occlusion and chewing function (**Figure 12**) [47].

In 1908, Max Ballin (1869–1934) proposed removing teeth at the site of the planned ostectomy months before surgery to minimize infection risk. This idea, presented at the American Society of Orthodontists and published in Ottolengui's journal, sparked noteworthy discussion (**Figure 13**) [48].

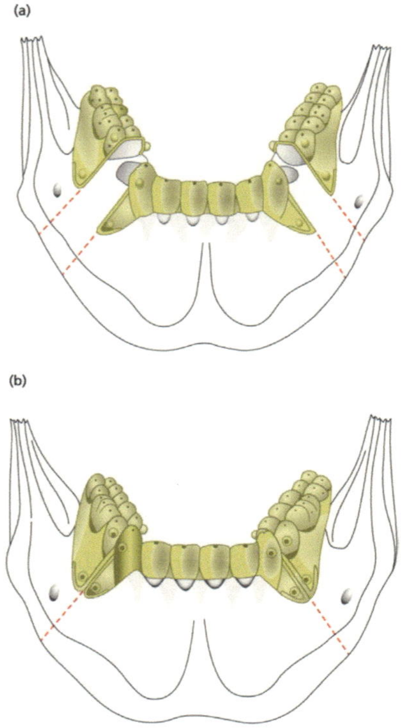

Figure 10.
Cast gold splints for postoperative fixation suggested by Edward Angle. (a) Pre-mandibular body ostectomy. (b) Postoperative [19].

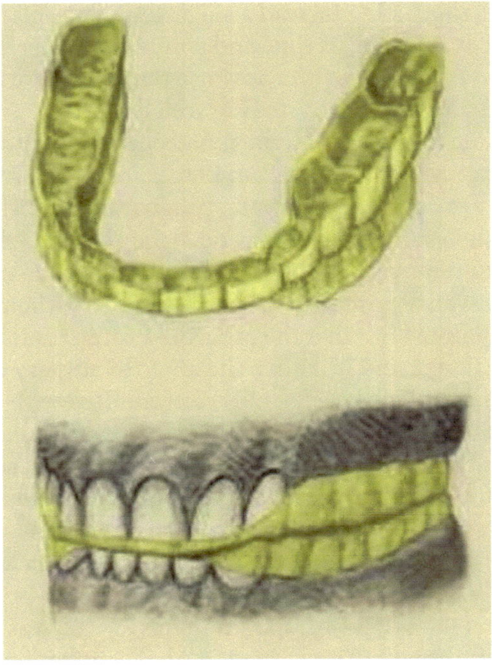

Figure 11.
Ottolengui surgical splint [43].

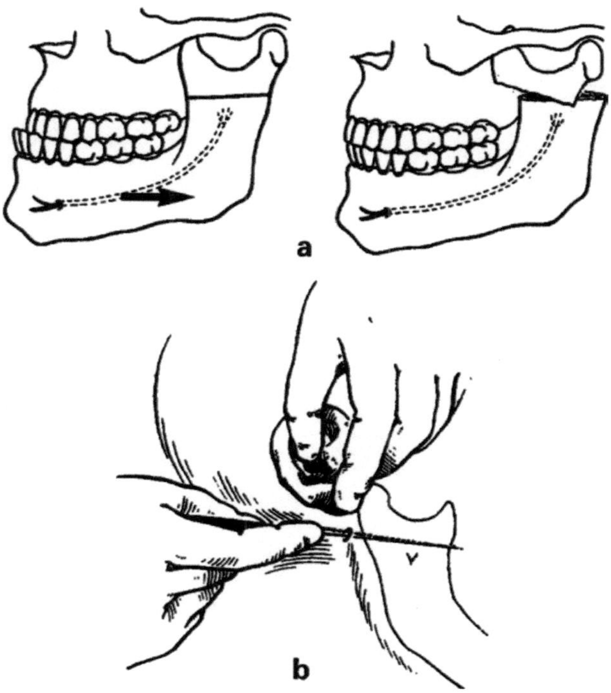

Figure 12.
(a) The technique of condylectomy for the correction of mandibular prognathism as described by Berger in 1897, by Babcock in 1909, and later by Bruhn in 1921. (b) Blind technique of horizontal osteotomy of the ramus according to Bruhn-Lindemann [2].

Between 1906 and 1917, several key advancements were made in orthognathic surgery. In 1906, Anton Freiherr von Eiselsberg introduced the osteotomy in progressive levels to increase bone contact, later refined by Pichler and Trauner. In 1912, William M. Harsha improved surgical outcomes by preserving the neurovascular bundle during extraoral mandibular resection. In 1917, Thomas G. Aller proposed an intraoral approach to remove a bony wedge for mandibular deformities, emphasizing the need for orthodontic involvement to optimize occlusion and treatment results [19]. During this period, the horizontal osteotomy of the ramus and condylar osteotomy were initially considered relatively simple procedures, but they yielded unsatisfactory results [2]. Common complications included relapse and open bite problems, primarily due to small bony contact areas and fragment dislocations caused by muscle pull. Efforts were made to improve the procedures between 1920 and 1940 with numerous proposals: Several renowned maxillofacial surgeons in Austria and Germany, including Perthes (1922) from Tübingen, Pichler (1928) from Vienna, Wassmund (1935) from Berlin, and Hofer (1936) from Linz, introduced new methods and bone cuts to address skeletal mandibular deformities [2]. During this period, progress in orthognathic surgery in the USA and other European countries was minimal. In 1928, Limberg, a Russian surgeon trained in part by Ivy in the United States, introduced new surgical techniques for treating jaw deformities [49]. In 1931, at the Second International Orthodontic Congress in London, Kazanjian presented a technique for treating mandibular prognathism with extraoral body ostectomies using a Gigli saw and surgical bur, emphasizing postoperative immobilization with an intraoral orthodontic appliance. This approach was published in 1932 (**Figure 14**) [50].

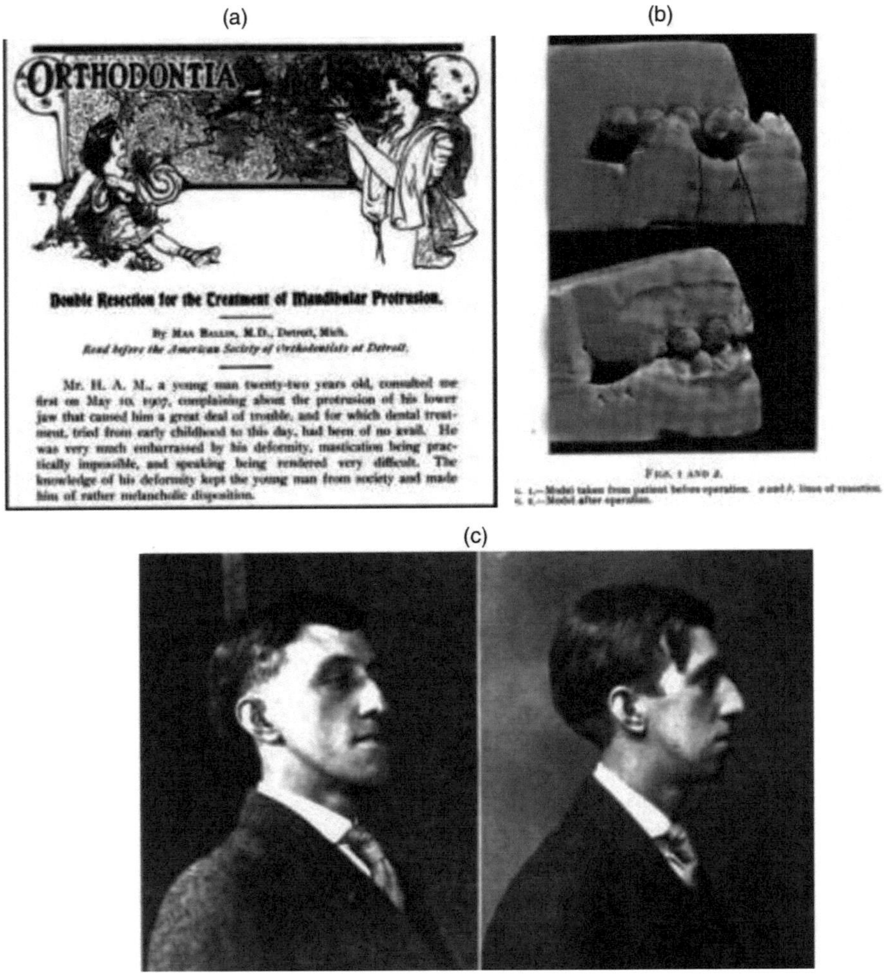

Figure 13.
(a) Ballin's paper from 1908. (b) Patient's dental models. (c) Patient's preoperative and postoperative facial appearance [47].

Between 1932 and 1940, Matthew Henry Cryer developed an electrically operated surgical engine for bone cutting and proposed a semicircular osteotomy for vertical mandibular rotation, although it led to posterior open bite and was not widely adopted [51]. In the 1950s, Ben Fickling and Gordon Fordyce [52] suggested using cancellous bone from the iliac crest or resected mandibular bone to promote bony union. While these advances improved outcomes, Hovell warned about potential complications related to bony healing [53]. However, progress in orthognathic surgery stagnated during World War II, as most surgeons were focused on treating facial injuries and reconstructive procedures. It was not until the early 1950s that orthognathic surgery began to emerge as a distinct specialty, leading to global success [2].

The foundations of modern orthognathic surgery were established in central Europe, particularly in Vienna and Graz, as well as Berlin and Hamburg. The "Vienna School" of maxillofacial surgery was founded by Pichler [54], who was succeeded by his pupil Trauner in 1955. Trauner advocated the inverted L osteotomy of the ramus

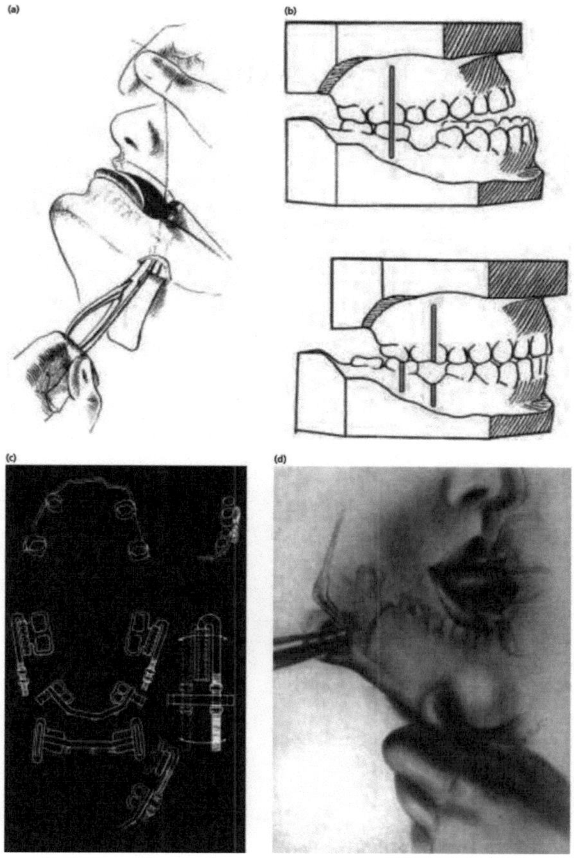

Figure 14.
(a) Kazanjian's use of a Gigli saw for a mandibular body ostectomy and setback. (b) Measurement of the amount of bone removal required using study models. (c) Orthodontic splint, cemented preoperatively. (d) Use of a surgical bur for an ostectomy. (e) Preoperative anterior open bite. (f) Postoperative result [19, 50].

for the correction of mandibular prognathism [54, 55]. He also trained Heinz Kölle and Hugo Obwegeser, who played pivotal roles in advancing orthognathic surgery (**Figure 15**) [56].

The real breakthrough in orthognathic surgery, however, came from Kölle and Obwegeser, the latter of whom was appointed chair of oral and maxillofacial surgery in Zurich in 1956, significantly advancing the field.

On February 17, 1953, Obwegeser performed the first sagittal split osteotomy of the mandibular ramus unilaterally *via* an intraoral approach [57]. Interested in collaborating, Trauner suggested they operate together: On one side, his reverse L-shaped osteotomy with the combined extraoral-intraoral approach, and on the other, Obwegeser's sagittal split of the ramus performed transorally.

The case involved a 27-year-old edentulous woman with a protruding mandible (**Figure 16**). Acrylic splints were placed on the jaws for postoperative intermaxillary fixation. The procedure was carried out with the patient in a half-sitting position and under local anesthesia, with Trauner and Obwegeser as the primary surgeons and H. Köle assisting. Trauner completed his part of the surgery first. Obwegeser then instructed the patient to open her mouth wide and made a mucosal incision along the left ascending ramus. Using a Stichsäge (keyhole) saw, he cut through the cortical plates.

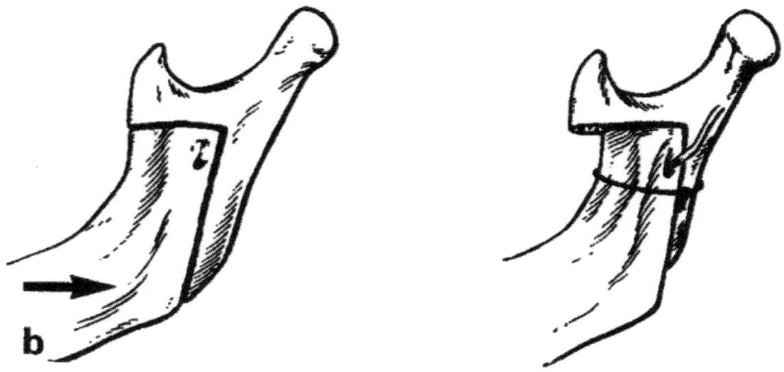

Figure 15.
Inverted L osteotomy of the ramus for the correction of mandibular prognathism by Trauner [54, 55].

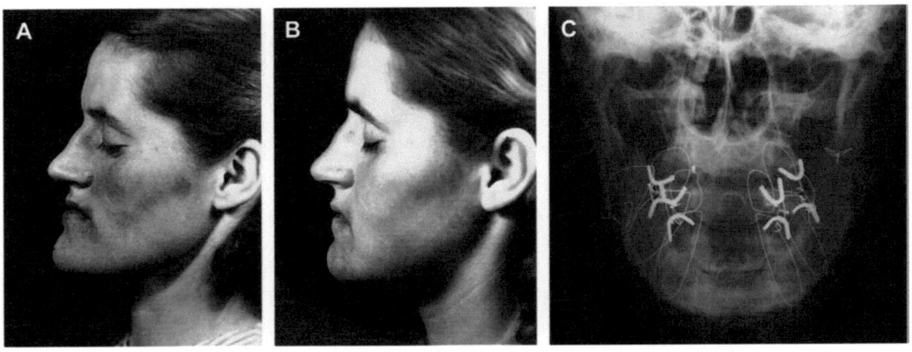

Figure 16.
The first attempt of the transoral sagittal split of the left ramus on February 17, 1953, by H. Obwegeser and a transcutaneous inverted L procedure on the right side by R. Trauner. Patient's profile (A) before and (B) after the procedure. (C) The postoperative radiograph [57].

First, he cut the lateral cortical plate from the inner to the outer angle of the jaw and then the medial cortical plate above the lingula, extending back to the posterior border. He connected these cuts along the anterior border of the ramus with a fissure bur. However, when he attempted to split the ramus with an osteotome, it unexpectedly shattered instead of splitting. The mandible was repositioned with splints, and the patient was kept in intermaxillary wire fixation for the postoperative period (**Figure 17**).

For the sagittal splitting of the rami procedure, the next variation involved repositioning the lateral corticotomy to increase the surface area of bony contact, thereby improving union and accommodating a wider range of advancement for the distal segment. This change entailed orienting the lateral corticotomy of the ramus horizontally, as opposed to the vertical corticotomy typically performed on the mandibular body [58].

In 1957, G. Dal Pont arrived in Zurich as a trainee under Professor Schmuziger and assisted both Schmuziger and Obwegeser in all cases. By observing the procedure, Dal Pont conceived the idea of shifting the lateral corticotomy from the horizontal ramus to the vertical mandibular body. They tested this approach with Dal Pont's assistance, and it proved successful [58].

In late 1958, Dal Pont returned to Italy and independently published the modification in 1959 in Italian [59] and in 1961 in the American literature [60] without

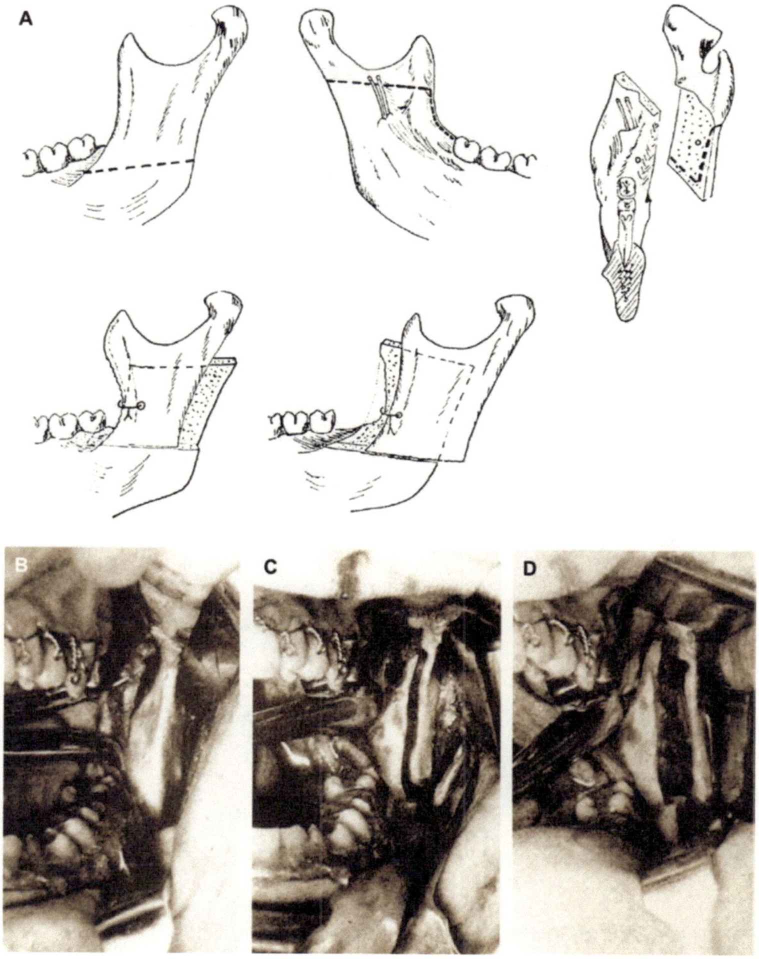

Figure 17.
Illustration from the publication of the sagittal splitting procedure in the 1957 English article by Trauner and Obwegeser [58].

including Obwegeser as a coauthor or acknowledging that the case shown in his article was Obwegeser's patient or that the modification was based on Obwegeser's original technique (**Figure 18**) [58–60].

Obwegeser continued to refine his sagittal split technique with minor modifications. Later, further adjustments were proposed by American military oral surgeon Ervin Eugene Hunsuck in 1968 [61]. He recommended performing an incomplete horizontal osteotomy on the medial side of the ramus, stopping behind the lingula instead of extending to the posterior border of the ramus. This approach relied on vertical cleavage lines within the mandible to complete the split. This modification minimized the risk of inadvertently severing vessels at the posterior region and thereby reduced the potential for bleeding [19, 61].

In 1977, Bruce Epker further modified the Hunsuck approach, advocating for minimal soft tissue dissection to reduce postoperative edema. He recommended that the periosteum and masseter muscles should not be reflected laterally from the

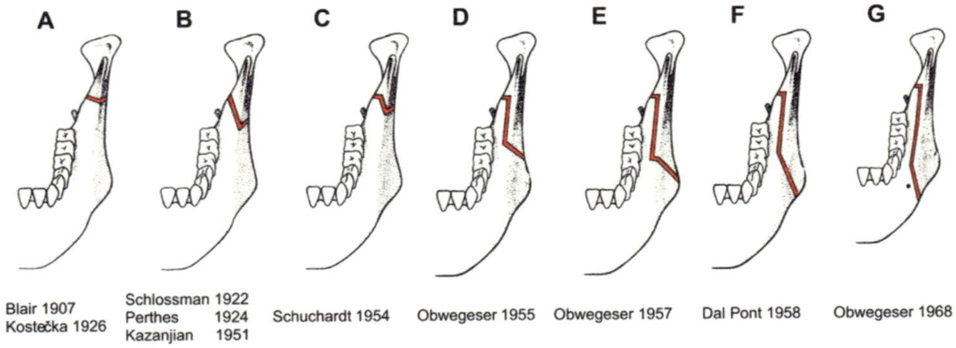

Figure 18.
Evolution of the mandibular osteotomies. (A) Blair, 1907 (B) Schlössmann-Perthes-Kazanjian, 1922–1951 (C) Schuchardt, 1954 (D) Obwegeser, 1955 (E) Obwegeser, 1957 (F) Dal Pont, 1958 (G) Obwegeser, 1968 [58]. The dates indicate the publication and not the date of the first procedure by the surgeon.

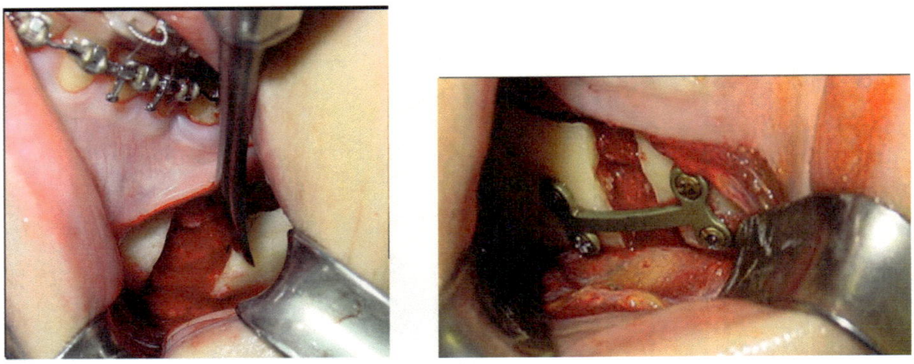

Figure 19.
Clinical illustrations of a sagittal osteotomy of the ascending ramus (Original figure).

mandibular ramus and that stripping the pterygomasseteric sling at the inferior-posterior border of the mandible was unnecessary, as the proximal segment was not being repositioned (**Figure 19**) [62].

4. Genioplasty

Until the mid to late 1950s, the correction of retrogenia was primarily done through onlay techniques *via* a submental incision, using autogenous bone or cartilage grafts, or alloplastic implants (like titanium, Silastic, and acrylic) to create chin prominence. While bone grafts initially yielded good results, they were often temporary due to resorption, requiring secondary procedures. Alloplastic materials, though permanent and easy to shape, were prone to complications such as infection, displacement, and erosion into the dental roots [58].

The first recorded surgical procedure to advance a recessive chin dates back to 1942, performed by Otto Hofer, who had trained under Hans Pichler (1887–1949) in Vienna [63]. Pichler, a distinguished oral surgeon, was the founder of the "Vienna School" of maxillofacial surgery succeeded by his pupil Trauner [2]. He was also notably known for performing over 30 operations on Sigmund Freud between 1923 and 1939 [64].

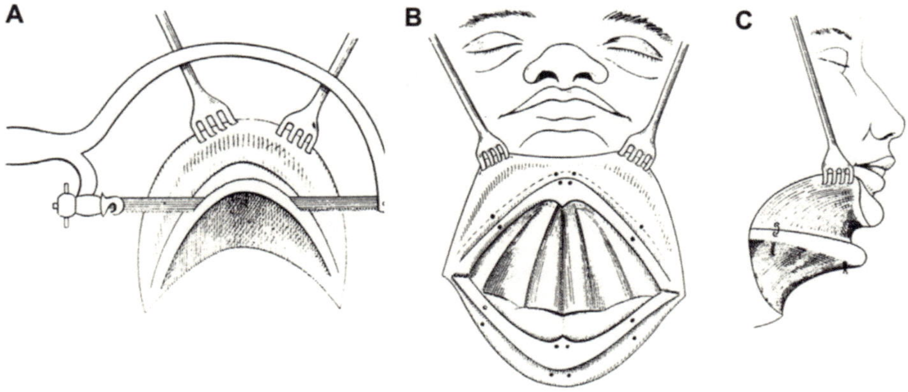

Figure 20.
Hofer's advancement genioplasty of the osseous chin, undertaken via *an extraoral approach on a cadaver [63].*

Hofer advanced the chin using an extraoral approach, though his paper did not mention that the procedure had been performed on a cadaver (**Figure 20**) [58].

The term "genioplasty" and the intraoral advancement approach were introduced by Obwegeser in 1957 [58].

In 1964, John Marquis Converse and Donald Wood-Smith published an article detailing various modifications of osseous genioplasty, including chin advancement, as well as the simultaneous reduction or augmentation of chin height and correction of asymmetry [65].

Following these developments, many variations of the procedure emerged: In 1947, Gillies and Millard reported a jumping genioplasty for a patient with Treacher-Collins syndrome *via* an external incision [66].

In 1957, Trauner and Obwegeser were the first to describe an intraoral approach to advance the chin, utilizing the anterior labial sulcus for access and circumandibular wires for stabilization [58].

In 1965, Otto Neuner introduced an intraoral advancement technique, while Obwegeser described a triple-step advancement in 1970 [67].

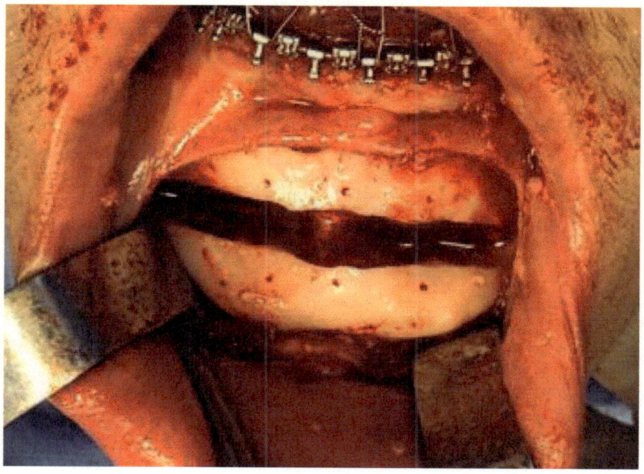

Figure 21.
Clinical illustrations of a genioplasty (Original figure).

Hinds and Kents first recognized the significance of preserving soft tissue attachments along the inferior segment in 1969 [66].

Over the years, various authors have contributed additional modifications in surgical access, osteotomy design, and fixation methods for genioplasty, noting that since 2007, genioplasty has been used to reposition and advance the genioglossus muscle for obstructive sleep apnea-hypopnea syndrome (**Figure 21**) [68].

5. Segmental maxillar osteotomy

5.1 Anterior segmental maxillar osteotomy

The first segmental maxillary osteotomy performed to correct a malocclusion, and thus considered the first maxillary orthognathic procedure, was carried out by the German surgeon Gunther Cohn-Stock in 1920 and published in 1921 [69]. In this paper, he presented two cases that were carried out in May and June of 1920 (**Figures 22** and **23**).

His technique involved the bilateral extraction of a maxillary premolar, a palatal approach to the anterior maxillary dentoalveolus, the removal of a wedge-shaped segment of bone, and retroclination of the dentoalveolus. This approach was effective for retroclining a proclined anterior maxillary dentoalveolus but was not suitable for bodily retrusion of a prominent dentoalveolus, as the maxillary incisors would inevitably retrocline [19, 69].

In his book [70], Martin Wassmund acknowledges Gunther Cohn-Stock as the first to perform this operation. However, many subsequent authors have overlooked Cohn-Stock's contribution and instead attributed the procedure to Wassmund. Some of these authors vaguely suggest that Cohn-Stock's operation was not entirely successful due to partial relapse (**Figure 24**) [69].

Martin Wassmund, as mentioned before, was a towering figure in maxillofacial surgery, known for being the first to perform a Le Fort I osteotomy for malocclusion correction, authoring several major textbooks, and playing a pivotal role in the establishment of the German Society of Maxillofacial Surgery after World War II.

In 1935, he introduced his renowned segmental setback of the anterior maxillary dentoalveolus. The procedure was carried out in two stages: initially, palatal bone was removed *via* the palate, and a month later, bone was removed through a buccal approach to facilitate the setback of the anterior maxilla (**Figure 25**).

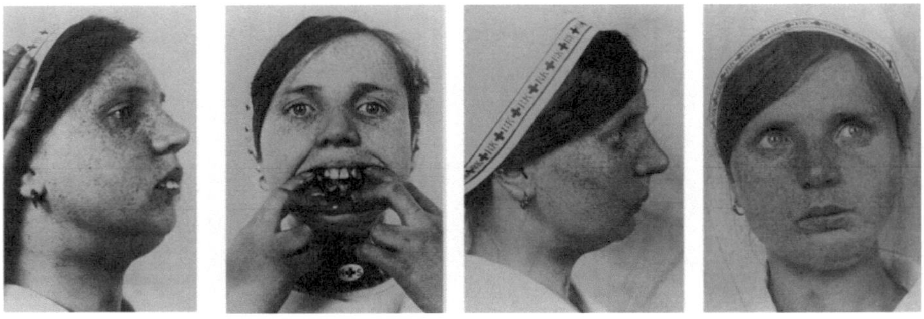

Figure 22.
Before and after photographs of Case l in Cohn-Stock's paper. (Dental models and X-rays not available) [69].

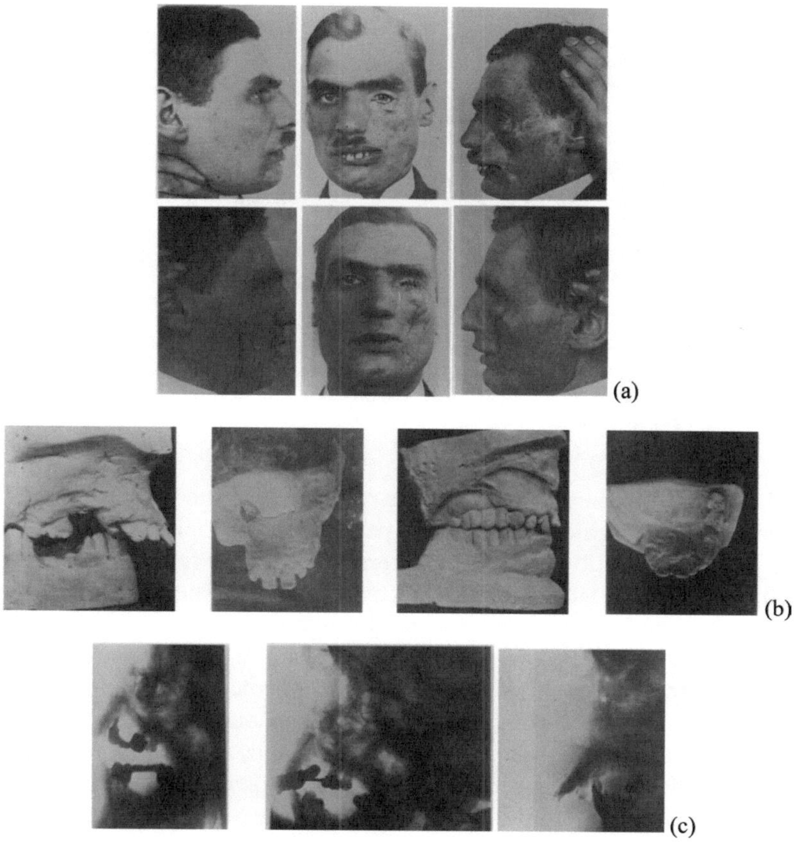

Figure 23.
Case II in Cohn-Stock's paper. (a) Before and after photographs. (b) Dental models. (c) Radiographs [69].

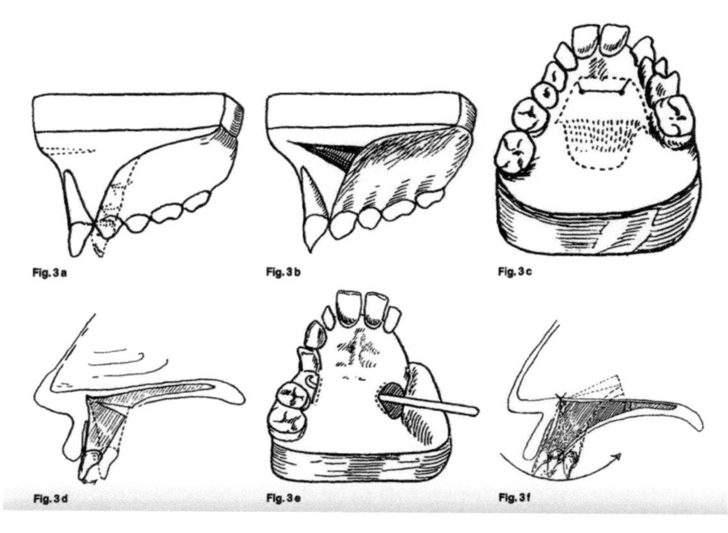

Figure 24.
Diagrams from Cohn-Stock's paper. Fig. 3a Cohn I, a first idea Figs. 3b-d Cohn II, leaving only a vestibular pedicle, as later described by Wunderer. Figs. 3e, f Cohn Ill, the definitive version, leaving the palatal artery intact [69].

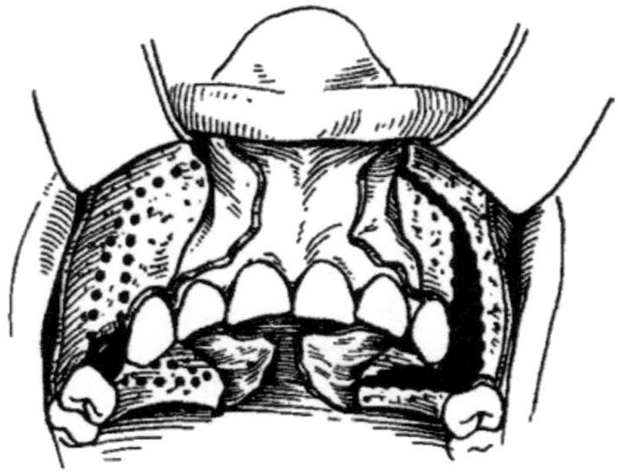

Figure 25.
Diagram of Wassmund procedure [69].

In 1954, Cupar from Zagreb described an osteotomy of the maxillary labial segment (from canine to canine), utilizing the palatal blood supply [19]. The Cupar osteotomy involved a vestibular incision extending from the first premolar to the first premolar on the opposite side, with the mucoperiosteum being elevated through this incision. The mucoperiosteum was elevated through the vestibular incision to expose the piriform aperture and the anterior wall of the maxilla, extending up to the canine fossa. Bilateral extraction of the maxillary first premolars was performed. Palatal tunneling was then carried out through the extraction sockets, converging at the midline. With the gingivoperiosteal flap intact and well retracted, a maxillary osteotomy was performed from the extracted premolar sockets to the piriform aperture on both sides, followed by the palatal osteotomy. After completing the osteotomy, the anterior maxillary segment was downfractured and repositioned superiorly and posteriorly [71].

In 1959, Köle outlined several variations of segmental maxillary osteotomies aiming to aid subsequent orthodontic treatment, involving a subapical osteotomy to move the alveolar bone along with the teeth as a single block (**Figure 26**) [72–74].

In 1962, Wunderer, based in Vienna, introduced a significant modification to Wassmund's segmental osteotomy technique. Wunderer's innovation involved performing the procedure as a single-stage operation using a palatal approach. A key feature of his modification was the preservation of a broad labial mucoperiosteal pedicle, which helped maintain blood supply and provided improved stability for the repositioned maxillary segment. This approach streamlined the procedure, reducing the need for multiple stages while also minimizing soft tissue disruption. Wunderer's technique, now widely recognized, is referred to by his name and remains a cornerstone in the evolution of maxillary osteotomy procedures [75].

5.2 Posterior segmental maxillar osteotomy

In 1935, Schuchardt introduced the concept of posterior segmental impaction of the maxillary dentoalveolus as a two-stage procedure [76]. The goal of Schuchardt's method was to achieve forward mandibular autorotation and close an anterior open bite, a challenge that was difficult to address with traditional techniques at the time. His approach involved bilateral impaction of the posterior maxillary dentoalveolar processes, which shifted the maxillary segment superiorly while allowing the mandible to rotate forward. This movement helped to correct the open bite by bringing the upper and lower teeth into better alignment.

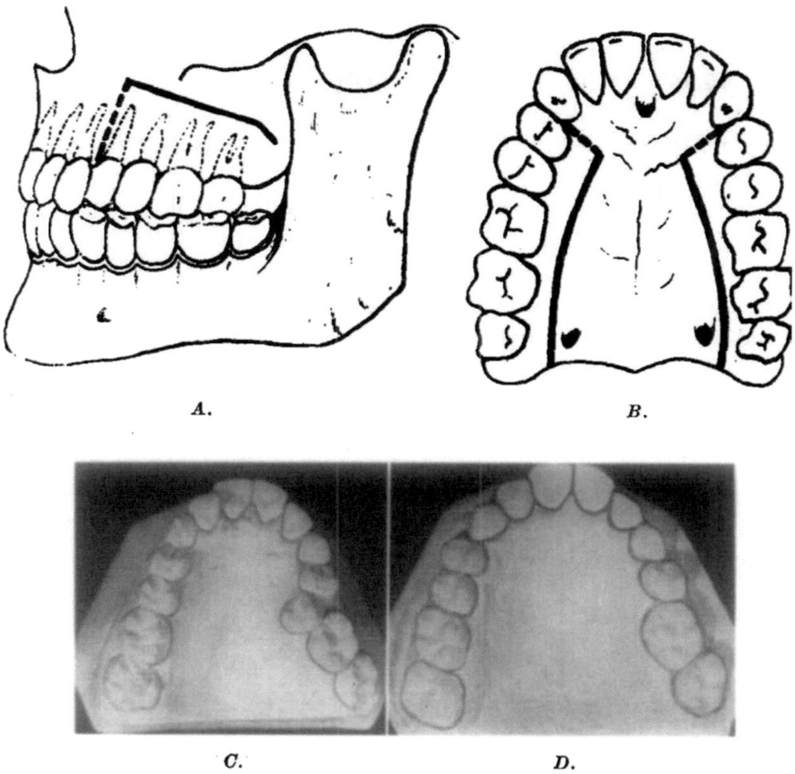

Figure 26.
Contraction of the maxilla. Sketch of the corticotomy (A and B), models before (C) and after (D) treatment for 3 months [71] traction of the maxilla. Sketch of the corticotomy (A and B) and models before (C) and after (D) treatment for 3 months [72].

The procedure was carried out in two distinct stages. In the first stage, Schuchardt performed an osteotomy of the hard palate, releasing the mucoperiosteum while ensuring that the greater palatine artery was preserved. This was critical for maintaining blood flow to the palate and avoiding necrosis of the soft tissue. The sagittal osteotomy was made bilaterally, starting behind the maxillary canine and extending along the palatal roots to the maxillary tuberosity. Once the osteotomy was completed, the mucoperiosteum was carefully sutured back into place, ensuring that the soft tissues were undisturbed.

Following a healing period of 3–6 weeks, the second stage of the procedure was performed. This involved making a horizontal incision in the buccal vestibule, through which a horizontal strip of bone was removed from the lateral wall of the maxilla, specifically above the roots of the premolar and molar teeth. The ostectomy extended vertically behind the terminal molar, exposing the posterior maxilla. After this, either finger pressure or a controlled stroke with a mallet was used to mobilize the alveolar process, which was then repositioned superiorly to close the open bite. Finally, dental splints and intermaxillary wiring were used to stabilize the repositioned segment and maintain proper occlusion during the healing phase.

Despite the innovative nature of Schuchardt's technique, several drawbacks emerged, particularly regarding the healing process [19]. By the time the second stage was initiated, the initial palatal osteotomy sites had often begun to fuse, making it challenging to achieve the desired movement of the maxillary segment. Additionally, the maxillary tuberosity area required additional manipulation and trauma to move the osteotomized segment into its new position, which led to longer recovery times and a higher risk of complications.

In response to the limitations of Schuchardt's two-stage technique, Kufner [77, 78] introduced a significant modification, transforming the procedure into a one-stage operation. Kufner's technique involved making a vestibular incision extending from the apex of the first premolar to the apices of the maxillary molars. Horizontal bony strips were removed from the lateral wall of the maxilla above the roots of the posterior teeth, eliminating the need for a palatal incision. By performing the entire osteotomy in one stage, Kufner reduced the trauma to the maxillary structures, sped up the overall procedure, and minimized the risk of complications that arose from the prolonged healing time between the two stages in Schuchardt's method.

Kufner's one-stage procedure streamlined the process, making it less invasive and more predictable in terms of recovery. Additionally, the reduction in surgical stages helped decrease the risk of infection and other postoperative complications, offering an important advancement over Schuchardt's original approach. This modification has been widely adopted and further refined over time, making Kufner's approach a standard method in the treatment of maxillary segmental impaction.

6. Segmental mandible osteotomy

6.1 Anterior mandibular subapical alveolar osteotomies

The mandibular subapical alveolar osteotomy, initially described by Hullihen in 1849, remained relatively unexplored until 1936 [19] when Hofer introduced an anterior mandibular subapical osteotomy aimed at advancing the mandibular labial dentoalveolar segment [79]. However, Hofer's procedure inadvertently severed the mental nerves, leading to potential complications.

In 1959, Köle made significant modifications to this approach. His refinement involved a vestibular incision that preserved the mental nerves, reducing the risk of nerve damage. He also introduced a horizontal osteotomy positioned 10 mm below the apices of the mandibular incisors, avoiding trauma to the incisor roots. This modification enabled the advancement of the dentoalveolar segment by up to 20 mm, providing improved bone contact for healing and better postoperative outcomes [72–74].

To stabilize the osteotomized segment, Köle used an intraoral splint secured with a circumferential wire that passed through a predrilled hole in the segment and was twisted over the splint. This technique allowed for controlled repositioning of the mandibular segment while minimizing the risk of complications associated with nerve damage and tooth involvement (**Figure 27**).

Several variations of anterior mandibular subapical alveolar osteotomies have been described over the years. In 1968, John Sowray [80] and Richard Haskell [81] introduced a technique to shorten the mandibular body by performing bilateral ostectomy of a first premolar and its associated socket, along with a vertical segmental ostectomy extending from the midline of the mandibular symphysis. This procedure not only reduced the length of the jaw but also narrowed the chin, helping to feminize the facial appearance (**Figure 28**).

In 1969, *Obwegeser* described a similar approach, but with the added step of elevating the osteotomized anterior dentoalveolus to close an anterior open bite. He also

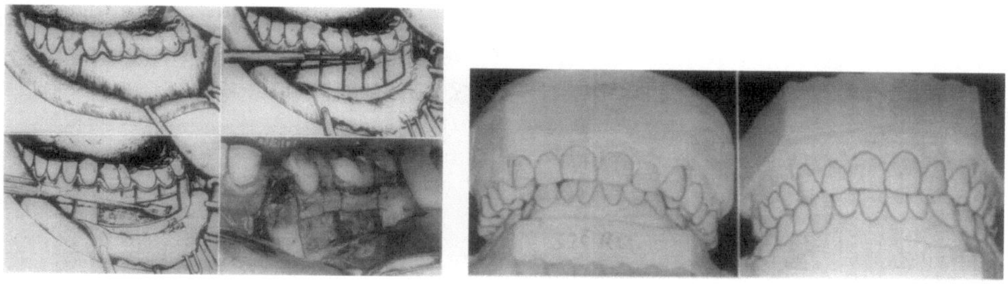

Figure 27.
Case of corticotomy for mandibular linguoversion. On the left, photographs of the operation. On the right, plaster models before treatment and after 2 months of treatment [72].

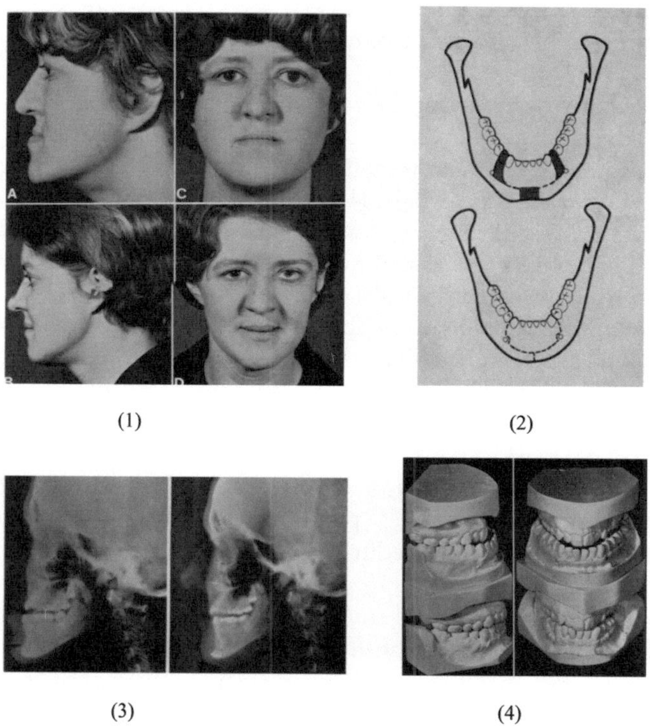

Figure 28.
Sowray's case of mandibular segmental osteotomy [80]. (1) A, Preoperative profile. B, Postoperative profile. C, Preoperative full-face appearance. D, Postoperative full-face appearance. (2) Diagrams showing by means of shading the sites of bone and tooth removal. The posterior fragments rotate medially, and the anterior fragment is moved posteriorly. (3) Lateral radiographs taken pre- and postoperatively. (4) Plaster models before and after treatment.

used a bone graft from the inferior border of the chin to fill the space created beneath the dentoalveolar segment [24].

6.2 Total mandibular subapical osteotomy

A further advancement in anterior mandibular subapical osteotomies was the total mandibular subapical (alveolar) osteotomy, introduced by *MacIntosh* in 1974 [82].

This technique allows for the mobilization and repositioning of the entire mandibular dentoalveolar process. MacIntosh identified three key indications for this procedure:

1. *Infantile apertognathia* (open bite extending from the molars forward), which is difficult to address with traditional ramus osteotomies due to the impact on molar occlusion.

2. *Relapse after prior ramus osteotomies*, where the anterior alveolar osteotomy provides an alternative solution.

3. *Condylar agenesis/hypoplasia*, where maintaining the functional relationships of the condyle and ramus without disturbing the masticatory muscles is crucial.

These variations have expanded the scope of subapical mandibular osteotomies, allowing for more flexible and effective treatment options in complex cases.

6.3 Surgical procedures involving the condyle and condylar neck

The first documented condylar resection was performed by *Humphry* in 1856 at Addenbrooke's Hospital in Cambridge. He treated a 21-year-old female with temporomandibular joint (TMJ) "chronic rheumatic arthritis," which appeared to be a case of right-sided condylar hyperplasia causing progressive mandibular asymmetry [47]. Humphry successfully resected the right condyle *via* an extraoral approach, improving the patient's dental occlusion, mandibular symmetry, and chewing ability, with stability maintained at a 9-month follow-up.

The first bilateral condylectomy for mandibular prognathism was performed by *Berger* in 1897. *Berger,* a pioneering surgeon from Paris, is also credited with introducing the use of surgical masks in 1897 to reduce postoperative infection, as mentioned before. A year later, French surgeons *Jaboulay* and *Bérard* reported similar successful outcomes from removing the condyles "piece by piece" using tooth forceps through a preauricular incision [83]. This procedure was primarily used to correct mandibular asymmetry or prognathism resulting from condylar pathology.

Ivy later noted that while bilateral condylectomy could help set back a prognathic mandible, it often led to less-than-optimal dental occlusion [45].

In 1921, *Dufourmentel* in Paris introduced the osteotomy of the condylar neck to correct mandibular prognathism [84].

Kostecka, a surgeon from Prague, in 1928 further refined and popularized the technique, using an extraoral approach with minimal incisions and a Gigli saw [85].

Kostecka's procedure made its way to the UK through Major *C. Konig*, the chief dental surgeon of the Czechoslovak Armed Forces.

This method involved constructing cast metal interdental cap splints for each jaw separately. A rod-and-tube device was used to lock the two splints together when the jaw had been repositioned to the desired position. The splints were fitted to the teeth the day before the operation. After anesthetizing the patient with a mandibular block and subcutaneous infiltration, Kostecka's needle was passed behind the posterior border of the left ramus, emerging near the angle of the zygomatic arch.

The Gigli saw wire was attached, and with only a few strokes, the condylar neck was bisected. The same procedure was performed on the right side. Afterward, the jaw could be pushed back and the splints locked into place. Kostecka recommended keeping the splints in place for 12 weeks to ensure proper healing.

Additional modifications were suggested, mainly the one by *Smith* in 1940 from Los Angeles [86]. His approach involved removing a small rectangle of bone from the sigmoid notch, followed by a horizontal osteotomy of the condylar neck to achieve mandibular setback. This illustrated the ongoing exploration of different mandibular techniques, with surgeons continuously striving for effective solutions to correct mandibular prognathism.

7. Current concepts in orthognathic surgery

One of the most transformative innovations in orthognathic surgery is virtual surgical planning (VSP). Advances in imaging technology have significantly enhanced diagnosis and treatment planning by providing better visualization of preoperative, intraoperative, and postoperative phenotypic changes. High-resolution, low-radiation computed tomography (CT) imaging has made the practical application of computer-aided design/computer-aided modeling (CAD/CAM) possible, allowing for detailed preoperative planning of osteotomies, fabrication of cutting guides to improve surgical precision, and the creation of both intermediate and final splints.

While these advancements have greatly enhanced craniofacial visualization, we must remain mindful of their limitations, as many commercial systems offer limited clinical utility.

More reliable techniques, such as 3D laser scanning, can capture soft tissue details and be superimposed onto Cone Beam Computed Tomography (CBCT) images. However, challenges persist, particularly in accounting for individual variations in how soft tissues respond to hard tissue movements: While CBCT proves valuable for presurgical planning and the development of craniofacial implants, further refinement is needed before these technologies can be fully integrated into routine orthognathic surgery (**Figure 29**).

Other techniques, such as model surgery, serve as a critical step in simulating the planned surgical procedures on the patient's preoperative dental models, which are

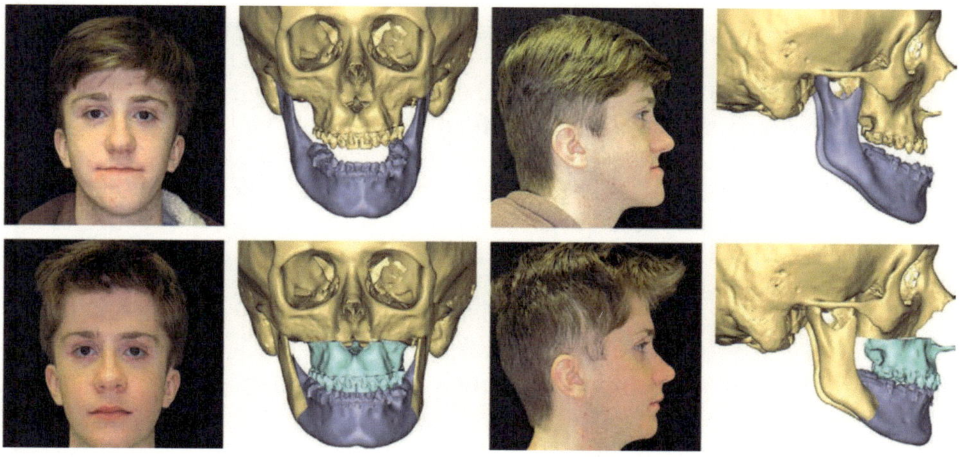

Figure 29.
Virtual plan of an orthognathic surgery [87].

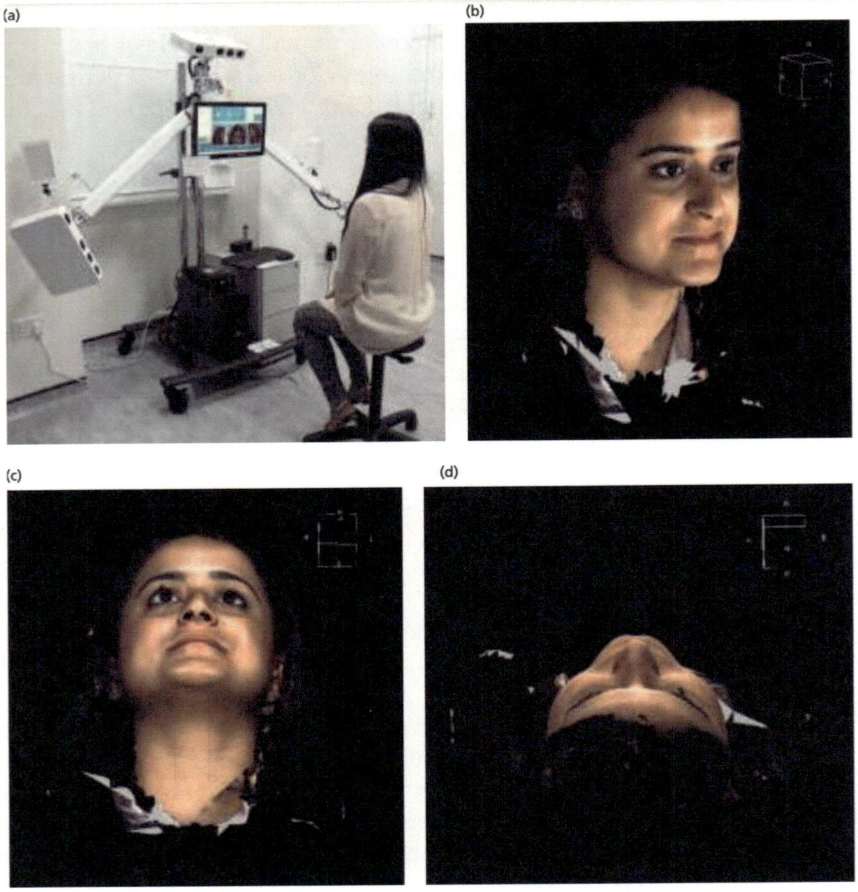

Figure 30.
3D stereophotogrammetry. (a) Multiple cameras capture images of the face simultaneously. (b) An example of an image as viewed on a computer monitor, which may be rotated and viewed from different angles, such as (c) a worm's-eye view or (d) a bird's-eye view [19].

mounted on an articulator. Essentially, it functions as a trial run of the surgery using study models. The objectives of model surgery are two-fold (**Figure 30**) [19]:

1. To ensure that the planned surgical procedures, based on clinical evaluation and predictive planning, are realistic and feasible.

2. To facilitate the fabrication of the surgical wafer splints. In cases of bimaxillary surgery, the maxillary cast is repositioned in relation to an unmoved mandibular cast to create the intermediate wafer. Then, the mandibular cast is repositioned to produce the final wafer.

8. Orthognathic surgery and orthodontic collaboration

The close collaboration between orthodontists and surgeons in orthognathic surgery dates back to the origins of the field in St. Louis, Missouri, during the late nineteenth century. At that time, Vilray Blair worked alongside Edward Angle, who is often regarded as the Father of Modern Orthodontics. Together, they performed the first documented ostectomy of the mandible in a patient with mandibular prognathism (Chapter 2).

An orthodontist's involvement in orthognathic surgery can be divided into several key phases: initial evaluation, presurgical orthodontics, surgical planning, and post-surgical orthodontics [88]. At each of these stages, effective collaboration between the orthodontist and the surgeon is crucial: a lack of coordination between the two professionals can lead to suboptimal outcomes.

Orthognathic surgery is generally approached in two ways: *surgery intermediate*, where surgery is performed between pre- and post-orthodontic phases, and *surgery first*, where surgery occurs before orthodontic treatment [88].

Orthodontic preparation aims to decompensate the malocclusion and restore the true skeletal discrepancy, ensuring that the jaws are positioned optimally for surgery. This process involves transitioning to heavier surgical wires, which should be fully expressed before taking occlusal impressions to prevent any changes in tooth position that could affect splint fit and surgical alignment. The success of orthognathic surgery heavily depends on proper orthodontic preparation, as it corrects dental compensations and facilitates the resolution of skeletal discrepancies.

At the start of treatment, it is important to establish clear presurgical orthodontic goals, which may not always involve complete arch leveling, space closure, or perfect interdigitation.

The extent of orthodontic preparation directly influences the skeletal movements achievable during surgery. Each type of malocclusion has its own set of dental compensations, which can be identified and addressed accordingly. Effective orthodontic preparation requires thorough planning, careful monitoring, and strong communication between the surgeon and orthodontist to avoid complications and ensure optimal results.

Concerning the sequence of osteotomies is planned in advance, with a final splint (for single-jaw surgery) or an intermediate and final splint (for bimaxillary surgery) guiding the repositioning of the maxilla. The maxilla is usually repositioned first, although the order can be reversed with the appropriate splint. After final jaw positioning, osseous genioplasty is performed if necessary [89].

Recent literature has highlighted several advantages to bypassing presurgical orthodontics and opting for a "surgery first" approach in orthognathic surgery. In this protocol, skeletal deformities are corrected initially, followed by the establishment of a transitional occlusion. Orthodontic appliances are then applied to finalize the occlusion. The benefits of the "surgery first" approach include [88, 89]:

- Addressing the patient's chief complaint early in the treatment process
- Immediate improvement in both dental function and facial aesthetics
- Potentially shorter overall treatment times
- Faster dental movement due to postoperatively accelerated orthodontic tooth movement
- The ability to achieve challenging dental movements, such as maxillary incisor torque, through segmental osteotomies and repositioning of skeletal segments

The feasibility of this approach is largely attributed to the increased stability provided by rigid fixation. With rigid fixation, the need for postoperative orthodontic elastics to stabilize skeletal movements is significantly reduced. However, the success of this protocol depends on careful coordination between the orthodontist and the surgeon. Overall, "surgery first" represents a promising new direction in orthognathic surgery.

As for the postoperative orthodontic phase, its primary goals are to stabilize skeletal movements and finalize the dental occlusion. Before surgery, full-dimension stainless steel arch wires are placed to support heavy interarch elastics, which are used postoperatively to refine minor skeletal adjustments and counteract soft tissue pull that may lead to relapse. The duration of the postoperative orthodontic phase depends on the amount of presurgical orthodontics performed, allowing for adequate skeletal consolidation.

9. Conclusion and future direction

As we look back on the evolution of orthognathic surgery and its integration with orthodontics, it is essential to recognize the pioneering work of those early surgeons and orthodontists who laid the foundation for the field. These trailblazers, through their dedication, ingenuity, and occasional challenges, developed the fundamental techniques and protocols that continue to serve as the backbone of modern practice. Their ability to adapt, innovate, and learn from both their successes and obstacles has shaped the methods we use today, and their contributions remain at the heart of orthognathic surgery.

Looking ahead, the field of orthognathic surgery is set to experience significant advancements, largely driven by the continued evolution of technology. One of the most notable of these innovations is the integration of virtual surgical planning, which has already transformed the practice. This shift toward digital methodologies not only enhances the accuracy of osteotomies but also enables highly individualized treatment plans, offering a level of customization that was once unimaginable.

Another promising area is the use of robotics in orthognathic surgery. The integration of robotic technology, whether in direct or remote surgery, holds the potential to make these procedures more accessible and efficient. Robots could assist in performing highly precise movements, reducing human error, improving surgical outcomes, and shortening recovery times. Furthermore, remote surgery could extend specialized care to underserved regions, increasing access to advanced orthognathic treatments worldwide.

While the future is full of potential, the core principles of orthognathic surgery and its close collaboration with orthodontics remain unchanged. The partnership between orthodontists and surgeons, as demonstrated by the pioneers in the field, continues to be fundamental. As we move forward with new technologies and techniques, it is essential to build upon the strong foundation established by our predecessors, honoring their contributions while expanding the possibilities for the future. Ultimately, the continued evolution of orthognathic surgery promises to improve the lives of countless patients, bringing life-changing results to more individuals than ever before.

DOI: http://dx.doi.org/10.5772/intechopen.1011702

Author details

Farid Bourzgui*, Zineb Safi-Eddine and Farid El Quars
Orthodontics Department, Dental School, Hassan II University of Casablanca
Morroco, Morocco

*Address all correspondence to: farid.bourzgui@etu.univh2c.ma

References

[1] Bourzgui F, Diouny S, Tougui I, Omari A, Serhier Z, Othmani M. Assessement of the nasal shape after orthognathic maxillary surgery. Integrative Journal of Medical Sciences. 2021:8. DOI: 10.15342/ijms.2021.552

[2] Steinhäuser EW. Historical development of orthognathic surgery. Journal of Cranio-Maxillofacial Surgery. 1996;**24**(4):195-204

[3] Ambrecht EC. Hullihen, the oral surgeon. International Journal of Orthodontia and Oral Surgery. 1937;**23**:377, 511, 598, 711

[4] Phillips BJ, Turco LM. Le Fort fractures: A collective review. Bulletin of Emergency and Trauma. 2017;**5**(4):221-230. DOI: 10.18869/acadpub.beat.5.4.499

[5] Noffze MJ, Tubbs RS. René Le Fort 1869-1951. Clinical Anatomy. 2011;**24**(3):278-281. DOI: 10.1002/ca.21091

[6] Kaul RP, Sagar S, Singhal M, Kumar A, Jaipuria J, Misra M. Burden of maxillofacial trauma at level 1 trauma center. Craniomaxillofacial Trauma & Reconstruction. 2014;**7**(2):126-130. DOI: 10.1055/s-0034-1371539

[7] Cesmebasi A, Oelhafen K, Shayota BJ, Klaassen Z, Tubbs RS, Loukas M. A historical perspective: Bernhard von Langenbeck German surgeon (1810-1887). Clinical Anatomy. 2014;**27**(7):972-975. DOI: 10.1002/ca.22433

[8] Halvorson EG, Mulliken JB. Cheever's double operation: The first Le Fort I osteotomy. Plastic and Reconstructive Surgery. 2008;**121**(4):1375-1381. DOI: 10.1097/01.prs.0000304442.15532.40

[9] Cheever DW. Displacement of the upper jaw. Medical and Surgical Report of the Boston City Hospital. 1870;**1**:156

[10] Drommer RB. The history of the "Le Fort I osteotomy". Journal of Maxillofacial Surgery. 1986;**14**(3):119-122. DOI: 10.1016/s0301-0503(86)80275-2

[11] Wassmund M. Frakuren und Luxationen des Gesichtsschadels. Leipzig: Meusser; 1927

[12] Moorhead A, Winters R, Serra M. Le Fort osteotomy. In: StatPearls [Internet]. Treasure Island (FL): StatPearls Publishing; 2024

[13] Axhausen G. Zur Behandlung veralteter disloziert geheilter Oberkieferbruche. Deutsche Zeitschrift für Zahn-, Mund- und Kieferheilkunde. 1934;**1**:334

[14] Axhausen G. Ueber die korrigierende Osteotomie am Oberkiefer. Deutsche Zeitschrift für Chirurgie. 1936;**248**:515-522

[15] Axhausen G. Die operative Orthopadie bei den Fehlbildungen der Kiefer. Deutsche Zeitschrift für Zahn-, Mund- und Kieferheilkunde. 1939;**6**:582-600

[16] Schuchardt K. Ein Betrag zur chirurgischen Kieferorthopadie unter Beruckssichtigung ihrer Bedeutung fur die Behandlung angeborener und erworbener Kieferdeformitaten bei Soldaten. Deutsche Zahn-, Mund-, und Kieferheilkunde mit Zentralblatt. 1942;**9**:73-89

[17] Moore FT, Ward TG. Complications and sequelae of untreated fractures of the

facial bones and their treatment. British Journal of Plastic Surgery. 1949;**1**:257-267

[18] Gillies HD, Rowe NL. L'osteotomie du maxillaire supérieur enoisagée essentiellement dans le cas de bec-de-lièvre total. Revue de Stomatologie. 1954;**55**:545-552

[19] Naini FB, Gill DS. Orthognathic Surgery Principles, Planning and Practice. London: Wiley-Blackwell; 2017. pp. 23-82, 944 p. ISBN: 978-1-118-64997-8

[20] Obwegeser H. Cirurgia del "mordex apertus". Revista de la Asociación Odontológica Argentina. 1962;**50**:430

[21] Obwegeser H. Eingriffe am Oberkiefer zur Korrektur des progenen Zustandsbildes. Schweizerische Monatsschrift für Zahnheilkunde. 1965;**75**:356

[22] Obwegeser H. Zur Behandlung der veralteten Oberkieferfrakturen. In: Fortschr Kiefer- u Gesichtschir. Stuttgart: Thieme; 1967

[23] Obwegeser H. Surgical correction of small or retrodisplaced maxillae. Plastic and Reconstructive Surgery. 1969;**43**:351

[24] Obwegeser H. Die bewegung des unteren alveolarfortsatzes zur korrektur von kieferstellungsanomalien. Deutsche Zahnärztliche Zeitschrift. 1969;**24**:5-15

[25] Bell WH. Revascularization and bone healing after anterior maxillary osteotomy: A study using adult rhesus monkeys. Journal of Oral Surgery. 1969;**27**:249-255

[26] Bell WH, Levy BM. Revascularization and bone healing after anterior mandibular osteotomy. Journal of Oral Surgery. 1970;**28**:196-203

[27] Bell WH, Levy BM. Healing after anterior maxillary osteotomy. Journal of Oral Surgery. 1970;**28**:728-734

[28] Bell WH, Levy BM. Revascularization and bone healing after posterior maxillary osteotomy. Journal of Oral Surgery. 1971;**29**:313-320

[29] Bell WH, Levy BM. Revascularization and bone healing after maxillary corticotomies. Journal of Oral Surgery. 1972;**30**:640-648

[30] Bell WH. Biologic basis for maxillary osteotomies. American Journal of Physical Anthropology. 1973;**38**:279-289

[31] Bell WH, Fonseca RJ, Kenneky JW, Levy BM. Bone healing and revascularization after total maxillary osteotomy. Journal of Oral Surgery. 1975;**33**:253-260

[32] Bell WH, Schendel SA, Finn RA. Revascularization after surgical repositioning of one-tooth dento-osseous segments. Journal of Oral Surgery. 1978;**36**:757-765

[33] Bell WH, You ZH, Finn RA, Fields RT. Wound healing after multisegmental Le Fort I osteotomy and transection of the descending palatine vessels. Journal of Oral and Maxillofacial Surgery. 1995;**53**:1425-1433; discussion 1433-4

[34] Marchac D, Arnaud E. Midface surgery from Tessier to distraction. Child's Nervous System. 1999;**15**(11-12):681-694. DOI: 10.1007/s003810050458

[35] Gillies HD, Harrison SM. Operative correction by osteotomy of recessed malar maxillary compound in a case of oxycephaly. British Journal of Plastic Surgery. 1950;**2**:123

[36] Tessier P. Osteotomies totales de la face: Syndrome de Crouzon, syndrome

d'Apert, oxycephalies, scaphocephalies, turricephalies. Annales de Chirurgie Plastique. 1967;**12**:273

[37] Tessier P, Guiot J, Rougerie JP, et al. Ostéotomies cranio-naso-orbito-faciales: Hypertelorisme. Annales de Chirurgie Plastique. 1967;**12**:103

[38] Wolfe SA. A Man from Heric: The Life and Work of Paul Tessier, MD, Father of Craniofacial Surgery: Volumes I and II. Raleigh, NC: Lulu.com; 2012

[39] Hullihen SP. Case of elongation of the under jaw and distortion of the face and neck, caused by a burn, successfully treated. American Journal of Dental Science. 1849;**9**(2):157-165

[40] Whipple JW. Double resection of the inferior maxilla for protruding lower jaw. Dental Cosmos. 1899;**41**(3):242-247

[41] Angle EH. Double resection of lower maxilla. Dental Cosmos. 1898;**40**:635-638

[42] Blair VP. Operations on the jaw-bone and face. Surgery, Gynecology & Obstetrics. 1907;**4**:67

[43] Ottolengui RD. A friendly criticism of Dr Angle's proposed technique in surgical correction of mandibular protrusion. Dental Cosmos. 1903;**45**:454-457

[44] Berger P. Du traitement chirurgical du prognathisme. Lyon: Med Thèse; 1897

[45] Ivy RH. Surgery in relation to orthodontia and facial harmony. International Journal of Orthodontia and Dentistry for Children. 1933;**19**:888-898

[46] Strasser BJ et al. A history of the medical mask and the rise of throwaway culture. Lancet. 2020;**396**(10243):19-20

[47] Humphry GM. Excision of the condyle of the lower jaw. Association Medical Journal (BMJ). 26 Jan 1856;**4**(160). Available from: https://www.jstor.org/stable/i25496964

[48] Ballin M. Double resection for the treatment of mandibular protrusion. The Dental cosmos; A Monthly Record of Dental Science. Apr 1903;**45**(4):268-274

[49] Limberg AA. Oblique osteotomy of the ramus for mandibular prognathism. Journal of the American Dental Association (1939). 1928;**15**:851

[50] Kazanjian KH. Surgical correction of mandibular prognathism. International Journal of Orthodontics. 1932;**18**:1224

[51] Cryer MH. Studies of the anterior and posterior occlusion of the teeth, with suggestions as to treatment. Dental Cosmos. 1913;**55**:673-691

[52] Fickling BW, Fordyce GI. Mandibular osteotomy for facial asymmetry. Proceedings of the Royal Society of Medicine. 1955;**48**:989

[53] Hovell JH. The surgical construction of variations in the facial skeletal pattern. Proceedings of the Royal Society of Medicine. 1956;**49**:546-556

[54] Pichler H, Trauner R. Mund- und Kieferchirurgie, Part I. Vol. 1 and 2. Vienna: Urban Schwarzenberg; 1948

[55] Trauner R. Zur Progenieoperation. Österreichische Zeitschrift für Stomatologie. 1955;**52**:361

[56] Trauner R, Obwegeser H. Zur Operationstechnik bei der Progenie und anderen Unterkieferanomalien. Deutsche Zahn-, Mund-, und Kieferheilkunde. 1955/56;**23**:1

[57] Obwegeser HL. Surgical procedures to correct mandibular prognathism and

reshaping of the chin. In: Trauner R, Obwegeser H, editors. The Surgical Correction of Mandibular Prognathism and Retrognathia with Consideration of Genioplasty. Vol. 10. Oral Surg Oral Med Oral Pathol; 1957. pp. 677-689

[58] Obwegeser HL. Orthognathic surgery and a tale of how three procedures came to be: A letter to the next generations of surgeons. Clinics in Plastic Surgery. 2007 Jul;**34**(3):331-355

[59] Dal Pont G. L'osteotomia retromolare per la correzione della progenia. Minerva Chirurgica. 1959;**14**:1138-1141

[60] Dal Pont G. Retromolar osteotomy for the correction of prognathism. Journal of Oral Surgery. 1961;**19**:42-47

[61] Hunsuck EE. A modified intraoral sagittal splitting technique for correction of mandibular prognathism. Journal of Oral and Maxillofacial Surgery. 1968;**26**:250-253

[62] Epker BN. Modifications in the sagittal osteotomy of the mandible. Journal of Oral Surgery. 1977;**35**:157-159

[63] Hofer O. Operation der prognathie und mikrogenie. Deutsche Zahn-, Mund-, und Kieferheilkunde. 1942;**9**:121-132

[64] Trauner R. In memory of professor Otto Hofer, D.D.S. Österreichische Zeitschrift für Stomatologie. 1972;**69**:112-113

[65] Converse JM, Wood-Smith D. Horizontal osteotomy of the mandible. Plastic and Reconstructive Surgery. 1964;**34**:464-471

[66] Mortazavi H, Tabrizi R, Mohajerani H, Ozkan T. Evaluation of stability in advancement genioplasty: An 18-month follow-up. Journal of Dentistry. 2009;**10**(Suppl 2009):61-64. DOI: 10.30476/dentjods.2019.43609

[67] Neuner O. Chirurgische Orthodontie. Schweizerische Monatsschrift für Zahnheilkunde. 1965;**75**:940-944

[68] Chkadua TZ, Libin PV, Sufiomarov NS. Surgical treatment of a patient with mandibular micrognathia accompanied by obstructive sleep apnea syndrome using extended genioplasty. Stomatologiia (Moskva). 2023;**102**(6):48-51

[69] Wolfe SA. Günther Cohn-Stock, M.S., D.D.S., father of maxillary orthognathic surgery. Journal of Cranio-Maxillofacial Surgery. Oct 1989;**17**(7):331-334. DOI: 10.1016/s1010-5182(89)80065-4

[70] Wassmund M. Lehrbuch der praktischen Chirurgie des Mundes und der Kiefer. Leipzig: Meusser; 1935

[71] Cupar I. Die chirurgische behandlung der form und stellungsveranderungen des oberkiefers. Österreichische Zeitschrift für Stomatologie. 1954;**51**:565-577

[72] Köle H. Surgical operations on the alveolar ridge to correct occlusal abnormalities. Oral Surgery, Oral Medicine, and Oral Pathology. 1959;**12**(3):277-288

[73] Köle H. Surgical operations on the alveolar ridge to correct occlusal abnormalities. Oral Surgery, Oral Medicine, and Oral Pathology. 1959;**12**(4):413-420

[74] Köle H. Surgical operations on the alveolar ridge to correct occlusal abnormalities. Oral Surgery, Oral Medicine, and Oral Pathology. 1959;**12**(5):515-529

[75] Wunderer S. Die prognathie-operation mittels frontal gestielten

maxillafragment. Österreichische Zeitschrift für Stomatologie. 1962;**59**:98-102

[76] Schuchardt K. Experiences with the surgical treatment of some deformities of the jaws: Prognathia, micrognathia, and open bite. In: Wallace AB, editor. Transactions of Second Congress, International Society of Plastic Surgeons. London: E&S Livingstone Ltd.; 1961

[77] Kufner J. Nové metody chirurgického léceni otevreného skusu. Cs Stomatol. 1960;**60**:387-392

[78] Kufner J. Experience with a modified procedure for correction of open bite. In: Walker RV, editor. Oral Surgery: Transactions of the Third International Conference on Oral Surgery. Edinburgh and London: E&S Livingstone; 1970. pp. 18-23

[79] Hofer O. Die vertikale osteotomie zur verlagerung des einseitig verkürzten aufsteigenden unterkieferastes. Atschr Stomatol. 1936;**34**:826

[80] Sowray JH, Haskell R. Ostectomy at the mandibular symphysis. The British Journal of Oral Surgery. 1968;**5**:97-102

[81] Henry TC. Localized osteotomy in cases of mild inferior protrusion. In: Walker RV, editor. Oral Surgery: Transactions of the Third International Conference on Oral Surgery. Edinburgh and London: E&S Livingstone; 1970. pp. 80-92

[82] MacIntosh RB. Total mandibular alveolar osteotomy: Encouraging experiences with an infrequently indicated procedure. Journal of Maxillofacial Surgery. 1974;**2**:210-218

[83] Jaboulay M, Berard L. Traitement chirurgical du prognathisme inferieur. Presse Médicale, Paris. 1898;**6**:173-176

[84] Dufourmentel L. Le traitement chirurgical du prognathisme. Presse Médicale. 1921;**29**:235

[85] Kostecka F. Surgical correction of protrusion of the lower and upper jaws. Journal of the American Dental Association (1939). 1928;**15**:362

[86] Smith AE, Johnson JB. Surgical treatment of mandibular deformations. Journal of the American Dental Association (Chicago, IL). 1940;**27**:689-700

[87] Naran S, Steinbacher DM, Taylor JA. Current concepts in orthognathic surgery. Plastic and Reconstructive Surgery. 2018;**141**(6):925e-936e

[88] Wirthlin JO, Shetye PR. Orthodontist's role in orthognathic surgery. Seminars in Plastic Surgery. 2013;**27**(3):137-144

[89] Liou EJ, Chen PH, Wang YC, Yu CC, Huang CS, Chen YR. Surgery-first accelerated orthognathic surgery: Orthodontic guidelines and setup for model surgery. Journal of Oral and Maxillofacial Surgery. 2011;**69**(3):771-780

Chapter 2

Craniomaxillofacial Surgery: An Overview of Techniques and Procedures

Yanko Castro-Govea, Melissa Fernanda Ochoa Cortez and Cynthia Minerva Gonzalez-Cantu

Abstract

The use of flaps is a recurring, constant and quite useful practice in the area of plastic surgery. Its use is so prevalent that new surgical techniques are constantly being devised with the aim of optimizing each tissue used. Particularly in patients after treatment for some type of cancer, the recipient areas are a therapeutic challenge, for which new and more ingenious ways of covering and repairing defects are increasingly being designed. There are various options for reconstructing defects in both the floor of the mouth and the neck, but in cases of recurrence or when the patient receives radiotherapy, many of these are not feasible. In this chapter, we review the techniques described and also propose a new coverage technique developed by our surgical team.

Keywords: plastic surgery, reconstructive surgery, facial surgery, maxillofacial surgery, craniofacial surgery, minimally invasive surgery

1. Introduction

Craniomaxillofacial surgery (CMFS) encompasses a wide range of conditions, from functional problems affecting vital capacities such as breathing, chewing, and speech, to esthetic alterations that modify facial symmetry and proportion. Highly complex reconstructions required after trauma or oncological procedures are also part of the vast field of CMFS. This specialty, which is in fact a subspecialty, integrates knowledge from various areas such as plastic surgery, orthognathic surgery, traumatology, and neurosurgery. Therefore, it stands at the intersection of functional and esthetic medicine.

Its multidisciplinary approach allows for the treatment of complex cases that demand surgical precision, a deep understanding of craniofacial anatomy, and the use of advanced technologies such as computer-assisted surgical planning and 3D printing with bio-printer assistance for various purposes. The continuous advancement in biocompatible materials and surgical techniques has expanded therapeutic options, improving both functional and esthetic outcomes for patients. The perspective of treating the craniofacial complex, particularly the face, demands striving for perfection.

CMFS addresses a broad spectrum of congenital and acquired pathologies, making an interdisciplinary approach essential to ensuring satisfactory functional and esthetic results. For this reason, developing an artistic sensibility is highly beneficial to restoring lost form with natural-looking standards. Among the most notable congenital anomalies are craniofacial deformities that affect both function and appearance [1].

2. Cleft lip and palate

Undoubtedly, the most common congenital craniofacial condition is cleft lip and palate (CLP), caused by a failure in the partial or complete fusion of the embryonic frontonasal and maxillary facial processes during the first weeks of development. This condition can disrupt communication between the oral and nasal cavities, affecting feeding, speech, and facial esthetics [2].

The etiology of cleft lip and palate is multifactorial; in general, it can be caused by genetic and environmental factors. Other contributing factors may include smoking, alcohol consumption, maternal nutritional deficiencies, and parental age [3].

In this congenital malformation, structures such as the lip, alveolar process, hard palate, and soft palate are affected. The incisive foramen (IF) is the key anatomical landmark for all classifications of CLP, distinguishing between the primary and secondary palate. Primary palate clefts are located anterior to the incisive foramen, involving the lip, premaxilla, anterior nasal septum, and the hard palate in front of the incisive foramen. In contrast, secondary palate clefts are posterior to the IF, affecting the hard palate, soft palate, and uvula. Additionally, minor alterations such as microform cleft lip and submucous cleft palate may also be present [4].

Various classification systems categorize the different forms of CLP involvement. These classifications must specify the affected structure, whether the cleft is partial or complete, the affected side or both sides, and even midline involvement. The Victor Veau and Kernahan and Stark classifications are the most widely used [4]. The integration of a multidisciplinary team is essential, including specialists in plastic surgery, dentistry-orthodontics, pediatrics, otolaryngology, and genetics (providing genetic counseling to parents and prospective parents), as well as speech therapy, neurology, and other specialties [1].

3. Surgical treatment sequence

There are certain differences in the sequence of surgical treatment, but the most standardized approach follows this timeline:

- Lip reconstruction is performed between 3 and 6 months of age.
- Palate reconstruction is carried out at approximately 1 year of age.
- Follow-up surgeries may take place between 2 and 21 years of age.

During lip closure, it is highly desirable to perform a gingivoperiosteoplasty with bone grafting. Three-dimensional orthopedic treatment is fundamental for guiding the growth of the dental arches, promoting a better vertical and transverse relationship, ensuring maxillary development, and consequently improving facial symmetry and growth.

The most commonly used techniques for lip cleft repair include the modified Millard II technique. Skilled use of the flap system in this technique allows for the reconstruction of the philtrum and Cupid's bow, which are key esthetic elements of the upper lip. Lip closure must be accompanied by rhinoplasty, as nasal cartilage remodeling is often required for an optimal esthetic outcome. Currently, nasal anatomy can be further shaped using nasal conformers, even before lip closure.

The most commonly used techniques for palate closure are Push Back and Wardill-Kilner. It is crucial to reposition the muscles from the abnormal insertions of the palate to suture them at the midline. The goal is to reconstruct a competent velopharyngeal sphincter to achieve proper speech in the patient. For very wide palatal clefts, the Von Langenbeck technique, with relaxing incisions, allows the mobilization of mucoperiosteal flaps to join them at the midline of the palate.

The purpose of the therapeutic approach is to provide the patient with optimal ability for swallowing and suction and improve language development, and, from our perspective, it is also essential to achieve a high esthetic outcome, not only for the lip but also for the nose, which is often deformed.

4. Orthognathic surgery

Another fascinating field is orthognathic surgery, which addresses skeletal growth disorders of the midface and mandible, leading to occlusal discrepancies. This, in turn, affects chewing, and for some patients, the primary concern is facial appearance. These dysmorphic alterations can be caused by genetic factors, acquired as a consequence of trauma, or be part of Craniofacial Syndromes. Prognathism and maxillary hypoplasia are among the most common conditions [5].

Craniofacial trauma, resulting from accidents and traumatic injuries, often causes complex fractures of specific structures such as the mandible, maxilla, zygomatic bone, orbit, and skull. These injuries, often accompanied by severe damage to the surrounding soft tissues, require extensive reconstructions that demand a highly specialized multidisciplinary approach. The challenge is not only assembling bone fragments, similar to a puzzle, but success is directly related to restoring essential functions such as vision, olfaction, breathing, and mastication.

5. Hemifacial microsomia

Hemifacial microsomia (HFM) is a congenital disorder and the second most common craniofacial malformation. It is characterized by hypoplasia of the tissues derived from the first and second branchial arches, affecting both soft and skeletal tissues on one side of the face, leading to varying degrees of facial asymmetry depending on the disease's penetrance. The small size of the maxilla and mandible can affect the orbit, the temporomandibular joint (TMJ), and, logically, dental occlusion. Its manifestation is highly variable, sometimes presenting defects at the cardiac, vertebral, and central nervous system levels.

In 1969, Samuel Pruzansky [6] classified the different degrees of mandibular hypoplasia in patients with HFM. In his classification, he identified three types of mandibular hypoplasia: a relatively small but complete mandible (Grade I); the condyle, ramus, and sigmoid notch present but with greater alteration (Grade II); and a very small or absent mandibular ramus (Grade III). This classification focuses solely on the description of the mandible.

Years later, Kaban et al. modified Pruzansky's classification by adding a description of the deformities observed in the TMJ. The major difference lies in Grade II, which is further subdivided based on the position of the glenoid fossa. It can either be normal (IIA) or altered (IIB).

Due to the great variability in phenotypic expression and its frequency, the OMENS classification [7] was introduced in 1991 based on three criteria. First, it needed to be inclusive and versatile. Second, anatomical components had to be analyzed separately. Third, data had to be expressed in a numerical scale to be clinically useful. The acronym OMENS [7] corresponds to the five main manifestations of HFM:

- O: Orbital asymmetry (Orbit)
- M: Mandibular hypoplasia (Mandible)
- E: External ear deformity (Ear)
- N: Nerve involvement (Nerve)
- S: Soft tissue deficiency (Soft Tissue)

6. Mandibular distraction osteogenesis

Mandibular distraction osteogenesis (MDO) is an excellent, effective, and versatile alternative for all conditions involving mandibular hypoplasia. Using the MDO technique, it is possible to gradually lengthen bones through specialized devices, promoting tissue formation *via* induced osteogenesis.

The main approach consists of performing complete osteotomies, followed by the placement of distraction devices. Once mechanical traction is activated, bone growth occurs at a rate of 1 mm per day. When the desired elongation is achieved, these devices remain in place as space maintainers to allow the consolidation of newly formed bone tissue. Subsequently, the distractors are removed [8].

This approach has proven to be an effective solution for treating severe skeletal deformities, offering a less invasive alternative compared to traditional procedures. By combining functional and esthetic improvements, this technique significantly contributes to the comprehensive rehabilitation of the patient.

Mandibular distraction osteogenesis is perhaps the most widely used, but elongation can also be performed in the midface and upper facial third. Collectively, these innovations reflect how technology has raised the standards in craniomaxillofacial surgery, transforming medical care into a more precise, safe, and efficient process.

7. Progressive hemifacial atrophy

Progressive hemifacial atrophy (PHA), also known as Parry-Romberg Syndrome, is a rare condition of unknown etiology. It is characterized by atrophy of the skin and soft tissues on one side of the face, often involving skeletal tissue as well. This condition progresses slowly, is irreversible, and stabilizes at a certain point in life. Craniofacial asymmetry is linked to the severity of the disease.

A notable case involves a 35-year-old patient with a 10-year progression of the disease and 5 years of stabilization. This case was treated using cell-assisted lipotransfer (CAL), an innovative technique that utilizes autologous fat enriched with adipose-derived stem cells (ASCs) from the patient's own tissue. ASCs are pluripotent cells capable of differentiating into adipocytes to restore volume, promote angiogenesis through the release of growth factors, and act as stem cells, contributing to long-term tissue regeneration [1].

The use of autologous fat as a filler has proven effective in patients with mild to moderate Parry-Romberg syndrome (**Figure 1**). The CAL technique has gained recognition for its ability to reduce fat resorption and maintain graft stability over time, making it a promising solution for correcting defects associated with this and other soft tissue atrophies [9].

At the same time, oncologic reconstruction is another key pillar of craniofacial surgery, addressing the challenges of tumor resection and reconstructing affected areas using autologous bone grafts or microvascular flaps, restoring both function and structure after major oncologic surgeries.

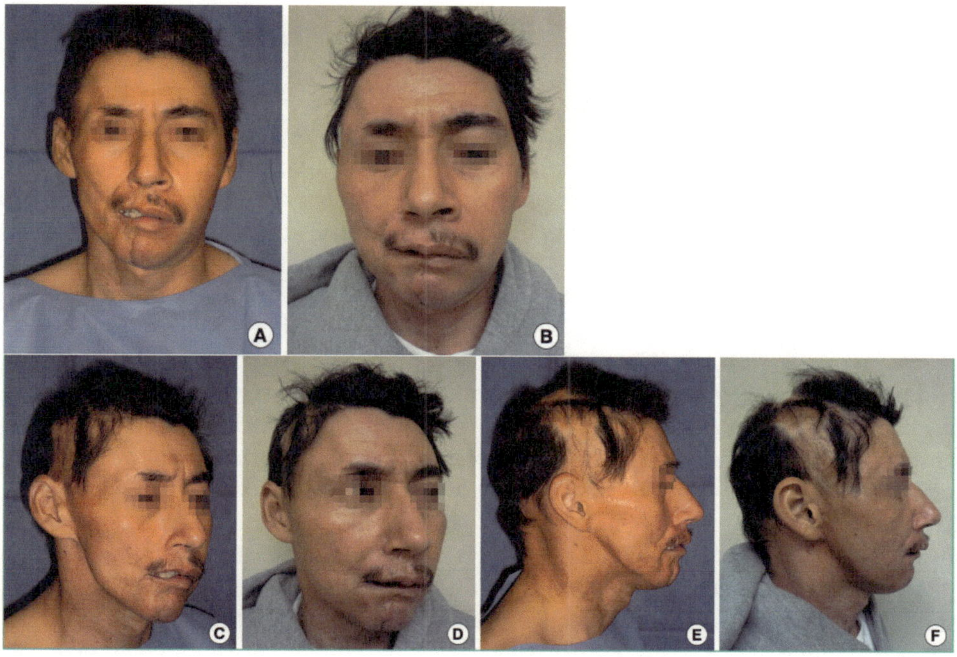

Figure 1.
(A, C, E) Preoperative view. (B, D, F) Postoperative view 12 months after lipoinjection enriched with stem cells and elements of the stromal vascular fraction.

8. Craniosynostosis

Craniosynostoses (CS) are characterized by the premature fusion of one or more cranial sutures. They can occur in isolation, without being part of any other condition, or they may be associated with a range of abnormalities classified within craniofacial syndromes. The dynamic growth of the brain promotes the expansion and shaping of the cranial vault, as the pressure exerted by the brain allows the skull to grow through the connections between its bones. When one or more sutures are fused, brain pressure is redirected, causing the malleable cranial bones to develop unique deformities. This condition can alter natural brain development and cognitive ability. Craniofacial syndromes such as Crouzon and Apert involve skeletal abnormalities combined with other complications that require a comprehensive surgical and medical approach [10].

Isolated, non-syndromic craniosynostosis causes varying degrees of craniofacial asymmetry, especially in cases affecting the coronal and frontal sutures. To date, several surgical techniques have been developed to treat this condition, with fronto-orbital advancement and frontal remodeling, along with their variations, being the most commonly used [11].

Regardless of the technique chosen, some types of asymmetry persist or recur, particularly when the cranial base is asymmetric. Persing observed that irregularities continued even after fronto-orbital contour advancement and proposed a second intervention between the ages of 3 and 5 years. This approach could reduce the severity of the deformity and help young patients attract less attention from their peers during their early school years.

9. Craniofacial malformations and their psychosocial impact

Craniofacial malformations have a significant psychosocial impact, as preschool and primary school children are often victims of bullying due to their appearance. Childhood and adolescence are critical stages in which the social environment is essential for psychological well-being and the development of self-esteem. Lovegrove and Rumsey reported that children in this vulnerable stage are particularly susceptible to comments about their appearance, teasing, ridicule, and bullying [12]. Similarly, recent studies have indicated that facial asymmetry can lead to psychological disorders that affect academic performance and personality development [10].

In response to this, a minimally invasive technique has been described to treat mild to moderate asymmetries that may occur after cranioplasty in pediatric patients. Specifically, these asymmetries involve depressions in the fronto-orbital and temporal complex, which can be corrected through volumetric lipoinjection using fat enriched with ASCs (**Figures 2–5**). This treatment helps boost patients' self-esteem from an early age. Achieving proper facial symmetry in patients with craniofacial sequelae positively influences their psychological development and social integration [10, 12].

Adipose tissue collected *via* suction not only contains adipocytes but also a significant number of cells from the stromal vascular fraction, including endothelial cells, pericytes, fibroblasts, and ASCs. ASCs and other regenerative cells present in aspirated fat play a crucial role in graft viability [8]. Studies have demonstrated that one of their main advantages is their ability to produce growth factors with angiogenic and anti-apoptotic properties, enhancing graft survival. These growth factors increase capillary density and improve graft quality, contributing to better long-term survival [13].

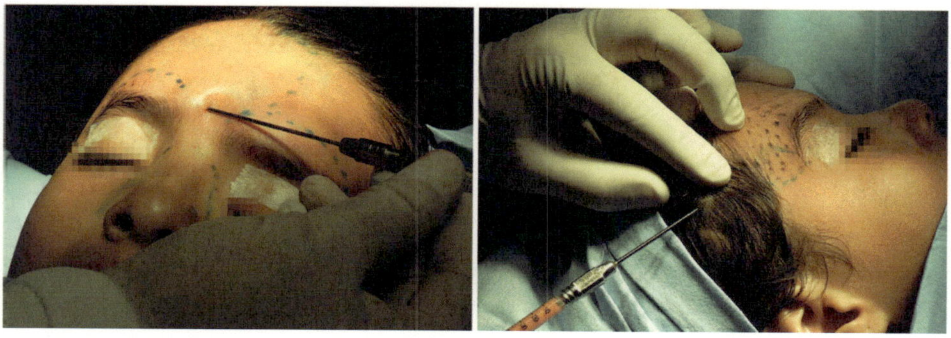

Figure 2.
Five-year-old girl with sequelae of craniosynostosis. Intraoperative view of the lipoinjection of adipose stem cells. (A) Glabellar approach. (B) Temporal approach (behind the hairline).

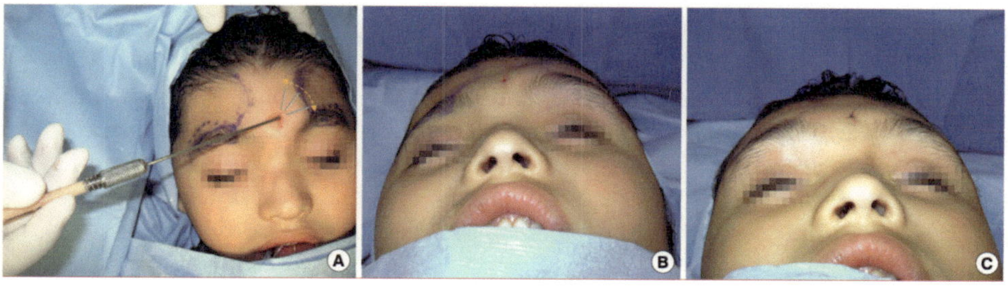

Figure 3.
Five-year-old boy with sequelae of craniosynostosis. Intraoperative view. (A) The glabellar lipoinjection was performed in a fan shape until adequate symmetry was achieved. (B) The treated left area. (C) Both treated areas.

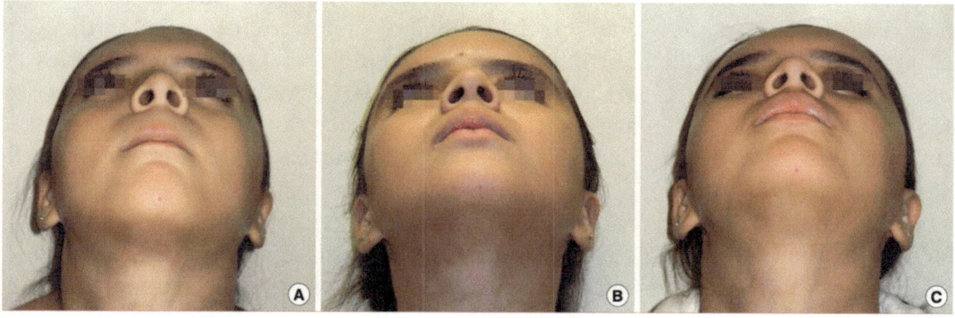

Figure 4.
Five-year-old girl with sequelae of right plagiocephaly. (A) Preoperative view. (B) One month after adipose stem cell lipoinjection. (C) Eighteen months after adipose stem cell lipoinjection.

Undoubtedly, ASC-enriched lipoinjection has become an excellent volumetric filler alternative in the vast field of craniofacial surgery, particularly for conditions that share soft tissue atrophy or hypoplasia as a common denominator [7–12].

In summary, our perspective is that craniofacial surgery will continue to evolve. Advances in technology and cutting-edge surgical techniques, combined with the incorporation of regenerative medicine to address complex pathologies in an increasingly personalized and effective manner, will represent the most promising approach to significantly improving patients' quality of life.

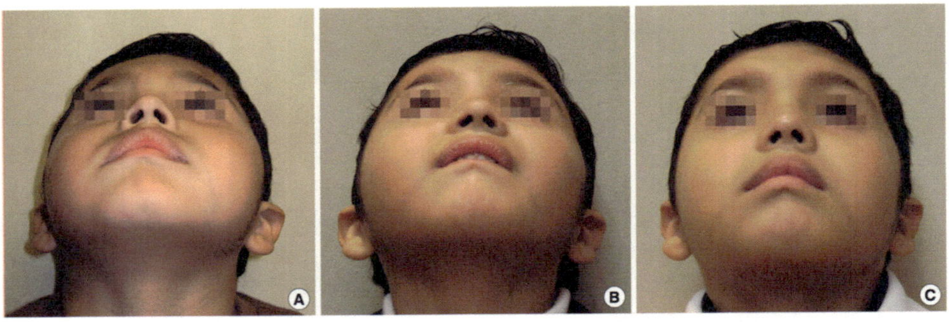

Figure 5.
Five-year-old boy with sequelae of brachycephaly. (A) Preoperative view. (B) One month after adipose stem cell lipoinjection. (C) Eighteen months after adipose stem cell lipoinjection.

10. Modern techniques and procedures in craniomaxillofacial surgery

The advancement of knowledge and technology has revolutionized craniomaxillofacial surgery (CMFS), optimizing both functional and esthetic outcomes while transforming the surgical experience for both patients and professionals. These innovations have enabled greater precision, significantly reducing risks and surgical times, resulting in comprehensive improvements in the planning and execution of procedures.

11. Clinical use of adipose-derived stem cells

As previously mentioned, autologous fat grafts supplemented with adipose-derived stem cells (ASCs) have become one of the most widely used procedures today. For example, nasal reshaping with autologous fat, enriched or not with ASCs, represents an excellent option for camouflaging dorsal nasal irregularities both during and after surgical rhinoplasty. Additionally, it is a valuable resource for thickening the skin, particularly in secondary or tertiary rhinoplasties, where tissue thinness often exposes irregularities in the bony and cartilaginous framework of the nasal dorsum [14].

We believe that non-surgical nasal reshaping using ASC-enriched micrografts could be an innovative alternative. Its versatility offers significant advantages for esthetic nasal contouring as well as correcting other types of nasal asymmetries. However, to date, we have not found specific information on the use of ASC-enriched autologous fat in rhinoplasty procedures.

12. 3D printing

Computer-assisted planning, based on CAD/CAM technology, has redefined the therapeutic approach and surgical planning for complex procedures. By generating personalized three-dimensional models, surgeons can anticipate, with millimeter precision, the necessary movements and adjustments in procedures such as orthognathic surgery and advanced reconstructions. This level of accuracy not only ensures better functional and esthetic outcomes but also facilitates communication with the medical team and the patient, ensuring a collaborative and highly effective treatment plan.

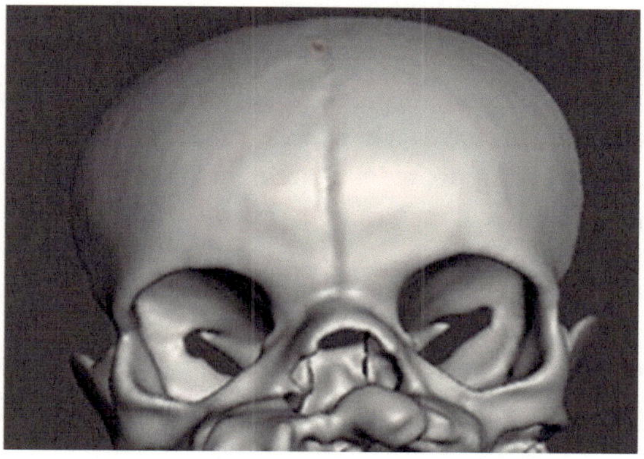

Figure 6.
Computed tomography scan and three-dimensional (3D) virtual image reconstruction. Frontal view of 3D image reconstruction with the residual tumor occupying the hard palate with extension to the nasopharynx.

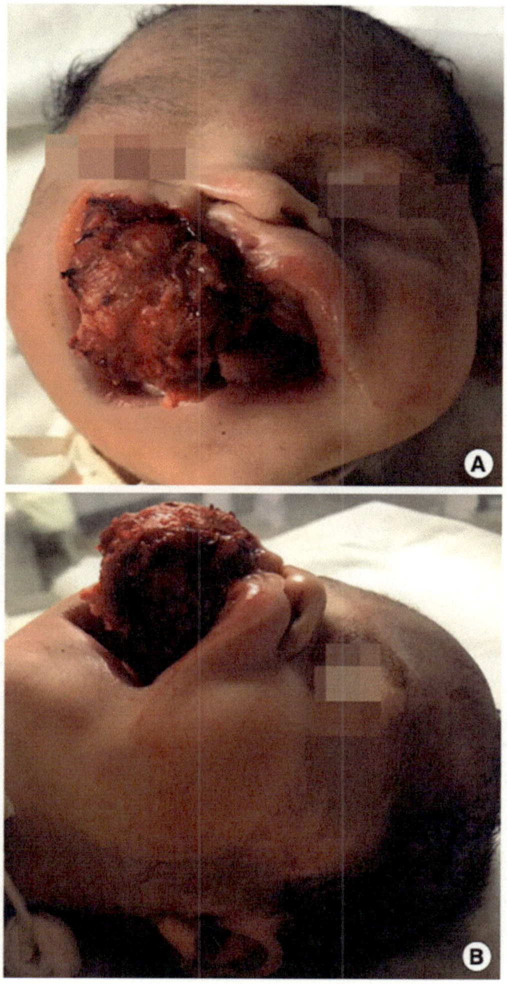

Figure 7.
Residual tumor protruding through the mouth. (A) Frontal and (B) oblique view of the tumor after extraoral resection.

3D printing has become an essential tool, allowing for the creation of surgical guides, implants, and customized prostheses like never before. This technology enables more precise and efficient surgical execution while also reducing operating room times. In highly complex cases where specific adjustments to anatomical structures are necessary, 3D printing provides personalized solutions that maximize results and minimize complications. This technology is of utmost importance in procedures requiring precise resections. The surgical treatment of an epignathus, a rare orofacial teratoma in a newborn, is an excellent example of the utility of 3D printing [14] (**Figures 6–10**).

Minimally invasive approaches, such as the use of mini endoscopes and laparoscopic techniques, represent another significant advancement. These techniques reduce damage to surrounding tissues, minimizing postoperative complications, pain, and recovery times. They are particularly effective in procedures such as facial

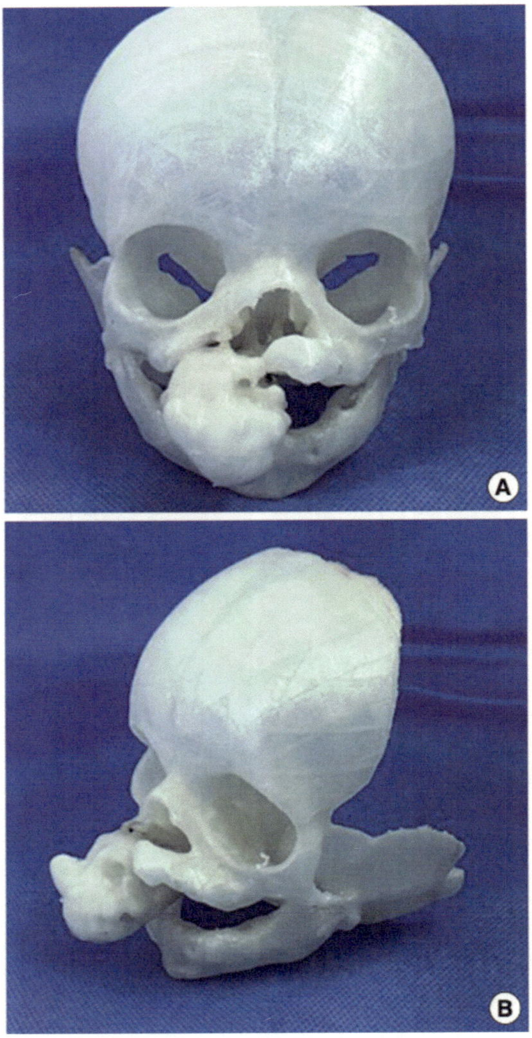

Figure 8.
Stereolithographic three-dimensional (3D) model of the facial skeleton to scale. (A) Frontal view of the 3D model and (B) right oblique view of the 3D model.

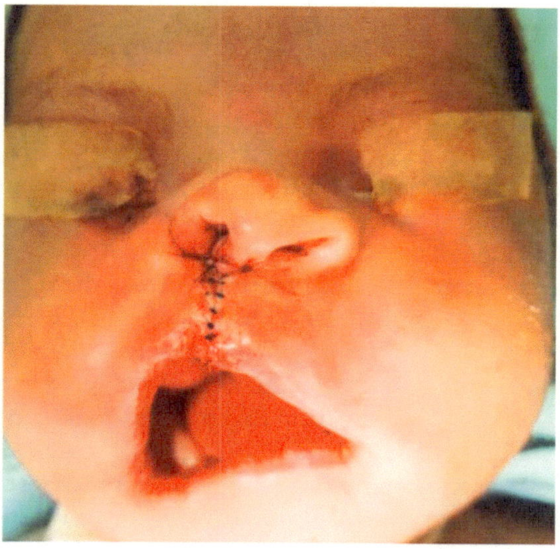

Figure 9.
Intraoperative view of epignathus resection. Final appearance after a bloc resection of the intraoral tumor and lip adhesion.

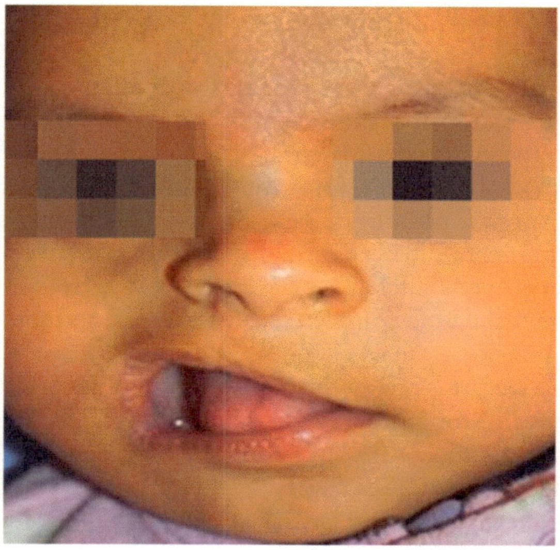

Figure 10.
Postoperative view of the patient. General appearance of the face at 6 months.

fracture repair and temporomandibular joint interventions, ensuring a faster and less traumatic recovery for the patient [15].

The use of biocompatible materials, such as titanium, collagen meshes, and bone matrices, has elevated the standards in reconstructive surgeries. These materials offer high compatibility with natural tissues, facilitating tissue and bone integration while providing safe, durable, and esthetically satisfactory solutions in complex surgical procedures.

Together, these modern techniques and procedures position CMFS as a constantly evolving subspecialty, capable of offering innovative and personalized solutions that transform patients' quality of life and optimize outcomes in every intervention.

13. Challenges and future of the specialty

Despite remarkable advances in craniomaxillofacial surgery (CMF), this sophisticated field of knowledge still faces persistent challenges that limit its ability to expand and evolve. These obstacles highlight the need for investments in infrastructure, improvements in professional training, and a constant focus on innovation to overcome structural and technical barriers. Logically, all of this must be closely linked to best clinical practices and evidence-based medicine.

Limited access to advanced technology remains one of the main challenges, especially in regions with scarce resources. The lack of specialized equipment and modern tools prevents the application of cutting-edge techniques, creating significant disparities in treatment quality, particularly in developing countries. Reducing this technological gap is crucial to ensuring that more patients can benefit from the advances in this specialty.

Another critical aspect is specialized training. Given the inherent complexity of craniomaxillofacial surgery, professionals require rigorous and continuous education. The rapid incorporation of new technologies and surgical approaches necessitates ongoing medical education programs to keep surgeons up to date. However, in low-resource settings, access to advanced training can be a significant challenge.

Finally, surgical complications represent an ongoing challenge, especially in highly complex procedures. These inherent risks demand not only a high level of sophisticated technical expertise but also robust protocols for complication prevention and management. Enhancing the capabilities of surgical teams and optimizing postoperative outcomes are essential objectives to address this challenge.

We believe that the future of craniomaxillofacial surgery is shaping up as a field of revolutionary advancements, thanks to the integration of emerging technologies such as augmented reality (AR), 3D bioprinting, and artificial intelligence (AI). AR will transform both surgical training and execution by providing interactive simulations and real-time guidance during procedures, optimizing precision and safety. Meanwhile, 3D bioprinting will facilitate the creation of personalized tissues and bone structures, revolutionizing complex reconstructions and reducing implant wait times.

From our perspective, AI is one of the most relevant aspects of modern computing innovation, creating value for individuals and businesses alike. There is enormous potential in the field of medicine and, undoubtedly, in CMF. AI will enable more precise surgical planning, improved diagnosis and prognosis, and personalized adaptation to patient needs, among many other potential applications.

CMF is undergoing a transformative evolution, marked by rapid technological advancements and the refinement of surgical techniques. This progress not only redefines medical practice standards but also opens new therapeutic possibilities for treating complex craniomaxillofacial conditions. Beyond technical advancements, the primary goal of CMF is to improve patients' quality of life by restoring essential functions such as chewing, speaking, and breathing while also restoring confidence and self-esteem through favorable esthetic outcomes.

As previously mentioned, many of these patients undergo treatment at an early age. Therefore, incorporating extensive knowledge and experience, along with a high level of artistic sensitivity, is essential to restoring both function and facial symmetry. This impact is particularly significant for patients with congenital deformities, severe trauma, or oncological sequelae, who see craniomaxillofacial surgery as an opportunity to rebuild their lives.

14. Conclusion

CMF is an exciting and highly specialized field of knowledge. Due to the nature of its practice, it is undeniably subject to constant refinement, driven by the continuous generation of new knowledge that balances technological innovation with a deep commitment to human well-being. Overcoming current challenges and continuing to adopt innovative approaches will ensure a more inclusive and promising future. The ultimate challenge is to bring the benefits of this discipline to an increasing number of patients worldwide. If we can bring a smile to a child's face, then we have made progress.

Author details

Yanko Castro-Govea*, Melissa Fernanda Ochoa Cortez
and Cynthia Minerva Gonzalez-Cantu
Hospital Universitario Dr. José Eleuterio González, Monterrey, Mexico

*Address all correspondence to: goveayanko@hotmail.com

References

[1] Castro-Govea Y, De La Garza-Pineda O, Lara-Arias J, Chacón-Martínez H, Mecott-Rivera G, Salazar-Lozano A, et al. Cell-assisted lipotransfer for the treatment of parry-romberg syndrome. Archives of Plastic Surgery. 2012;**39**(6):659-662. DOI: 10.5999/aps.2012.39.6.659. Epub 2012 Nov 14

[2] Tolarova MM, Cervenka J. Classification and birth prevalence of orofacial clefts. American Journal of Medical Genetics. 1998;**75**:126-137

[3] Croen LA, Shaw GM, Wasserman CR, Tolarova MM. Racial and ethnic variations in the prevalence of orofacial clefts in California, 1983-1992. American Journal of Medical Genetics. 1998;**79**:42-47

[4] Houkes R, Smit J, Mossey P, Don Griot P, Persson M, Neville A, et al. Classification systems of cleft lip, alveolus and palate: Results of an international survey. The Cleft Palate-Craniofacial Journal. 2023;**60**(2):189-196. DOI: 10.1177/10556656211057368. Epub 2021 Nov 23

[5] Reyneke JP. Surgical cephalometric prediction tracing for the alteration of the occlusal plane by means of rotation of the maxillomandibular complex. The International Journal of Adult Orthodontics and Orthognathic Surgery. 1999;**14**(1):55-64

[6] Kaye CI, Rollnick BR. Samuel Pruzansky and the center for craniofacial anomalies. Journal of Craniofacial Genetics and Developmental Biology. Supplement. 1985;**1**:25-30

[7] Vento AR, LaBrie RA, Mulliken JB. The O.M.E.N.S. classification of hemifacial microsomia. The Cleft Palate-Craniofacial Journal. 1991;**28**(1):68-76; discussion 77. DOI: 10.1597/1545-1569_1991_028_0068_tomens_2.3.co_2

[8] Castro-Govea Y, Cervantes-Kardasch VH, Borrego-Soto G, Martínez-Rodríguez HG, Espinoza-Juarez M, Romero-Díaz V, et al. Human bone morphogenetic protein 2-transduced mesenchymal stem cells improve bone regeneration in a model of mandible distraction surgery. The Journal of Craniofacial Surgery. 2012;**23**(2):392-396. DOI: 10.1097/SCS.0b013e318240fe9b

[9] Yoshimura K, Sato K, Aoi N, Kurita M, Inoue K, Suga H, et al. Cell-assisted lipotransfer for facial lipoatrophy: Efficacy of clinical use of adipose-derived stem cells. Dermatologic Surgery. 2008;**34**(9):1178-1185. DOI: 10.1111/j.1524-4725.2008.34256.x. Epub 2008 May 29

[10] Castro-Govea Y, Vela-Martinez A, Treviño-Garcia LA. Volumetric lipoinjection of the fronto-orbital and temporal complex with adipose stem cells for the aesthetic restoration of sequelae of craniosynostosis. Archives of Plastic Surgery. 2018;**45**(2):128-134. DOI: 10.5999/aps.2017.00997. Epub 2018 Mar 15

[11] Taylor JA, Paliga JT, Wes AM, et al. A critical evaluation of long-term aesthetic outcomes of fronto-orbital advancement and cranial vault remodeling in nonsyndromic unicoronal craniosynostosis. Plastic and Reconstructive Surgery. 2015;**135**(1):220-231

[12] Lovegrove E, Rumsey N. Ignoring it doesn't make it stop:

Adolescents, appearance, and bullying. The Cleft Palate-Craniofacial Journal. 2005;**42**(1):33-44. DOI: 10.1597/03-097.5.1

[13] Zhang B, Wu Y, Mori M, Yoshimura K. Adipose-derived stem cell conditioned medium and wound healing: A systematic review. Tissue Engineering. Part B, Reviews. 2022;**28**(4):830-847. DOI: 10.1089/ten.TEB.2021.0100. Epub 2022 Jan 10

[14] Gonzalez-Cantu CM, Moreno-Peña PJ, Salazar-Lara MG, García PPF, Montes-Tapia FF, Cervantes-Kardasch VH, et al. Surgical management of palatal teratoma (epignathus) with the use of virtual reconstruction and 3D models: A case report and literature review. Archives of Plastic Surgery. 2021;**48**(5):518-523. DOI: 10.5999/aps.2021.00318. Epub 2021 Sep 15. Erratum in: Arch Plast Surg. 2021 Nov;48(6):723. DOI: 10.5999/aps.2021.01984

[15] Xing Z, Ren R, Xia X, Yang L. Supra-temporalis approach for treating zygomaticomaxillary complex fracture. The Journal of Craniofacial Surgery. 2021;**32**(3):1087-1089. DOI: 10.1097/SCS.0000000000007463

Section 2

Techniques and Procedures

Chapter 3

Orthofacial Surgery, the Esthetic Surgery of the Facial Skeleton: Techniques, Approaches, and Outcomes

Joan Birbe

Abstract

The field of esthetic surgery of the facial skeleton combines the principles of cranio-maxillofacial reconstruction with advanced techniques to enhance facial harmony, symmetry, and function. By addressing the skeletal framework that supports soft tissues, these procedures significantly improve both esthetics and functionality, transforming patient outcomes. Key procedures include orthognathic surgery, which corrects jaw discrepancies while improving facial balance, and genioplasty, which reshapes the chin to achieve proportionality and alignment. Facial feminization surgery (FFS) tailors craniofacial features to align with gender identity, emphasizing softer, more delicate contours for a feminine appearance. Modern advancements, such as 3D printing and CAD/CAM-guided implants, enable patient-specific solutions, ensuring precision and long-lasting results. The integration of esthetic skeletal procedures with soft tissue modifications further enhances outcomes, addressing aging-related changes or specific contour deficiencies. This chapter explores the principles, surgical techniques, and technologies driving innovations in esthetic facial skeletal surgery, alongside case studies that illustrate its transformative impact. Additionally, it highlights the importance of patient-centered care and the ethical considerations of balancing realistic expectations with surgical possibilities. Future directions in robotics, AI-driven planning, and biomaterials promise to refine outcomes and expand possibilities in this dynamic field.

Keywords: esthetic facial surgery, orthognathic surgery, facial feminization surgery, genioplasty, custom implants, orthofacial surgery

1. Introduction

The field of esthetic surgery within cranio-maxillofacial practice has undergone a significant transformation in recent decades. Initially focused on reconstructive techniques to correct congenital anomalies, trauma, and pathology, this specialty now integrates esthetic goals to enhance harmony and balance in facial appearance [1].

This evolution mirrors broader societal trends, where facial esthetics are increasingly recognized as central to identity, confidence, and quality of life.

1.1 The shift toward esthetic enhancements

Cranio-maxillofacial surgery has traditionally prioritized restoring function, such as correcting malocclusions or addressing structural deformities. However, the growing understanding of facial proportions and symmetry has catalyzed a paradigm shift toward achieving esthetic goals alongside functional corrections. Today, procedures like orthognathic surgery and genioplasty are not only functional but are widely sought after for their transformative esthetic potential [2].

This dual-purpose approach has opened the doors to patient-centered care, where improving facial harmony, proportion, and symmetry is as important as correcting structural abnormalities. For example:

- *Orthognathic surgery*: Initially designed to correct malocclusions, this procedure now addresses esthetic concerns such as jaw asymmetry and facial projection.

- *Genioplasty*: Once a secondary adjunct to jaw surgery, genioplasty now plays a pivotal role in sculpting the chin and jawline, crucial for gender-specific esthetics and overall facial balance.

1.2 The role of facial skeletal aesthetics

Facial skeletal esthetics serve as the structural framework for the overlying soft tissues, dictating the contours, proportions, and overall appearance of the face. This foundation is critical in determining beauty, attractiveness, and individuality. Key elements of facial esthetics include symmetry, proportion, sexual dimorphism, and youthfulness, all of which guide planning in esthetic surgical interventions [3].

1.2.1 Symmetry

Symmetry is universally recognized as a key determinant of facial beauty. The balance between the left and right sides of the face influences visual appeal and is often the goal of many esthetic procedures. While perfect symmetry is rare in nature, subtle corrections to improve facial balance significantly enhance attractiveness.

1.2.2 Proportions

Facial proportions are evaluated using horizontal and vertical divisions:

- *Vertical proportions*: The face is divided into thirds: the forehead (trichion to glabella), midface (glabella to subnasale), and lower face (subnasale to menton). These proportions must be balanced for a harmonious appearance.

- *Horizontal proportions*: The face is divided into fifths, with equal widths between the lateral edges of the eyes, the nasal base, and the distance from the eyes to the ears.

1.2.3 Sexual dimorphism

Sexual dimorphism refers to the distinct differences in facial skeletal structure between males and females. These differences are fundamental to perceived gender identity and are central to many esthetic surgeries, especially facial feminization and masculinization procedures.

- *Male facial aesthetics*:
    - Strong, angular jawlines with prominent mandibular angles.
    - A broader chin that is often more squared.
    - Pronounced brow ridges and thicker zygomatic arches.
    - Heavier skeletal contours contribute to a rugged, masculine appearance.
- *Female facial aesthetics*:
    - Softer, rounded contours in the chin and jawline.
    - Narrower mandibles with less pronounced angles.
    - A more delicate zygomatic projection with smoother transitions.
    - Reduced brow prominence and a flatter frontal bone.

Esthetic surgeries, such as genioplasty, mandibular contouring, and zygomatic augmentation, aim to enhance or modify these features to align with patient goals, particularly in cases of facial feminization or masculinization.

1.2.4 Youthful appearance

Youthfulness is a desirable esthetic quality, often associated with volume, defined contours, and smooth transitions between skeletal and soft tissue structures. Over time, facial aging affects both the soft tissue and the underlying skeletal framework:

- *Bone resorption*: Aging leads to bone loss in the mandible, maxilla, and orbital rims, resulting in diminished support for soft tissues and a hollowed appearance.
- *Contour changes*: The jawline becomes less defined, and the midface appears flatter due to the resorption of the zygomatic bones.
- *Volume loss*: Combined with skeletal changes, the reduction in soft tissue volume exacerbates the aged appearance.

Surgical techniques such as cheek augmentation, orbital rim enhancement, and combined skeletal and soft tissue procedures restore youthful facial proportions. The integration of skeletal modifications with soft tissue rejuvenation (e.g., face lifts) ensures a comprehensive approach to reversing signs of aging.

1.3 Social and psychological impacts

Beyond physical transformation, esthetic surgery of the facial skeleton has profound psychological and social implications. The face is central to self-identity and interpersonal interactions. Procedures that enhance facial structure often lead to improved self-esteem, confidence, and social engagement. For example:

- *Facial feminization surgery (FFS)*: This set of procedures has become a cornerstone for transgender individuals seeking to align their appearance with their gender identity. By reshaping the forehead, jawline, and chin, FFS enables patients to achieve both esthetic and psychological congruence.

- *Orthognathic surgery for aesthetics*: Patients with facial asymmetries or retruded jawlines often report improved self-image and social confidence post-surgery.

1.4 Objectives of the chapter

This chapter seeks to provide a comprehensive exploration of the techniques, approaches, and outcomes of esthetic facial skeletal surgery. Key focus areas include:

- *Orthognathic surgery*: Its transformation from a functional correction to a cornerstone of esthetic enhancement.

- *Genioplasty*: Its versatility in reshaping the chin and defining the jawline.

- *Facial feminization surgery*: A nuanced approach to achieving gender-specific facial esthetics.

- *Custom implants*: The role of advanced materials like PEEK and the integration of CAD/CAM technology in tailoring patient-specific solutions.

- *Other facial osteotomies*: Beyond orthognathic surgery, procedures such as:

    - *Zygomatic osteotomies*: Used to refine cheekbone projection or width, enhancing midface proportions.

    - *Segmental maxillary osteotomies*: For detailed transverse and vertical corrections of the upper jaw, addressing asymmetries or localized deformities.

    - *Mandibular angle osteotomies*: Contouring the lower jaw to soften angularity or create a more defined esthetic.

    - *Forehead osteotomies*: Reshaping the frontal bone to reduce prominence in masculinized foreheads or enhance contour in feminization cases.

    - *Orbital rim osteotomies*: To address orbital asymmetry or enhance periorbital harmony as part of rejuvenation or feminization procedures.

1.5 Innovations and the future

The field continues to evolve with advances in imaging, surgical planning, and biomaterials. Virtual surgical planning (VSP) [4], custom implants, and minimally invasive techniques have set new benchmarks in precision and patient satisfaction. Looking ahead, technologies like artificial intelligence (AI) and robotic-assisted surgery hold promise for further refinements in technique and outcomes.

2. Anatomical and functional considerations

A thorough understanding of facial skeletal anatomy and its influence on esthetics is essential for achieving optimal outcomes in esthetic cranio-maxillofacial surgery. This chapter outlines the anatomical features, their role in overall facial appearance, and the variations influenced by ethnicity, gender, and aging. Additionally, it emphasizes the aging process of the facial skeleton and its implications for esthetic interventions.

2.1 Facial skeletal anatomy relevant to esthetic surgery

The facial skeleton provides the structural framework for soft tissue and dictates the contours and proportions of the face [5]. Key regions and their contributions to esthetics include:

- *Maxilla*: The maxilla forms the central support for the midface. It defines the nasolabial angle, contributes to midface projection, and supports the overlying soft tissue, such as the cheeks and upper lip. Maxillary deficiencies can result in flat midfaces, poor nasolabial contour, and malocclusion, all of which significantly impact facial harmony.

- *Mandible*: The mandible plays a critical role in shaping the lower face, particularly the jawline and chin. A well-defined mandible provides structural integrity to the lower facial contours, influencing the perception of youth, strength, and symmetry. Irregularities, such as a retruded or asymmetric mandible, can disrupt facial balance and esthetics.

- *Zygomatic arches*: The zygomatic arches are crucial for cheekbone prominence and midface width. A well-defined zygomatic structure enhances facial contours and creates a youthful, vibrant appearance. Diminished zygomatic projection leads to a flat midface and poor transition between the cheeks and the periorbital region.

- *Frontal bone and forehead*: The frontal bone, including the forehead, determines brow projection and forehead contour. Esthetic ideals for the forehead vary by gender, with softer, rounded contours preferred in feminine esthetics and stronger, more pronounced features favored in masculine profiles.

Understanding the intricate relationships between these skeletal regions and the overlying soft tissue is crucial for planning and executing esthetic surgeries.

2.2 Role of skeletal esthetics in overall facial appearance

The skeletal structure serves as the foundation for soft tissue, and its interplay dictates overall facial esthetics. Modifications to skeletal features can profoundly impact facial harmony and soft tissue contours. Key aspects include:

- *Facial balance*: Proportions between the maxilla, mandible, and zygomatic arches influence facial symmetry and balance. A well-proportioned skeletal framework enhances soft tissue appearance, improving nasolabial folds, cheek fullness, and jawline definition.

- *Cheek projection and zygomatic arches*: Enhancing zygomatic projection can improve cheek prominence, reduce midface hollowness, and create a more youthful appearance. Similarly, mandibular augmentations can sharpen the jawline, complementing soft tissue rejuvenation.

- *Soft tissue-skeletal interplay*: Surgical interventions on the skeleton, such as orthognathic surgery or custom implant placement, must account for their effects on overlying soft tissue. For example, advancing the maxilla enhances midface projection while improving nasolabial contours.

2.3 Ethnic, gender, and age variations

Facial skeletal anatomy varies significantly across populations, requiring a tailored approach to meet the unique esthetic goals of each patient [6].

2.3.1 Ethnic variations

Facial skeletal features are influenced by ethnicity, with variations in zygomatic prominence, mandibular angles, and maxillary projection:

- Patients of East Asian descent often have flatter midfaces and require enhanced zygomatic projection for balanced esthetics.

- Individuals of African descent frequently exhibit strong mandibular angles but may seek adjustments in nasal or midface contours.

- European facial features are typically characterized by pronounced cheekbones and angular jawlines, often requiring subtle refinements.

2.3.2 Gender variations

Sexual dimorphism in facial skeletal anatomy plays a pivotal role in gender-specific esthetics:

- *Masculine features*: Strong angular jawlines, broad chins, pronounced brow ridges, and wider zygomatic arches define male esthetics.

- *Feminine features*: Softer contours, narrower mandibles, rounded zygomatic structures, and reduced brow prominence are hallmarks of female facial features. Facial feminization and masculinization surgeries aim to align these features with the patient's gender identity.

2.3.3 Age-related changes

Age affects both the skeletal framework and soft tissue, contributing to an aged appearance:

- Skeletal resorption in the maxilla and mandible results in volume loss, flattened cheeks, and diminished jawline definition.

- Expansion of the orbital rim leads to hollowing and an aged periorbital appearance.

Addressing these variations requires a culturally sensitive and patient-centered approach.

2.4 Aging of the facial skeleton

Facial aging is not limited to soft tissue changes; the skeletal framework also undergoes significant transformations that affect the overall appearance of the face [7]. These skeletal changes are critical targets for comprehensive facial rejuvenation [8].

2.4.1 Bone resorption

- *Maxilla*: Aging leads to vertical shortening of the maxilla, resulting in midface volume loss, a flatter profile, and deepening of the nasolabial folds.

- *Mandible*: Resorption at the mandibular angle and chin reduce jawline definition, causing sagging soft tissues and prominent jowls.

- *Orbital rim*: Expansion of the orbital aperture contributes to a hollowed and aged periorbital appearance, exacerbating the appearance of eye bags and shadows.

2.4.2 Changes in facial contours

- *Midface changes*: Loss of skeletal support in the zygomatic arches results in a sunken appearance in the cheeks and temples, leading to midface flattening.

- *Lower face changes*: Reduced chin projection and mandibular angle resorption contribute to a diminished lower face and increased soft tissue sagging [9].

2.4.3 Clinical implications

Addressing the skeletal aspects of aging is essential for achieving comprehensive and lasting facial rejuvenation. Common interventions include:

- *Custom implants*: PEEK or CAD/CAM implants are used to restore volume and projection in the midface, orbital rim, and jawline.

- *Midface lifts*: These procedures reposition the soft tissue while restoring skeletal support.

- *Orbital rim augmentation*: Enhances the periorbital region to counteract hollowing and improve youthful contours.

By addressing the anatomical and functional considerations outlined in this chapter, surgeons can create personalized treatment plans that account for variations in ethnicity, gender, and age, while restoring structural support for soft tissue and resulting in esthetically pleasing and long-lasting outcomes.

3. Principles of esthetic facial skeletal surgery

3.1 Concept of facial balance and harmony

Facial balance is the alignment of skeletal proportions to achieve esthetic ideals, focusing on symmetry, proportionality, and harmony among the facial thirds (upper, middle, and lower). These ideals often rely on the golden ratio (1: 1.618), which is used as a guideline in surgical planning to create a natural and appealing appearance. For example, genioplasty (chin surgery) optimizes the projection and dimensions of the chin across anteroposterior, vertical, and transverse planes. This multidimensional approach ensures harmony between the chin and adjacent facial structures, enhancing the balance of the lower third of the face [10].

3.2 Patient evaluation and expectations management

Achieving successful outcomes in facial skeletal surgery hinges on a comprehensive patient evaluation and managing expectations effectively.

- *Assessment tools*:

  - *3D imaging*: Technologies like 3D imaging and virtual surgical planning (VSP) provide precise anatomical assessments, enabling accurate diagnoses and surgical previews.

  - *Profile analysis*: For procedures such as genioplasty or orthognathic surgery, a detailed evaluation of skeletal and soft tissue proportions is crucial. Considerations like labiomental angle, mentolabial competency, and chin projection are evaluated against normative data (e.g., lower dental height of 44 mm ± 2 mm for men and 40 mm ± 2 mm for women).

- *Communication*:

  - *Education*: Providing patients with realistic digital simulations and discussing limitations is key. Explaining the functional and esthetic benefits of surgical interventions (e.g., improved occlusion, and enhanced breathing with orthognathic procedures) promotes satisfaction.

- *Expectation management*: By aligning patient expectations with achievable results, surgeons foster trust and avoid dissatisfaction.

3.3 Planning the esthetic change

Surgical planning integrates esthetic and functional goals to deliver optimal results.

- *Digital simulations*: Advanced planning tools, such as virtual surgical planning (VSP), CAD/CAM surgical guides, and 3D-guided osteotomies, allow surgeons to visualize post-surgical outcomes. For instance, chin reshaping techniques (e.g., "wing-shield" or "inverted V"osteotomy) are simulated to refine chin proportions and symmetry.

- *Functional integration*: Esthetic facial surgery often overlaps with functional corrections:

  - *Orthognathic surgery*: Combines occlusal adjustments with facial skeletal repositioning to ensure both functional improvement and esthetic enhancement [11]. For example, addressing maxillary protrusion can simultaneously improve nasal base esthetics and occlusal relationships.

  - *Combined procedures*: Interventions such as genioplasty with rhinoplasty (profileplasty), orthognathic surgery with nasal, or a face-lift with genioplasty modifications offer comprehensive facial harmony.

3.3.1 Conclusion

Facial skeletal surgery requires a delicate balance between esthetics and function. By employing advanced evaluation tools, managing patient expectations, and leveraging modern surgical technologies, surgeons can deliver results that meet both cosmetic and functional goals while ensuring patient satisfaction.

4. Techniques and procedures

This part provides an in-depth exploration of the advanced surgical techniques employed in esthetic facial skeletal surgery. These include orthognathic surgery for functional and cosmetic improvements [12], genioplasty for chin contouring [13], and facial feminization surgery (FFS) for gender-specific facial refinement [14]. It also highlights the precision and customization afforded by modern technologies such as CAD/CAM-guided implants and discusses the integration of soft tissue and skeletal corrections for comprehensive results. Furthermore, the chapter underscores the importance of long-term stability in surgical outcomes and emphasizes the role of personalized planning in addressing the unique needs of gender-diverse patients. By adopting a patient-centered approach, surgeons can achieve long-lasting, transformative results that meet both esthetic and functional goals.

4.1 Orthognathic surgery for esthetic purposes: Orthofacial surgery

Orthognathic surgery plays a pivotal role in refining facial proportions by repositioning skeletal structures such as the maxilla, mandible, and chin. By addressing both functional and esthetic concerns, it enhances midface projection, jawline definition, and symmetry.

4.1.1 Stability, personalization, and gender considerations in orthognathic surgery

4.1.1.1 Stability and longevity

Ensuring stability is critical to the success of orthognathic surgery. Younger candidates, such as adolescents and young adults, particularly benefit from long-lasting corrections.

4.1.1.2 Gender-affirming surgery

Patients' gender identity significantly influences facial esthetic goals. For gender-diverse individuals, orthognathic surgery can address key gender-specific features, such as smooth foreheads, narrowed jawlines, or softened chin contours. Tailored surgical plans ensure the outcomes align with the patient's gender identity, reducing the need for subsequent corrective surgeries.

4.1.1.3 Integration with gender-affirming procedures

Orthognathic surgery can complement or replace other gender-affirming surgeries [15]. For example, narrowing the gonial angles or enhancing the malar projection can fulfill esthetic goals without requiring additional interventions.

Patient-Specific Esthetic Goals Orthognathic surgery's profound impact on facial esthetics necessitates a patient-centered approach that considers ethnicity, gender, and individual preferences. These factors play a pivotal role in defining a patient's perception of their own facial harmony and satisfaction with the surgical outcome. Recognizing these influences ensures that surgical plans are tailored to meet diverse needs while respecting cultural and personal values. Incorporating patient-specific goals, such as desired proportions or profiles, into the surgical plan promotes higher satisfaction and a more personalized outcome.

Gender Diversity and Orthognathic Surgery Gender diversity among orthognathic surgery candidates has introduced new dimensions of complexity and responsibility in treatment planning. With approximately 5.1% of individuals aged 18–25 identifying as gender-diverse in the United States, it is crucial for surgeons to consider the implications of gender identity when designing surgical plans. For this demographic, facial features that align with gender-affirming goals can have profound implications on psychological well-being and satisfaction. The surgeon must ensure that gender identity and preferences are explicitly addressed during pre-surgical evaluations to prevent unintended esthetic results that could exacerbate gender dysphoria.

4.1.1.4 Feminine and masculine esthetic characteristics in orthognathic surgery

Orthognathic surgery provides opportunities to shape craniofacial features in alignment with feminine or masculine ideals, supporting patients' gender-affirming goals [16].

- Feminine facial features: A feminine facial form often includes a smooth forehead without frontal bossing, a more obtuse nasofrontal angle, larger orbital apertures, a tapered chin, and a narrower jawline. Feminine features also involve increased anterior malar projection, creating the ogee curve, and greater incisor display at rest (2–4 mm). Re-establishing these characteristics through skeletal adjustments can often eliminate the need for additional soft tissue gender-affirming surgeries. Techniques such as high Le Fort I osteotomies, malar augmentation, and precise control of the nasolabial angle can refine these features.

- Masculine facial features: Masculine facial esthetics are characterized by stronger, more angular features, including a prominent jawline, a flatter mandibular plane angle, and reduced incisor show (1–2 mm). For example, counterclockwise rotation of the mandible may emphasize the jawline while addressing Class II malocclusion [16].

4.1.1.5 Avoiding gender dysphoria through informed surgical planning

In cases involving gender-diverse individuals, failing to align surgical outcomes with their gender identity can result in significant distress, including increased gender dysphoria. For instance, a transfeminine patient may require adjustments to achieve a feminine esthetic profile, such as narrowing of the gonial angles or reduction of chin width. If these preferences are not communicated or incorporated into the surgical plan, the patient may experience dissatisfaction or require additional corrective procedures. Surgeons must navigate sensitive situations, including cases where patients are exploring their gender identity or have not disclosed their preferences due to personal or familial concerns. This underscores the importance of creating a supportive, confidential environment where patients feel comfortable expressing their goals. Surgeons also have an ethical obligation to discuss the extent to which orthognathic surgery can meet gender-affirming objectives, particularly in scenarios where the surgical outcomes may inherently involve gender-related facial changes.

4.2 Techniques

4.2.1 Genioplasty (chin contouring)

Genioplasty focuses on reshaping the chin to harmonize the lower third of the face with other facial features.

- *Advancement or reduction*: Adjustments in chin projection help balance retruded or overly prominent profiles.

- *Vertical modifications*: Changes to chin height ensure proportional alignment with the upper and middle facial thirds.

- *Asymmetry correction*: Using 3D surgical planning, surgeons can correct transverse deviations, ensuring symmetry and enhancing facial esthetics.

4.2.2 Le Fort I osteotomy

Le Fort I osteotomy is utilized to reposition the maxilla and correct vertical and horizontal discrepancies. This procedure improves midface projection and nasolabial harmony, creating a more balanced and proportionate facial profile.

4.2.3 Bilateral sagittal split osteotomy (BSSO)

BSSO is employed to reposition the mandible and address retrognathia or prognathism. This technique harmonizes the lower third of the face with the upper and middle thirds, refining jawline contours and enhancing the overall profile.

4.2.4 Maxilla segmental osteotomies

Segmental osteotomies allow precise, localized adjustments to the maxilla or mandible. These are often integrated with other procedures to fine-tune facial symmetry and achieve optimal esthetic outcomes.

4.3 Facial feminization surgery (FFS)

Facial feminization surgery addresses the craniofacial characteristics associated with traditional feminine esthetics, helping patients achieve a softer, more feminine appearance (**Figures 1** and **2**) [17].

4.3.1 Key procedures

- *Forehead contouring*: Reduces the brow ridge and smooths the frontal bone, creating a more delicate profile.
- *Jawline and chin reshaping*: Narrowing mandibular angles and refining chin contours create a tapered, feminine lower face.
- *Cheek augmentation*: Enhances zygomatic projection, emphasizing the curves associated with feminine midfaces.

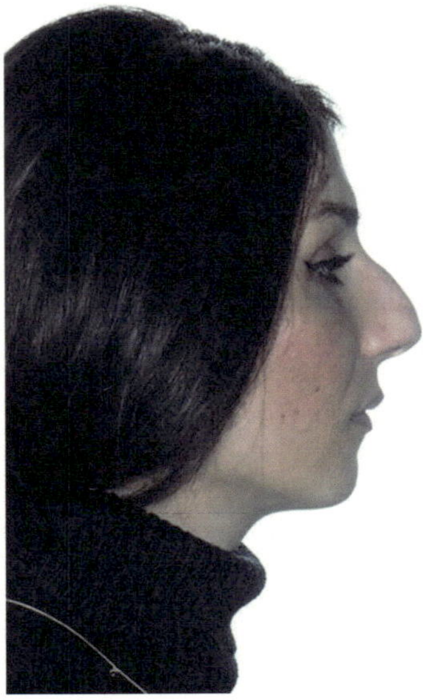

Figure 1.
Postop result after facial feminization surgery with rhinoplasty.

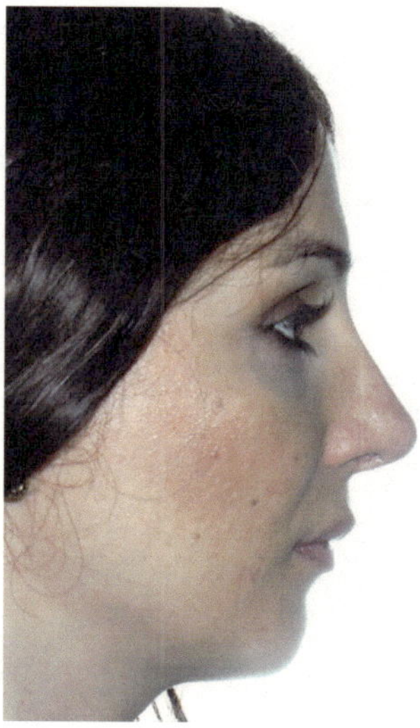

Figure 2.
Facial feminization surgery.

4.4 Custom facial implants

Custom implants provide precise solutions for skeletal deficiencies and asymmetries, offering long-term durability and patient-specific customization [18].

4.4.1 Materials and techniques

- *PEEK implants*: Polyetheretherketone (PEEK) implants, crafted using CAD/CAM technology, ensure anatomical precision and biocompatibility [18].
- *Applications*: These implants are used to enhance the jawline, cheeks, and chin, improving overall facial proportions and balance.

4.4.2 Advantages

Custom implants fit seamlessly with existing anatomy, minimizing complications and delivering natural, esthetically pleasing results.

4.5 Combined esthetic and soft tissue procedures

Integrating skeletal surgery with soft tissue corrections enhances the overall esthetic outcome by addressing both structure and surface features

4.5.1 Key combinations

- *Face-lift with genioplasty*: Combines chin contouring with skin tightening to rejuvenate the lower face.
- *Neck lift with mandibular augmentation*: Refines the jawline-neck angle while correcting structural deficiencies.

- *Orthognathic surgery with blepharoplasty*: Aligns skeletal repositioning with eyelid corrections for comprehensive facial harmony.
- *Orthognathic surgery with rhinoplasty:* Aligns skeletal repositioning with nasal function and harmony (**Figures 3** and **4**) [19, 20].

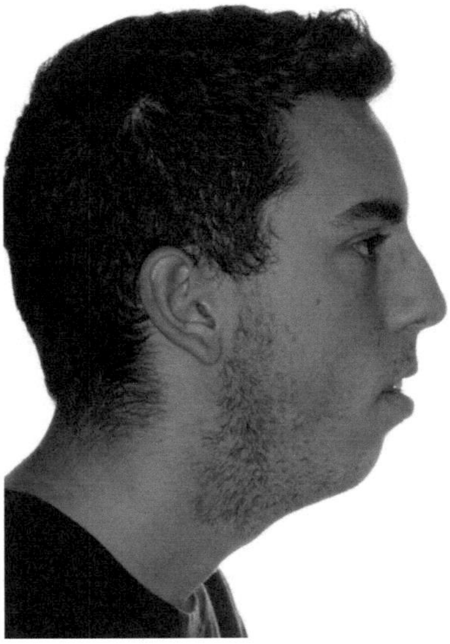

Figure 3.
Preop (above) and postop (below) facial changes of bimaxillary orthognathic surgery with simultaneous rhinoplasty and genioplasty.

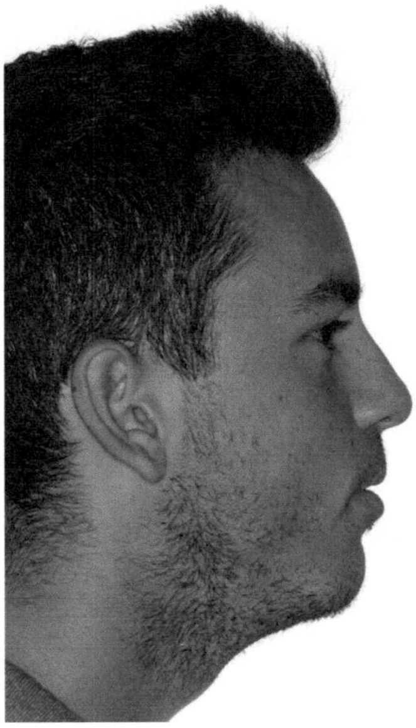

Figure 4.
Orthognathic surgery with rhinoplasty.

4.6 Orbital rejuvenation

Aging in the periorbital region often leads to changes that affect the appearance of youth and vitality. Orbital rejuvenation addresses these concerns by targeting skeletal, soft tissue, and skin changes [21].

4.6.1 Skeletal considerations in aging

Bone loss and enlargement of the orbital aperture contribute to hollowing and tear trough deformities. These changes require precise interventions to restore a youthful appearance.

4.6.2 Techniques

- *Infraorbital rim augmentation*: Custom implants or fat grafting restore volume and smooth transitions between the eyelids and cheeks.
- *Tear trough correction*: Combines skeletal augmentation with fillers or fat grafting to address hollows.
- *Lateral canthoplasty*: Tightens the outer eye corner to rejuvenate the periorbital area.
- *Blepharoplasty*: Refines the upper and lower eyelids, smoothing the eyelid-cheek transition.

4.6.3 Combining techniques

Midface lifts with skeletal augmentation correct both volume loss and soft tissue ptosis, while forehead and brow lifts elevate sagging tissues and improve symmetry.

5. Postoperative care and rehabilitation

5.1 Post-surgical management

The postoperative phase is critical for ensuring optimal recovery and achieving the intended surgical outcomes. Proper management of pain, swelling, and mobility is essential to support healing and prevent complications [22].

- *Pain control*: Effective pain management involves a combination of local anesthetics, oral analgesics, and anti-inflammatory medications tailored to the individual's needs. Regular assessment of pain levels helps to adjust treatment and improve patient comfort.
- *Swelling reduction*: Swelling is a natural response to surgical trauma, particularly in procedures involving skeletal manipulation or implants. Strategies such as criotherapy face mask, the elevation of the head during rest, and lymphatic drainage therapy can significantly reduce swelling and accelerate recovery.

- *Early mobilization*: Encouraging patients to resume light activities within a safe timeframe minimizes the risk of complications such as blood clots and promotes overall well-being.

5.1.1 Conclusion

The integration of advanced surgical techniques, personalized care, and meticulous postoperative management ensures the success of esthetic facial skeletal surgery. By addressing patient-specific needs and leveraging technological innovations, surgeons can achieve transformative results that enhance both functionality and esthetic appeal. A commitment to safety, education, and continuous monitoring fosters patient satisfaction and long-term stability, solidifying the role of these procedures in modern facial esthetic care.

6. Case studies

6.1 Case example 1: Facial feminization surgery (FFS)

A 32-year-old transgender woman sought facial feminization surgery to align her facial features with her gender identity. The patient exhibited prominent masculine characteristics, including a pronounced brow ridge, wide mandibular angles, and a dorsal nasal hump (**Figures 1** and **2**).

- *Surgical approach*: The comprehensive FFS procedure included forehead contouring to smooth the brow ridge, mandibular angle reduction to narrow the jawline, and rhinoplasty to refine the nasal dorsum and tip. These techniques were tailored to achieve a natural and feminine esthetic.

- *Outcome*: Postoperatively, the patient achieved a soft, feminized appearance with balanced facial proportions. Patient feedback indicated a marked improvement in self-confidence and satisfaction with the results.

6.2 Case example 2: Orthognathic surgery

A 24-year-old patient presented with mandibular deficiency characterized by a retrusive lower jaw, high mandibular plane angle lip incompetence, and ineffective pogonion, which affected both their facial balance lip and occlusal function. The treatment plan included a combination of bimaxillary advancement with counterclockwise rotation, genioplasty, and simultaneous preservation rhinoplasty (**Figures 3** and **4**).

- *Surgical approach*: The maxilla was repositioned using a Le Fort I osteotomy, the mandible was repositioned with bilateral sagittal split osteotmies, to enhance midface projection, while genioplasty was performed to advance the chin and balance the lower third of the face. These adjustments harmonized the facial profile and corrected the occlusal misalignment. A simultaneous rhinoplasty was also performed.

- *Outcome*: The procedure significantly improved jawline projection and overall facial balance, resulting in a balanced and esthetically pleasing profile. The patient reported high satisfaction with both the functional and cosmetic outcomes.

6.3 Case example 3: Combined procedures

A 39-year-old patient sought treatment for signs of aging, including facial sagging and volume loss, skin laxity, and diminished jawline definition. A combined approach of facial rejuvenation and skeletal enhancement with a rhinoplasty was recommended (**Figures 5–8**).

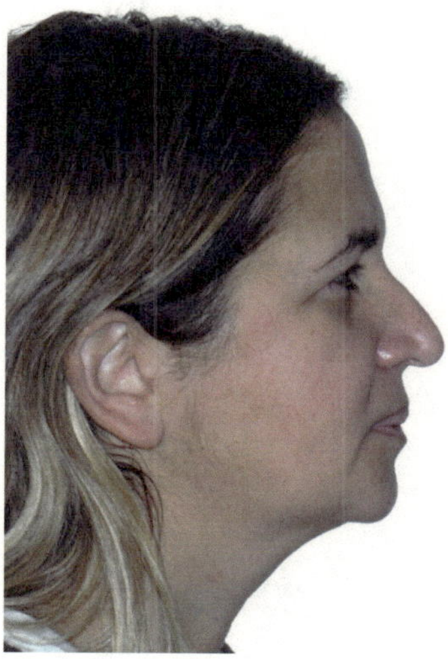

Figure 5.
Preop (above) and postop (below) facial changes of deep plane face and neck lift with upper blepharoplasty note improvement in jaw angle and neck angle definition with a natural soft tissue support.

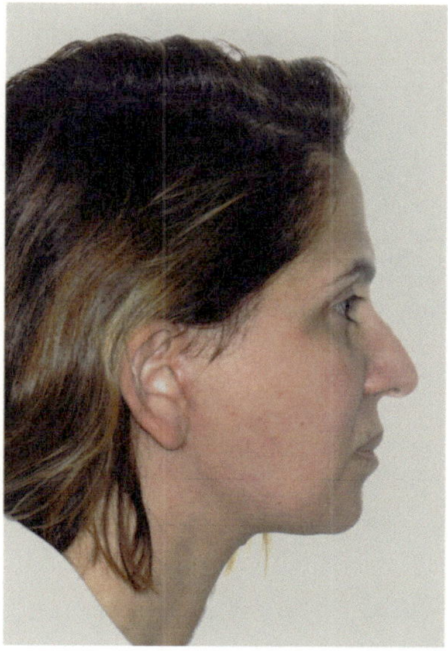

Figure 6.
Case example 3: Combined procedures.

- *Surgical approach*: The patient underwent a deep plane face and neck -lift to address skin laxity and restore midface volume, combined with rhinoplasty to enhance nasal breathing and treat dorsal excess. Lipofilling in the tear trough area was also performed with 1,5 cc of fat injected in a supraperiosteal plane.

- *Outcome*: The procedure achieved comprehensive rejuvenation, restoring youthful contours and improving facial harmony. The patient reported high satisfaction, highlighting both the natural appearance and the balanced esthetic results.

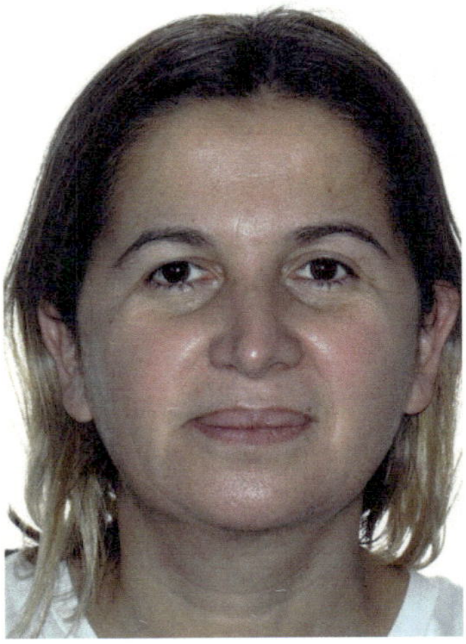

Figure 7.
Case example 3: Combined procedures.

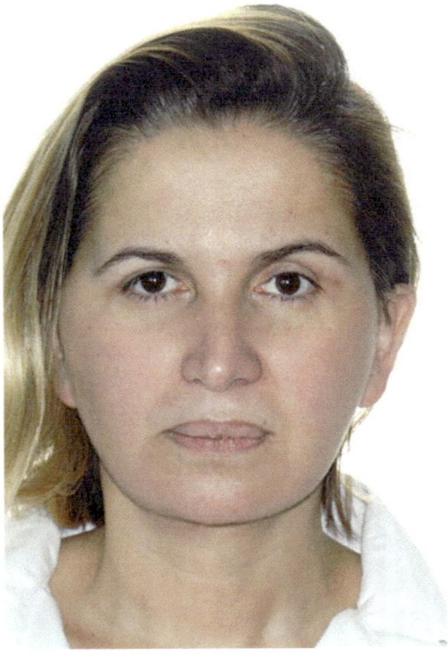

Figure 8.
Case example 3: Combined procedures.

7. Conclusion

Esthetic facial skeletal surgery represents a dynamic and transformative field that harmonizes form and function to improve patient quality of life. Through procedures such as orthognathic surgery, genioplasty, and facial feminization surgery, surgeons achieve tailored outcomes that address both structural and esthetic goals.

The integration of advanced technologies, including 3D printing, robotic assistance, and artificial intelligence, has elevated the precision and predictability of these procedures. Furthermore, the ethical responsibility of surgeons to balance patient desires with realistic outcomes underscores the importance of patient-centered care.

As innovations continue to shape the future of the field, including the development of new biomaterials and minimally invasive techniques, the potential for achieving natural, long-lasting, and transformative results will only grow. By combining technical expertise with compassion and attention to detail, surgeons can help patients achieve enhanced self-confidence, functionality, and facial harmony.

Author details

Joan Birbe
Private Practice, Clinica BIRBE, Barcelona, Spain

*Address all correspondence to: doctor@birbe.org

References

[1] Facial aesthetic surgery: Enhancing beauty through maxillofacial procedures. Journal of Oral Medicine, Oral Surgery, Oral Pathology and Oral Radiology. 2023;**9**(3)

[2] Rosen HM. Facial skeletal expansion: Treatment strategies and rationale. Plastic and Reconstructive Surgery. 1992;**89**:798-808. DOI: 10.1097/00006534-199205000-00006

[3] Faderani R, Singh P, Monks M, Dhar S, Krumhuber E, Mosahebi A, et al. Facial aesthetic ideals: A literature summary of supporting evidence. Aesthetic Surgery Journal. 2024;**44**(1):NP1-NP15. DOI: 10.1093/asj/sjad295

[4] Robiony M, Salvo N, Costa F. Virtual reality and stereolithographic models in maxillofacial surgical planning. International Journal of Oral and Maxillofacial Surgery. 2008;**37**(3):167-170. DOI: 10.1016/j.ijom.2007.07.01

[5] Johnson P, Tighe D. Modification of the facial skeleton in aesthetic facial surgery. In: Oxford Textbook of Plastic and Reconstructive Surgery. Oxford, UK; 2021. p. 1425-C12.11.S18. DOI: 10.1093/med/9780199682874.003.0118

[6] McCleary SP, Nirbhay J, Moghadam S, Le C, Roostaeian J. Racial perspectives on facelifts: Evaluating techniques and outcomes across diverse populations. Aesthetic Surgery Journal. 2024;**44**(8):785-796. DOI: 10.1093/asj/sjae046

[7] Shaw RB, Kahn DM. Aging of the facial skeleton: Implications for rejuvenation. Plastic and Reconstructive Surgery. 2007;**119**(1):1-10. DOI: 10.1097/01.prs.0000242500.80427.d6

[8] Mendelson BC, Wong CH. Changes in the facial skeleton with aging: Implications and clinical applications in facial rejuvenation. Aesthetic Plastic Surgery. 2012;**36**(4):753-760. DOI: 10.1007/s00266-012-9904-3

[9] Spiegel JH. Facial skeletal changes with aging and implications for facial rejuvenation. Facial Plastic Surgery Clinics of North America. 2005;**13**(3):371-380. DOI: 10.1016/j.fsc.2005.05.007

[10] Whitaker LA, Morales L. Aesthetic surgery of the facial skeleton. Clinics in Plastic Surgery. 1987;**14**(4):749-760. DOI: 10.1016/S0094-1298(20)31343-5

[11] Altaibi NM, Liu CH, Benington PC, Ayoub AF. Improvement in facial aesthetics of orthognathic patients after surgery-first approach. Aesthetic Surgery Journal. 2024;**44**(1):NP1-NP15

[12] Jansma J, Schepers RH. Adjunctive aesthetic procedures in orthognathic surgery. Oral and Maxillofacial Surgery Clinics. 2023;**35**(1):139-152

[13] Kim T, Lee J, Cho Y. Inverted V-shape osteotomy with central strip resection: A simultaneous narrowing and vertical reduction Genioplasty. Plastic and Reconstructive Surgery Global Open. 2014;**2**:e227

[14] Uranbey O, Kaygisiz OF, Ayrancı F, et al. Exploring the evolution of facial feminization and masculinization surgery: A bibliometric analysis and visualization study. Maxillofacial Plastic and Reconstructive Surgery. 2024;**46**:19

[15] Raffaini M, Magri AS, Agostini T. Full facial feminization surgery:

Patient satisfaction assessment based on 180 procedures involving 33 consecutive patients. Plastic and Reconstructive Surgery. 2016;**137**(2):438-448

[16] Fisher EL et al. Planning the cut: Gender-affirming considerations in orthognathic surgery. Journal of Oral and Maxillofacial Surgery. 2024;**82**(11):1343-1346

[17] Owusu JA, Boahene KD. Advances in facial feminization surgery. Current Opinion in Otolaryngology and Head and Neck Surgery. 2020;**28**(4):243-249

[18] Narciso R, Basile E, Bottini DJ, Cervelli V. PEEK implants: An innovative solution for facial aesthetic surgery. Case Reports in Surgery. 2021;**2021**:5518433. DOI: 10.1155/2021/5518433

[19] Birbe J. Cambios nasolabiales en cirugia ortognática maxilar. Revista Española de Ortodoncia: Birbe Journal. 2005;**35**:217-228

[20] Nasal dorsum reduction simultaneous to orthognathic surgery: A proof-of-concept report. Facial Plastic Surgery Birbe Journal. 2021;**37**:646-650

[21] Glat PM, Sykes JM, Stucker FJ. Aesthetic contours of the midface and periorbital region. Facial Plastic Surgery Clinics of North America. 1995;**3**(4):449-462

[22] Etemad SA, Poh MM. Enhanced recovery after gender-affirming surgery. Aesthetic Surgery Journal. 2024;**44**(Suppl. 1):S3-S14

Chapter 4

Mandibular Resection: Disabilities, Challenges, Reconstruction Techniques, Advances, and Quality of Life

Fadia Awadalkreem and Haifa Kamal

Abstract

Congenital anomalies, trauma caused by road traffic accidents, sports, and violence, cyst removal, and benign and malignant tumor eradication may require mandibular resection. A procedure that has many adverse effects, such as facial disfigurement, esthetic impairment, compromised masticatory efficiency, speech problems, bargained social interaction, and physiological circumstances that adversely affect the patient's quality of life. The rehabilitation of patients with mandibular resection still presents a challenge for both maxillofacial surgeons and prosthodontists and emphasizes the role of a multidisciplinary team approach for optimum treatment outcomes. This chapter aims to elucidate the different disabilities associated with mandibular resections, challenges encountered, the different surgical and prosthetic reconstructive techniques that can be used for rehabilitation, and their impacts on patient quality of life.

Keywords: mandibular resection, marginal mandibulectomy, prosthetic reconstruction, segmental mandibulectomy, surgical reconstruction

1. Introduction

Congenital anomalies; trauma from road traffic accidents, sports, and violence; and cyst removal and benign and malignant tumor resection may result in maxillofacial defects that have several adverse effects, including facial disfigurement, esthetic impairment, compromised masticatory efficiency, speech problems, limited social interaction, and physiological circumstances that hamper the patient's quality of life [1–8].

2. Oral cancer and mandibular defect

Head and neck cancers (HNC) pose a significant global issue, ranking as the seventh most common neoplasm worldwide, with over 900,000 new cases annually [9, 10]. Of these, 40% are oral cancers, accounting for 377,713 new diagnoses per year [9–12] .

Surgical irradiation of the tumor, alone or in combination with radiotherapy (RT) and/or chemotherapy (CT), is the most common treatment modality for oral cancers [9, 13].

Considering the mandibular oral cancer cases, two different surgical resection techniques can be performed according to the tumor extension: marginal mandibulectomy and segmental mandibulectomy [5, 8]. Marginal mandibulectomy is defined as the surgical removal of a segment of the mandible, without resulting in a continuity defect while segmental mandibulectomy is a type of mandibulectomy that involves the surgical removal of a portion of the mandible. Both techniques result in several disabilities that necessitate expeditious rehabilitation (**Figure 1**) [14].

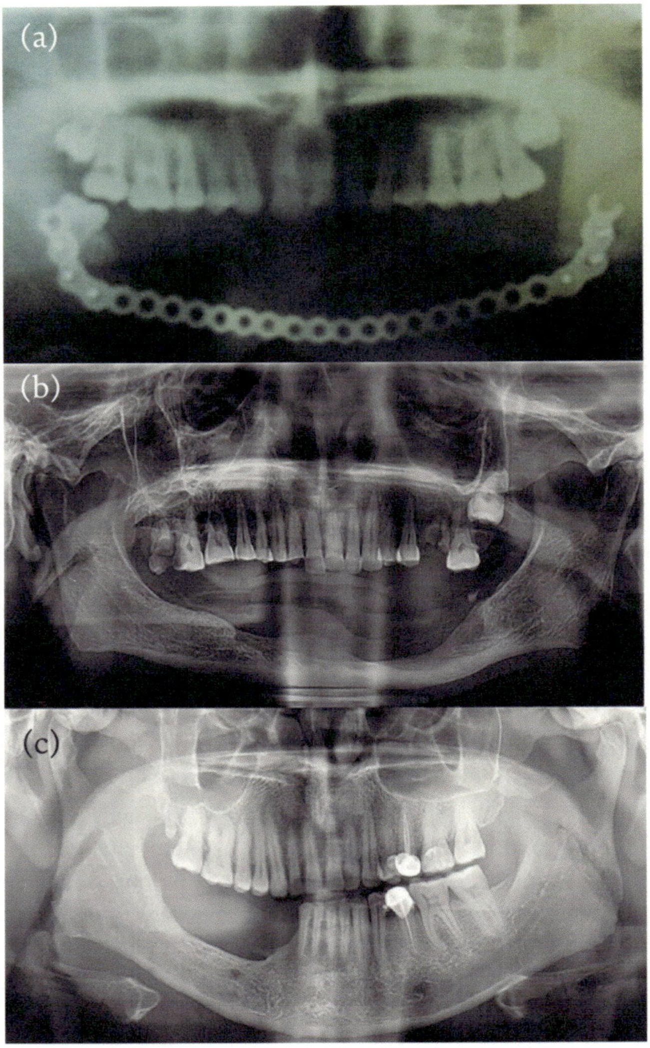

Figure 1.
Panoramic radiograph of a patient with (a) segmental mandibulectomy, (b) completely edentulous patient with marginal mandibulectomy, and (c) posterior marginal mandibulectomy showing inadequate vertical height above the mandibular canal.

3. Disabilities associated with mandibular resection

The geometrical U shape of the mandible defines the esthetic of the lower third of the face, supporting the tongue and the muscles of the mouth and facilitating the patient's mastication, deglutition, articulation, normal breathing, and salivary control [15]. Following mandibulectomy, the patient may encounter several disabilities, including cosmetic deformity, impaired speech and articulation, compromised control of salivary secretion, deviation of the mandible during opening, closing, and functional movement, difficulty in swallowing, chewing problems, diminished social activity, and reduced patient quality of life [1–8].

The main goals of mandibular reconstruction are to re-establish the form of the lower third of the face, ascertain the required alveolar bone height, establish the arch form and width, improve the patient's esthetics, mastication, swallowing, deglutition, and phonation; maintain the airway passage; control the saliva dropping; and improve the patient's psychology and quality of life (**Figure 2**) [1–8, 15, 16].

The selection between the different reconstructive modalities is significantly determined by many factors [1, 2, 5, 17, 18], such as the position and extension of the defects [1, 2, 5, 17], the depth of the vestibular sulci [6, 7, 15, 16, 19], the remaining soft and hard tissues [4, 5, 15–17], the degree of tongue impairment [5–7], the need for radio- and/or chemotherapy as adjunctive therapy and the associated circumstances [5–9], the cost [4, 15], the expertise of the maxillofacial surgeon, the presence of a specialized centre, and the patient's preference [1–7, 15, 20–22].

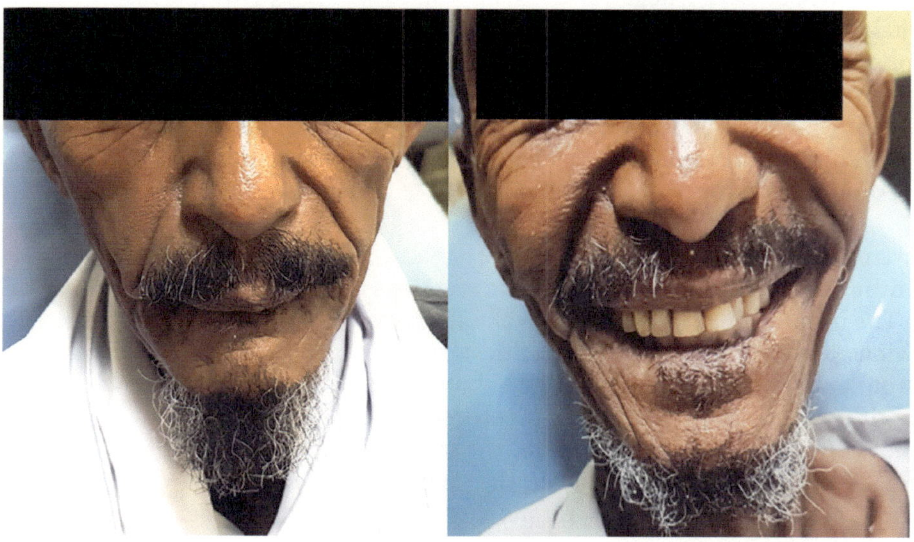

(a) (b)

Figure 2.
Extra-oral frontal view of anterior marginal mandibular resection patient. (a) Before reconstruction. (b) After reconstruction.

4. Classification of mandibular defects

The literature documented several classifications for mandibular defects. The mandibular defects are generally classified according to their positions into anterior, lateral, and ramus/condyle defects [8].

Jewer et al. [23] provide another classification based on the complexity of the restoration, with central defects extending between canine to canine, forming a C"-shaped defect, and lateral segments excluding the condyle in the form of "L." When the condyle is resected together with the lateral mandible, the defect is in the form of an "H," or hemi-mandibular defect [23, 24].

Boyd et al. [25] considered the mucosal and/or soft tissue component of the defect by adding characters o, m, and s as osseous only, mucosa, and/or external skin, respectively.

Another classification provided by Urken et al. [26] is based on functional considerations caused by the detachment of different muscle groups and difficulties with cosmetic restoration. C—condyle, R—ramus, B—body, S—total symphysis, and SH—hemisymphysis.

Petrovic et al. [21] classified the marginal mandibular resection patients from a prosthetic aspect into three subgroups, including completely edentulous patients, partially edentulous patients, and dentate patients with non-tooth-bearing area marginal mandibulectomy, that is, the ascending ramus of the mandible.

5. Timing of mandibular reconstruction (immediate/delayed)

Following mandibular resection, the defect can be immediately reconstructed, or after a while, using a delayed/staged approach, which provides an observational period of tumor recurrence. However, in benign cases, nowadays, the immediate reconstruction approach is widely acceptable with a high success rate and significant improvement in the patient's quality of life [23, 27–32].

5.1 The role of the maxillofacial team in the management of mandibular resection patients

Management of mandibular resection cases necessitates the interaction between the different oral and maxillofacial team members for successful rehabilitation [2, 21]. The primary objective of the maxillofacial team is to restore the patient to their previous state of health. The target of the treatment plan should be restoring the continuity of the mandibular bone, if possible, and replacing the soft and hard tissue loss with a stable, well-functioning prosthesis [2, 5, 21, 33, 34].

Seok H [35] emphasized the role of the multidisciplinary approach for the management of patients with oral cancer; the team can include the following specialists: oral and maxillofacial surgeons, plastic surgeons, otolaryngologists, radiation oncologists, hematology oncologists, prosthodontists, general dentists, and speech-language pathologists, depending on the case, extension, and tumor grading.

Wang et al. [36] reported a relatively lower risk mortality rate in patients treated with a multidisciplinary team. In the same line, de Boer et al. [37], Kutuk emphysized et al. [38], Ahmad et al. [39], Shah [40], and Suliman and Awadalkreem [41] underscore the role of interprofessional collaboration in optimizing the oral health management for head and neck cancer patients with and without radiation therapy.

6. Rehabilitation of mandibular resection defects

The rehabilitation of mandibular resection defects may follow two stages/approaches:

1. Surgical reconstruction of the mandibular defects.

2. Prosthetic reconstruction of the mandibular defects.

6.1 Surgical reconstruction of the mandibular defects

Through the past decades, several surgical techniques [2, 3, 8, 18, 21, 42–126] have been described in the literature for the reconstruction of mandibular defects, including primary closure of the defect (healing by primary intension), skin graft, the use of alloplastic metallic mesh and plate, regional flaps, non-vascularized flaps, free vascularized bone graft, distraction osteogenesis, bone substitutes, and advance technology (**Figure 3**).

6.1.1 Primary closure

Primary closure of the oral tissues is the simplest method as it does not involve replacing the defected bone and instead allows the mucosa to heal with secondary intention. Small defects less than 2 cm can be closed primarily by expanding the surrounding buccal or floor-of-mouth mucosa over the bony defect (**Figure 3**) [1, 3, 5, 8, 18, 55].

6.1.2 Skin graft

Reverdin first described the skin graft in 1869; later in 1972, Ollier highlighted its usage, which had been reviewed by Stele in 1870 and documented by Pai et al. [55]. The use of split skin grafts is a simple technique that allows close oncologic monitoring while ensuring excellent speech and swallowing function. Both spilt-thickness and full-thickness skin grafts can be used for small-defect mandibular reconstruction with the advantages of rapid healing, extended flaps with limited morbidity of the

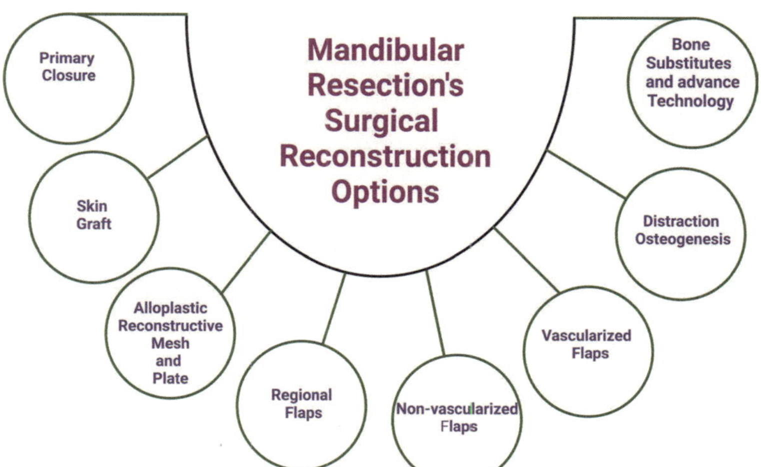

Figure 3.
Surgical mandibular reconstructive techniques.

donor site, and avoidance of the flap's bulk. The immobilization of the flap during the healing process plays a significant role in its success and can be facilitated by the construction of a surgical stent. However, in some cases, the intra-oral bulk of the skin graft may limit the use of a removable reconstructive prosthesis. Additionally, the preoperative radiation therapy may compromise the healing of the graft [127].

6.1.3 Alloplastic mandibular reconstructive mesh and plate

Reconstructive mesh and plate are the most commonly used alloplastic devices for mandibular reconstruction due to their low costs, reliability, and short intraoperative time, which require less surgical expertise than other surgical techniques [2, 15, 55–59]. Before completing the resection, surgeons commonly shape and place the plates to ensure correct segment alignment. Furthermore, it is crucial to exercise meticulous care in maintaining proper occlusion to ensure satisfactory joint function (**Figure 4**).

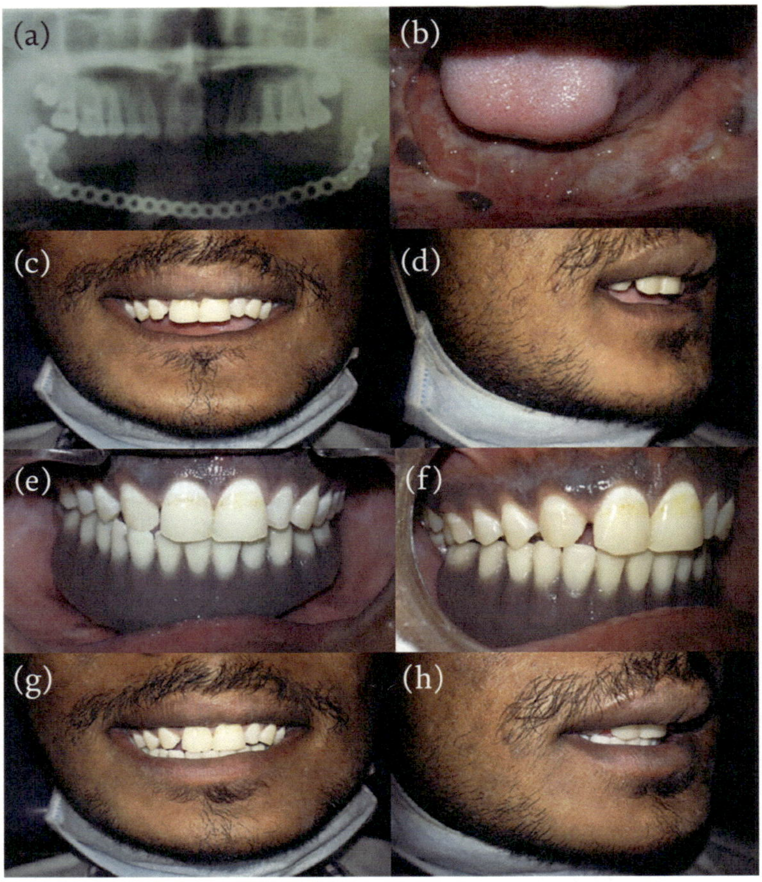

Figure 4.
Mandibular reconstruction with alloplastic reconstructive plate. (a) Postoperative patient's orthopantomography showing segmental mandibular resection reconstructed with alloplastic reconstructive plate. (b) Intra-oral view of the patient at the time of the presentation. (c) Extra-oral frontal view photograph of the patient showing compromised lower lip support. (d) extroral lateral view photograph of the patient. (e) Intra-oral frontal view of the patient showing reconstruction with tissue borne acrylic tissue-supported prosthesis. (f) Intra-oral lateral view of the reconstructive prosthesis (g) Extra-oral frontal view photograph of the patient after reconstruction showing improved lower lip support. (h) Extra-oral lateral view photograph of the patient after reconstruction showing improved lower lip support and patient's esthetic.

However, the compromised esthetic outcome, the limited support for the soft tissues, limited masticatory function, and the possibility of infection that may or may not result in plate exposure and painful sensation, especially in patients with radiotherapy, are the main drawbacks of this reconstructive modality [2, 15].

To improve the esthetic result of reconstructive plate combination with a soft tissue pedicle flap had been considered. Furthermore, this technique has the potential to alleviate tension and minimize the risk of plate exposure, particularly in patients who are radiated [2].

The most commonly used metals for reconstructive plates are stainless steel, vitallium, and titanium. Nowadays, a titanium hollow osseointegrated reconstruction plate (THORP) which is a specialized system has been used widely. It allows bone ingrowth, improving the stability of the bony interface and preventing the necrosis of the bone underneath, without reported adverse effects with radiation per se (**Figure 4**) [15, 56, 57].

6.1.4 Regional flap

The goals of the regional flap are to restore the form and function and minimize donor site morbidity. The buccal fat pad flap, the facial artery musculomucosal flap, the platysma, the pectoralis major, the temporalis muscle flap, and the trapezius flaps are some of the regional pedicle flaps that can be used for reconstruction inside the mouth [55].

The choices between the different regional flaps depend mainly on the size and anatomic position of the defect. Small to medium defects can be reconstructed using local mucosal or cutaneous flaps [55].

Moreover, the amount of the flap tissue needed and the arc of rotation are the main determinants for a regional flap's success. Therefore, it can be used with predictable success for smaller defects or as a salvage of partially failed reconstructions [55].

6.1.4.1 Autogenous bone reconstructed flap

6.1.4.1.1 Historical background

According to the literature [60, 61], the first reported successful bone transfer was performed by an unknown Russian surgeon and documented by van Meekeren in 1668. The graft was a xenograft correcting a cranial defect of a soldier. Von Walther documented the first autograft in 1821, while Bardenheuer in 1892 described the use of a pedicle graft of the mandible itself to restore continuity. However, this flap did not restore the bone tissue loss [60, 61]. Additionally, researchers have used several free, nonvascularized bone grafts from the tibia, iliac crest, or ribs, supported by metallic reconstruction plates [60, 62]. In 1950, Converse reported the use of 12 bone grafts and 14 bone and cartilage grafts for the reconstruction of maxillary and mandibular defects. Vascular surgery led to the use of pedicle osteomyocutaneous flaps [15], ribs with the pectoralis major (15), clavicles with the sternocleidomastoid [15, 50], and the scapula with the trapezius [15, 51], all of which had limited esthetic results.

Later, with the advancement in microsurgical flaps, Taylor et al. [62] and Sanders and Mayou [63] dissipated the use of a deep circumflex iliac artery and vein-free flap, while Swartz et al. [64] documented the use of a scapular osteocutaneous-free flap in 1986.

According the literature, bone grafting techniques have been categorized into the following:

1. The non-vascularized bone graft
2. The vascularized free bone flaps.

The choice between the two techniques is based on [15].

1. The soft tissue quality at the reconstruction site, along with the history of radiation and infection linked to or unrelated to prior graft failure, is crucial.
2. The quantity of soft tissue.
3. The contour and size of the defect.
4. Surgeon expertise and specialized centre availability.
5. Patient preferences.

6.1.5 The non-vascularised bone graft

Commonly utilized for small- to medium-sized defects with limited or no soft tissue loss (less than 5 cm long), it is usually used in cases of benign tumors rather than malignant ones, as well as in orthogenic cases [20].

The most common sites of non-vascularised bone grafting are the rib (whole rib graft/split rib graft) and the iliac crest, with an advantage of faster revascularisation with split rib graft. Despite the fact that the rib graft provides a favorable shape that matches the geometrical shape of the mandible, resulting in a high esthetic outcome, the limited quality and quantity (length and width) of the rib may compromise the use of osseointegrated implants (**Figure 5**) [2, 20].

On the other hand, iliac graft can be used in medium-sized defect sites as it is associated with an abundant amount of both cancellous and cortical bone with increased demand on sculpture and good planning to ensure the correct geometrical shape needed [15, 50].

The literature reported several drawbacks and contraindications for the use of autologous bone, including the increased cost compared to alloplastic plates, increased intraoperative and recovery time, the need for hospitalization, and physiologic resorption of the bone graft with a range from 15–20% [15, 65–69] that may hamper the successful use of osseointegrated dental implants, which require a minimum of 7 mm of bone height for stable anchorage [15, 69–74]. Some investigators reported an increased amount of this resorption, such as Johansson et al. [74], who documented an average of 49.5, and Pai et al. [55], who reported a physiological resorption up to 60%.

6.1.6 Vascularised free flaps

Microvascular free tissue transfer presents the greatest milestones in reconstructive surgery. This surgical approach ensures the transfer of the flap, including the blood anastomosis structures, and its harvesting with a cutaneous or muscular component, thereby increasing the possibility of soft tissue reconstruction. It facilitates the healing of the flap independent of a compromised recipient bed in antagonism to the non-vascularising flap. Moreover, it has advantages of early bone union (within 6 weeks), reduced bony

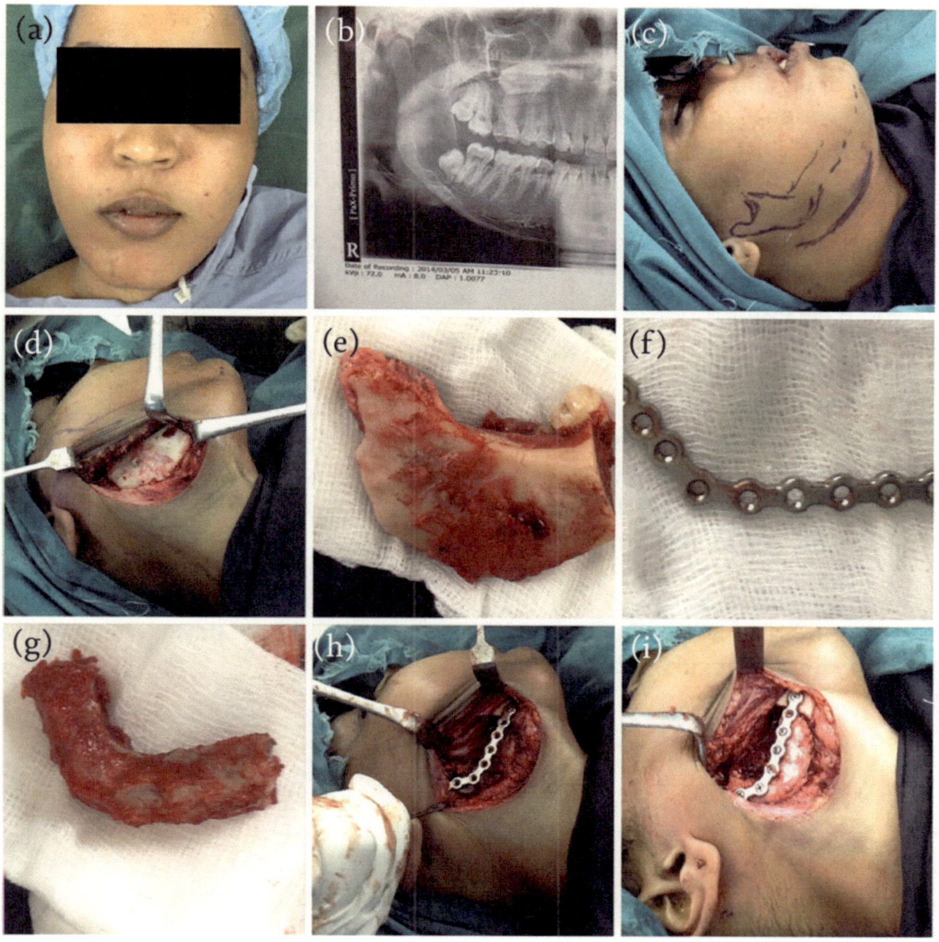

Figure 5.
Mandibular reconstruction with rib bone graft. (a) Preoperative patient's photograph. (b) Preoperative patient's orthopantomography. (c) Intraoperative photograph illustrating the demarcation of the proposed resected area. (d) Intraoperative photograph immediately before resection. (e) Intraoperative photograph of the resected mandibular portion. (f) Intraoperative photograph of the supporting reconstructive plate. (g) Intraoperative photograph of the rib bone graft. (h) Intraoperative photograph illustrating the attachment of the supporting reconstructive plate. (i) Intraoperative photograph of the rib graft and supporting reconstructive plate.

resorption rate, and better toleration for radiation therapy subject to complications such as resorption, fracture, necrosis, and extrusion [20, 75]. Hence, it is commonly used in cases associated with extensive segmental loss and/or compromising precipitant bed.

Several vascularizing free flaps have been documented based on the donor sites including free fibular flap, scapula free flap, anteriolateral thigh flap, the pectoralis major myocutaneous flap, the metatarsus osteocutaneous flap, iliac crest free flap, clavipectoral osteomyocutaneous free flap [20].

6.1.6.1 The fibula free flap

The free fibula osteocutaneous flap is the most frequently used free flap for mandibular reconstruction. It was first described by Hidalgo in 1989 [20, 76]. This flap can provide up to 22–25 cm of bony segment [20].

The use of a free fibula flap has the superiority of an abundant blood supply from the peroneal artery via both endosteal and periosteal branches, as well as a bicortical bone anchorage and a low donor site morbidity rate [20, 77, 78].

The limitation of the skin paddle is the primary disadvantage of the free fibula flap; hence, in larger soft tissue defects, a need may arise for a second soft tissue flap [15, 86].

Moreover, studies have highlighted the potential for donor-site morbidities, wound healing issues, compromised graft survival, and incomplete reconstruction goals such as persistent disfigurement, bone resorption, delayed or unsuccessful bone union, stress plate fracture, recurrent infection, and traumatic ulcer (**Figure 6**) [15, 20, 77, 78, 86].

6.1.6.2 The iliac crest free flap

This flap provides an abundant amount of cortical and cancellous bone for mandibular reconstruction with generous blood supply. It is characterized by natural curvature that facilitates its use for the replacement of lateral mandibular defects; however, for anterior defects, it requires more osteotomy for reshaping [15, 20, 81].

Donor site complications include the challenge of restoring the abdominal wall, the susceptibility of hernia formation, and the poor pliability of the overlying skin, which may limit its regular usage [15, 20, 82].

6.1.6.3 The radial forearm free flap

The radial forearm fasciocutaneous flap can provide 10–12 cm of bone with a thin, abundant amount of skin. This limited amount of bone may prevent the use of osseointegrated implants, thus restricting their use to cases of limited mandibular defects, after which a tissue bone reconstructive prosthesis can be constructed [15, 20, 96].

Additionally, the lack of curvature necessitates a lot of reshaping; the possibility of a pathological fracture of the remaining donor site and susceptible postoperative hand weakness or pain may limit its routine use [15].

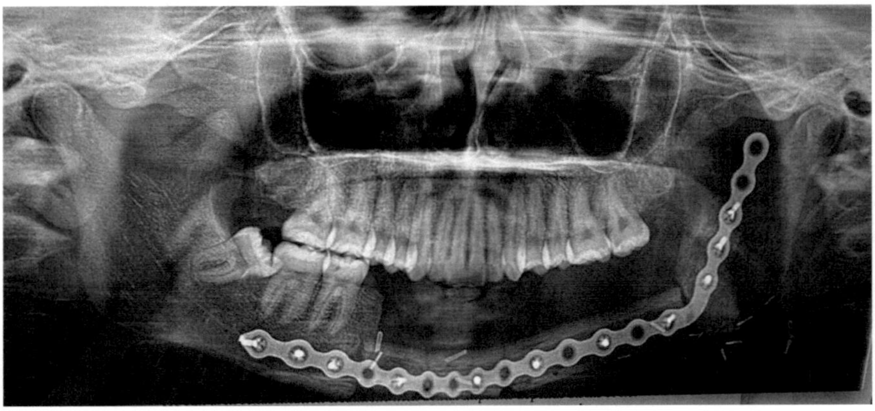

Figure 6.
Panoramic radiograph of a patient presented with segmental mandibulectomy reconstructed with free fibula bone graft supported with reconstructive plate.

6.1.6.4 The scapula free flap

In 1982, Gilbert and Teot [84] described the first use of a free scapular flap. Later, Teot et al. highlighted the use of an osteocutaneous scapular flap for mandibular reconstruction in one patient [85].

Although the scapula osteocutaneous free flap can provide a range of 11 to 14 cm tissue pedicle with acceptable soft tissue bulk and donor morbidity and deformity, its selection as a reconstructive flap for mandibular cases may be limited by the difficulty in positioning the patient to allow for simultaneous resection and microvascular anastomosis, extended intraoperative time, and post-operative shoulder stiffness [15, 20, 87].

The literature describes a number of other mucosal/cutaneous flaps, including the pectoralis major myocutaneous flap for reconstruction of the mandible, floor of mouth, upper neck, and lower one-third of the face when the defect is primarily mucosal or cutaneous [15, 20, 87].

The association between the use of various surgical reconstructive flaps and the different types of mandibular defect reconstruction is well established as follows:

6.1.6.5 Anterior mandibular defects

Reconstruction of anterior defects is commonly done using vascularizing bone grafts, with the free fibula flap reported superiority. Moreover, the use of supportive reconstructive plates guides the shaping of the mandible [20]. Nowadays, computer-generated cutting techniques guide precise treatment planning using computer-aided design software, leading to more acceptable esthetic and functional results.

6.1.6.6 Lateral mandibular defects

For lateral mandibular defect reconstruction, both vascularizing and non-vascularizing flaps can be considered, with a preference for vascularizing in large defect cases and non-vascularized bone grafts in small defects with healthy wound beds [20].

6.1.6.7 Posterior mandibular defects

Cases of posterior mandible reconstruction associated with limited condyle and subcondylar ramus present controversy with reported acceptable appearance, speech, and swallowing function with the use of soft tissue flaps [128, 129]. Other advantages of this flap may include potentially reduced operative time compared to bony flap harvest and shaping, faster recovery, and a low complication rate.

6.1.6.8 Condylar defects

Reconstruction of the condyle with titanium prostheses has been documented with some reported complications, including infection, plate fracture, and erosion into the middle cranial fossa [20].

Takushima et al. [87] emphasized that the selection of a suitable flap for mandibular reconstruction depends mainly on the type of soft and hard tissue defect. They categorized the mandibular defects into two categories: bony defects, which can be either lateral or anterior, and soft tissue defects, which are further subdivided into three categories: none, skin or mucosal, and through-and-through defects. Moreover, they recommended considering the bony defect for perfect flap selection, followed by the soft tissue defect. In addition, they highlighted the use of free fibula flaps for lateral defects with minor "skin or mucosal defects," the scapula flap for lateral defects with extensive skin, mucosal, or through-and-through soft tissue defects, and the fibula flap in conjunction with other soft tissue flaps for optimal outcomes in anterior defects with extensive skin, mucosal, or through-and-through soft tissue defects [87].

6.1.7 The use of distraction osteogenesis

Transport disc distraction osteogenesis is a well-known procedure where a segment of bone is cut contiguous to the defect and moved gradually across the defect by a mechanical device; hence, new bone will fill the space in between the two separated bone segments [2, 88, 89].

Despite the fact that distraction osteogenesis can be used successfully for marginal mandibular resection cases, the patient's advanced age, metabolic diseases, radiation therapy, extensive scar tissue, and tissue necrosis can prohibit the bone-promoting potential at the recipient site. Furthermore, a second surgery is required to remove the distraction device [2, 88, 89].

6.1.8 The use of bone graft substitutes and advance technology

Despite the reported success rates of the traditional surgical approaches, that is, autogenous bone grafting, vascularized free flaps, and alloplastic materials, these techniques may be associated with various limitations, including donor site morbidity, limited availability of graft material, and potential for infection or rejection, highlighting the need for a more conservative approach [5, 94].

Bone morphogenetic proteins (BMPs) are a group of growth factors characterized by their ability to induce bone formation. Their osteoinductive properties can stimulate new bone growth. Researchers have explored BMPs as alternatives to traditional bone grafts and associated donor site morbidity in mandibular reconstruction [94, 95].

Moghadam et al. [94] reported the first human application of BMPs in mandibular reconstruction in 2001, successfully using a BMP bioimplant to reconstruct a 6-cm mandibular defect following ameloblastoma resection. Radiographic evidence at 3 and 9 months postoperatively showed new bone formation, with histological confirmation at 9 months. Later, several studies reported the successful use of bone morphogenetic protein-2 (rhBMP-2) [95, 97–100], bioimplants containing BMP-7 [94, 96], and recombinant human bone morphogenetic protein-2 (rhBMP-2) [98, 99] for reconstruction of mandibular bone defects in humans; however, challenges still exist and limit its regular use, such as the determination of the optimal dosing, delivery methods, and cost.

In the same line, the successful use of a cancellous bone and marrow (PBCM) graft, researchers have documented the successful use of cancellous bone and marrow (PBCM) in conjunction with custom-made titanium mesh (TiMesh) [46, 77, 102–106]. Nevertheless, a skilled operator/technique is mandatory to achieve high esthetic and functional results; a limitation has been overcome with the use of computer-assisted virtual surgical simulation and a three-dimensional (3D) printed model [107–111].

Recent advances in tissue engineering documented the possibility of using patient autologous cells to regenerate functional tissues [15, 82, 100, 101].

Today, studies have highlighted the use of stem cells as a successful method for reconstructing and regenerating crucial-sized maxillofacial defects [112, 113]. Stem cells are characterized by their ability to self-renew and differentiate into various cell types. In the context of mandibular reconstruction, mesenchymal stem cells

(MSCs) are of particular interest due to their capacity to differentiate into osteoblasts, the bone-forming cells [112, 113, 115–126, 130]. MSCs can be sourced from various tissues, including dental pulp tissue [116, 120], bone marrow [121], umbilical-cord blood [122], and adipose tissue [123]. Isolating these cells, expanding them in vitro, and seeding them onto suitable scaffolds implanted into the defect site allows them to differentiate into osteoblasts, mimicking the biological process of natural bone development and bone regeneration, which can be a promising alternative to bone grafting procedures and associated risk factors [112–126, 130, 131].

Recent Advance Technology and mandibular reconstruction include 3D planning and 3D printing:

The historical background of 3D planning and 3D printing had been documented in 1986, when 3D printing technology, or rapid prototyping (RP) or additive manufacturing (AM), was introduced and used for the fabrication of objects with complex geometries and architecture. This technology is considered a major innovation in the medicine, dentistry, engineering, and education fields. Based on the literature, the most established 3D printing technologies are stereolithography (SLA), selective laser sintering (SLS), fused deposition modeling (FDM), and direct metal laser sintering (DMLS) [132].

Mandibular reconstruction has significantly advanced with the integration of 3D planning and 3D printing technologies. These innovations enhance surgical precision, reduce operative time, and improve patient outcomes [77, 110, 133]. The application of 3D printing in mandibular reconstruction has evolved to include the creation of patient-specific implants and surgical guides. Virtual surgical planning (VSP) allows the surgeons to meticulously plan mandibular reconstructions preoperatively and facilitate patient education. By creating detailed digital models from patient imaging data, surgeons can simulate osteotomies, design optimal bone grafts, and foresee potential challenges. This preoperative planning enhances surgical accuracy and efficiency while the 3D printing translates virtual plans into tangible tools and implants.

Nowadays, the applications of VSP in head and neck reconstruction continue to broaden and include anterior mandible, delayed mandible, maxillary, skull base surgery, trauma, and immediate dental implantation [133–136].

Despite improvements, achieving precise anatomical replication can be challenging. Virtual plans and actual surgical outcomes diverge [77]. The current 3D printing materials may not fully replicate the mechanical properties of natural bone. The lack of standardized protocols and regulatory guidelines, technical expertise, and high cost may present challenges. This underscores the necessity for additional research to improve the effectiveness and dependability of 3D-printed solutions in mandibular reconstruction [132, 137].

Recent studies have explored the combination of mixed reality, 3D printing, and robotic-assisted navigation technologies to enhance the accuracy of mandibular reconstructions. This multidisciplinary approach aims to further refine surgical outcomes and reduce operative times [37, 138–141].

Although the previously discussed surgical techniques can restore the hard and soft tissue deficiencies owing to mandibular resection, the restoration of the patient's ability to eat, chew, and speak requires the replacement of the patient's dentation with prosthetic restoration [90, 91].

6.2 Prosthetic rehabilitation in mandibular reconstruction

From a prosthetic reconstructive perspective, both marginal and segmental mandibulectomy patients can be further subdivided into three categories: complete edentulous patients, partial edentulous patients, and patients with non-tooth-bearing defects [1].

6.2.1 Prosthetic rehabilitation in marginal mandibular reconstruction cases

6.2.1.1 Completely edentulous cases

Completely edentulous cases with mandibular resection present a complex and challenging situation owing to the compromised ridge support, vital structure approximation (inferior dental and mental nerves), the large inter-ridge space, and the compromised tongue movement [5, 21]. Moreover, the obliterated vestibular sulci may aggravate the situation and necessitate the use of vestibuloplasty with or without stent incorporation [5, 19, 21].

Researchers have documented the use of implant-supported prostheses when sufficient bone height and width are available to ensure high primary stability [5, 6, 21]. Nevertheless, a bone graft is necessary in cases with compromised ridge support to provide the necessary bony foundation for implant anchorage.

6.2.1.2 Partial edentulous cases

For partial edentulism patients, both fixed or removable reconstructive prostheses supported by teeth or implants can be used. The selection is based mainly on the extent and location of the defect, the number and health status of the remaining teeth, the inter-occlusal distance, the tongue impartment, the specialist's expertise, and the patient's preference [5, 21].

In cases with anterior defects, the height and width of the remaining bone, as well as the health of the remaining teeth, play a critical role in treatment selection [5, 18, 21]. In cases where the bone height is satisfactory, both implant- and tooth-supported prostheses can be considered, leading to predictable results and significant satisfaction [5, 6, 17, 21, 126, 142].

Moreover, a clasp-retained partial reconstructive prosthesis can provide notable stability, retention and function in cases with compromised bone support and an adequate number of healthy teeth [5–7, 21].

On the other hand, telescopic partial reconstructive appliances may be the preferred treatment approach when the limited number of remaining teeth compromise the prosthesis' retention and support (**Figure 7**). Alternatively, implant-supported reconstructive prostheses can be considered with bone grafting [5, 21].

Cases with posterior defects and limited bone height and width are not suitable for endosseous implant-supported prostheses unless they proceed with bone grafting, a treatment modality that may be associated with many complications [5, 21, 142, 143]. Hence, the use of removable reconstructive appliances may be a feasible solution with limited or no complications [5, 9, 144].

6.2.2 Prosthetic rehabilitation in segmental mandibular reconstruction cases

Cases of segmental mandibulectomy may be associated with mandibular deviation toward the resected side, exhibiting rotation and angular path of jaw closure, which is challenging the prosthetic rehabilitation of the patient, especially in edentulous patients, and highlights the importance of using intermaxillary fixation at the time of surgery or mandibular/maxillary guidance appliances afterward (**Figure 8**) [145–162].

Additionally, the use of monoplane teeth in a neutrocentric concept is recommended to avoid restricted/deflective occlusal contacts. In cases where the

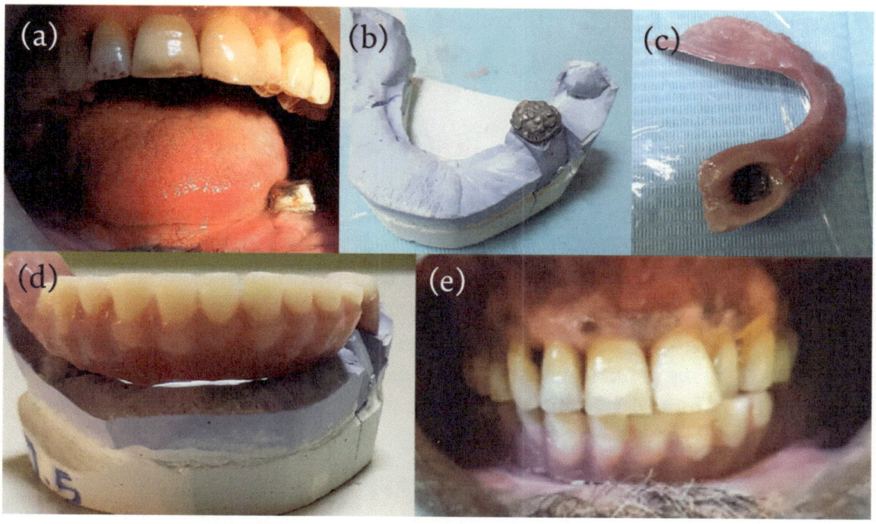

Figure 7.
Mandibular reconstruction with telescopic reconstructive prosthesis. (a) Postoperative patient's intra-oral view showing marginal mandibular resection and inner metal copping cemented over the left mandibular first molar tooth. (b) A photograph presenting the outer metal copping on the cast. (c) A photograph illustrating the fitting surface of the acrylic reconstructive prosthesis. (d) A photograph illustrating the polishing surface of the acrylic reconstructive prosthesis. (e) An intra-oral frontal view of the patient showing the acrylic reconstructive prosthesis after insertion.

mandibular deviation cannot be corrected, a twin occlusion (palatal row for occlusion and buccal row for check support) should be considered [153, 163–168].

Definitive dental rehabilitation of segmental mandibular resection cases without bone reconstruction is difficult and present a challenge for prosthodontists.

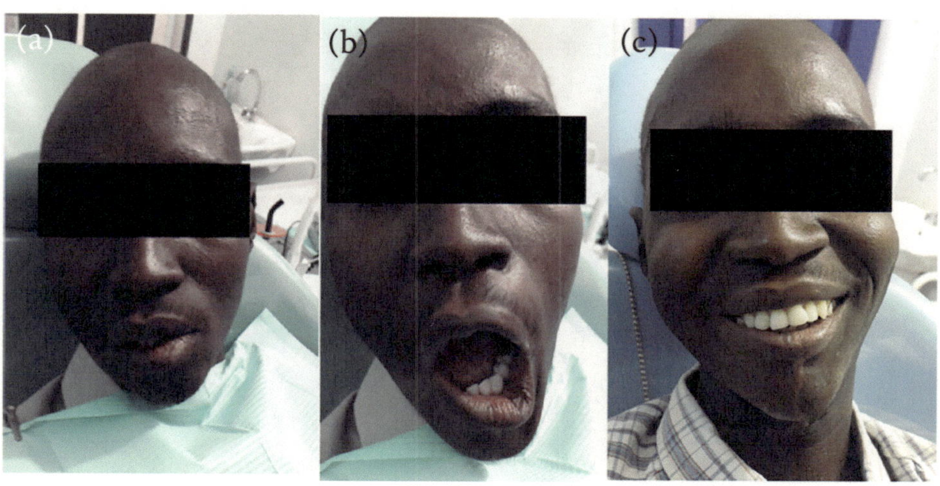

Figure 8.
(a) Extra-oral frontal view of the patient with lateral segmental mandibular resection. (b) Extra-oral frontal view of the patient illustrating mandibular deviation following mandibular resection. (c) Extra-oral frontal view of the patient showing the patient's esthetic improvement following reconstruction using mandibular reconstructed and guidance appliances at 1 month follow-up visit.

However, cases associated with corrected mandibular deviation, optimum soft tissue bulk, sufficient supporting natural dentition, and adequate space for replacement of teeth can be rehabilitated using removable and fixed prostheses (**Figure 9**).

Cases where the mandibular continuity is maintained using a reconstructive plate alone, a tissue-bone-removable reconstructive prosthesis can be used to improve the patient's esthetics, function, satisfaction, and quality of life (**Figure 10**).

On the other hand, when sufficient bone is available after reconstruction with bone grafting procedure, both conventional removable prostheses and implant supported prostheses including basal implants can be used with predictable success.

A non-tooth-bearing defect highlighted the use of free vascularizing flaps with the superiority of the fibula and iliac crest flap [5, 6, 9, 23].

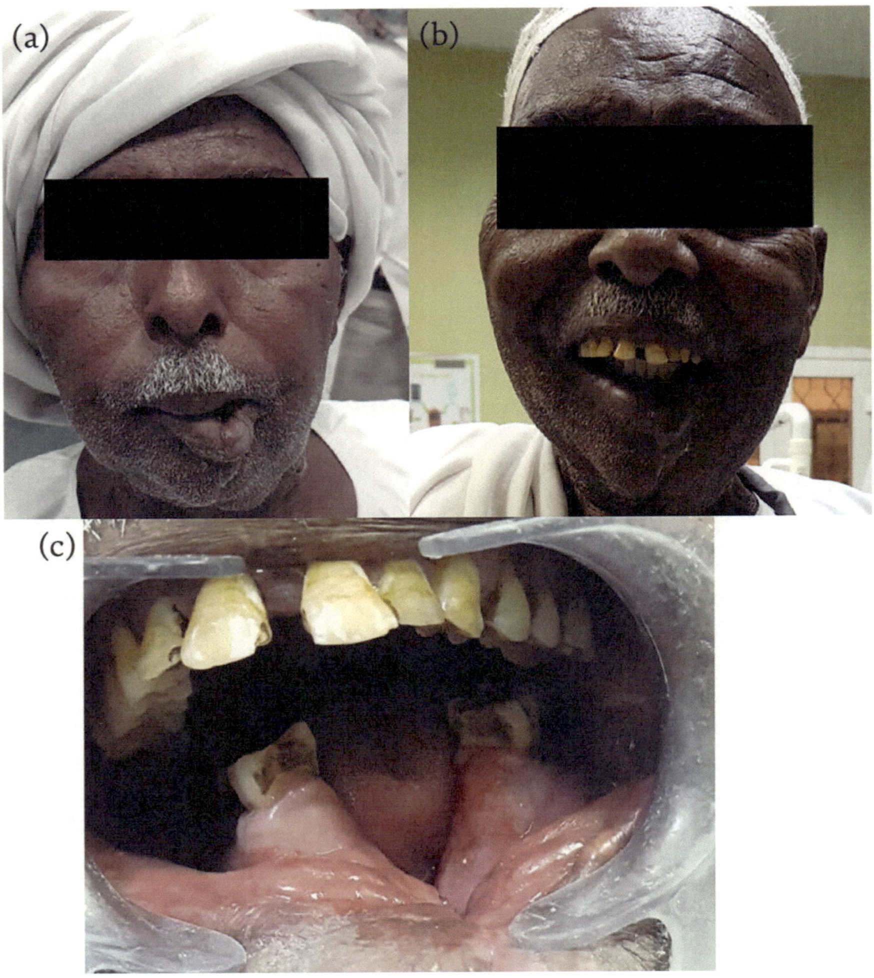

Figure 9.
(a) Extra-oral frontal view of the patient with anterior segmental mandibular resection. (b) Intra-oral frontal view of the patient illustrating the anterior segmental mandibular resection. (c) Extra-oral frontal view of the patient showing the patient after reconstruction with removable reconstructive prosthesis.

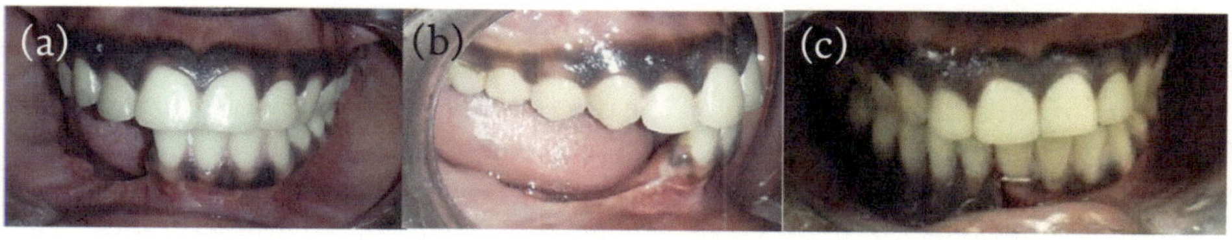

Figure 10.
(a) Intra-oral frontal view of the patient showing lateral mandibular resection. (b) Intra-oral lateral view of the patient illustrating the lateral mandibular resection. (c) Intra-oral frontal view of the patient after reconstruction with acrylic mandibular reconstructive prosthesis.

6.2.2.1 Mandibulectomy and basal implant-supported prosthesis

Today, with advancements in implant treatment, basal implants have become widely used due to their high reported survival and success rates, predictable biomechanical, prosthetic, esthetic, and phonetic outcomes, and improvements in patient satisfaction [3, 5, 18, 22, 86]. A treatment modality that has been described as an alternative option in cases of extensive ridge loss and maxillofacial defect rehabilitation with many advantages, including the following: implants utilize the strongest basal bone to gain satisfactory cortical engagement because of their high primary stability without the need for bone grafting and its vulnerable complications (**Figure 11**).

Moreover, implant splinting with a framework enhances the biomechanical force distribution, reduces the force per unit implant, and strengthens the possibility of immediate loading. Furthermore, there is the possibility of using acrylic veneer

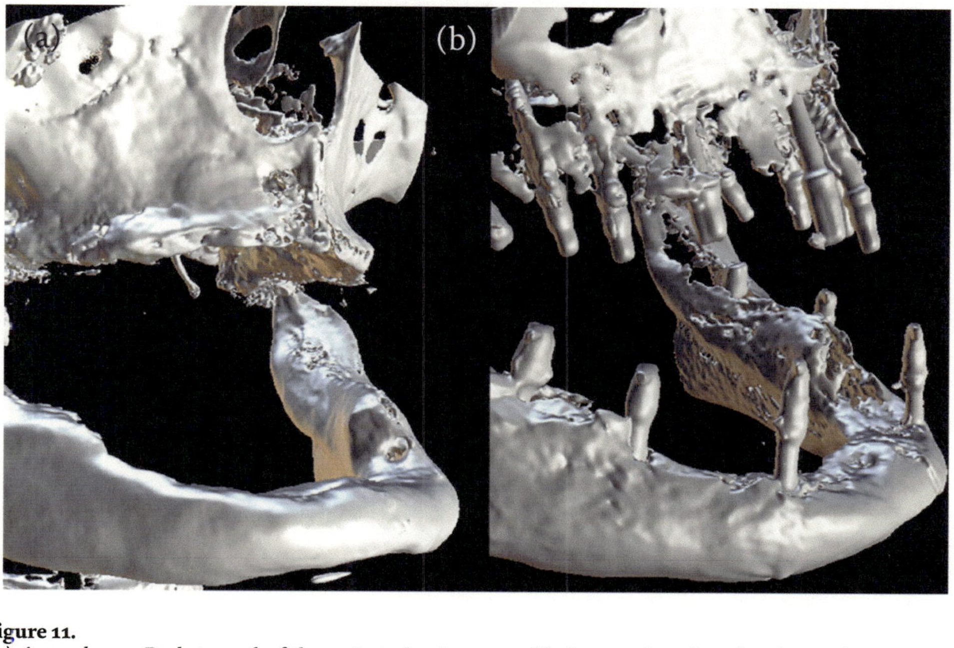

Figure 11.
(a) A cone beam 3D photograph of the patients showing a mandibular complete edentulous jaw with anterior marginal resection. (b) A cone beam 3D photograph of the patients showing a mandibular complete edentulous jaw with anterior marginal resection and basal implant insertion (Corticobasal® implant, BCS® implant design, Dr. Ihde Dental AG, Switzerland).

material to compensate for the tissue loss and restore the patient's esthetic (**Figures 12** and **13**) [3, 5, 18, 22, 86].

Awadalkreem et al. [5] investigated the use of basal implant-supported prostheses (BCS® implant design, Dr. Ihde Dental AG, Switzerland) in patients with marginal mandibulectomy for 5 years. The examined patients showed a 100% implant survival rate with optimum peri-implant soft tissue health, increased per-implant bone level, and high reported patient satisfaction concerning comfort, esthetics, mastication, and phonation. Only one patient reported an increase in the amount of teeth shown owing to midline lip splinting incision.

Recently, Akifuddin S and Awadalkreem F [86] described the successful use of a Corticobasal® implant reconstructive prosthesis following a free fibula flap after 5 years of function with a 100% implant survival rate with no implant loss or fracture, excellent peri-implant soft tissue health, complete union of the bone graft, and a very stable prosthesis.

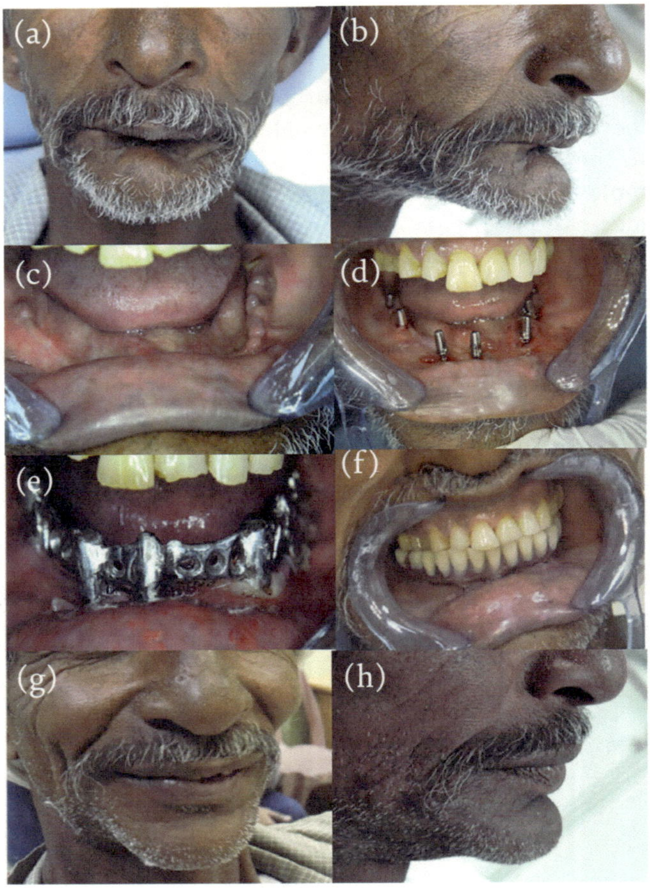

Figure 12.
(a) Extra-oral frontal view of a patient presenting with a complete mandibular edentulous arch with marginal mandibular resection. (b) Extra-oral lateral view of the patient. (c) Intra-oral view of the patient showing reduced ridge height after marginal mandibulectomy and obliterated mandibular sulci anteriorly. (d) Intra-oral view of the patient showing the Corticobasal® implant distribution using the flapless technique. (e) Intra-oral view of the patient illustrating metal framework connecting the implants. (f) Intra-oral view of the patient showing mandibular implant reconstructive prosthesis insertion. (g) Extra-oral frontal view of the patient. (h) Extra-oral lateral view of the patient (note the improvement of the patient's esthetic).

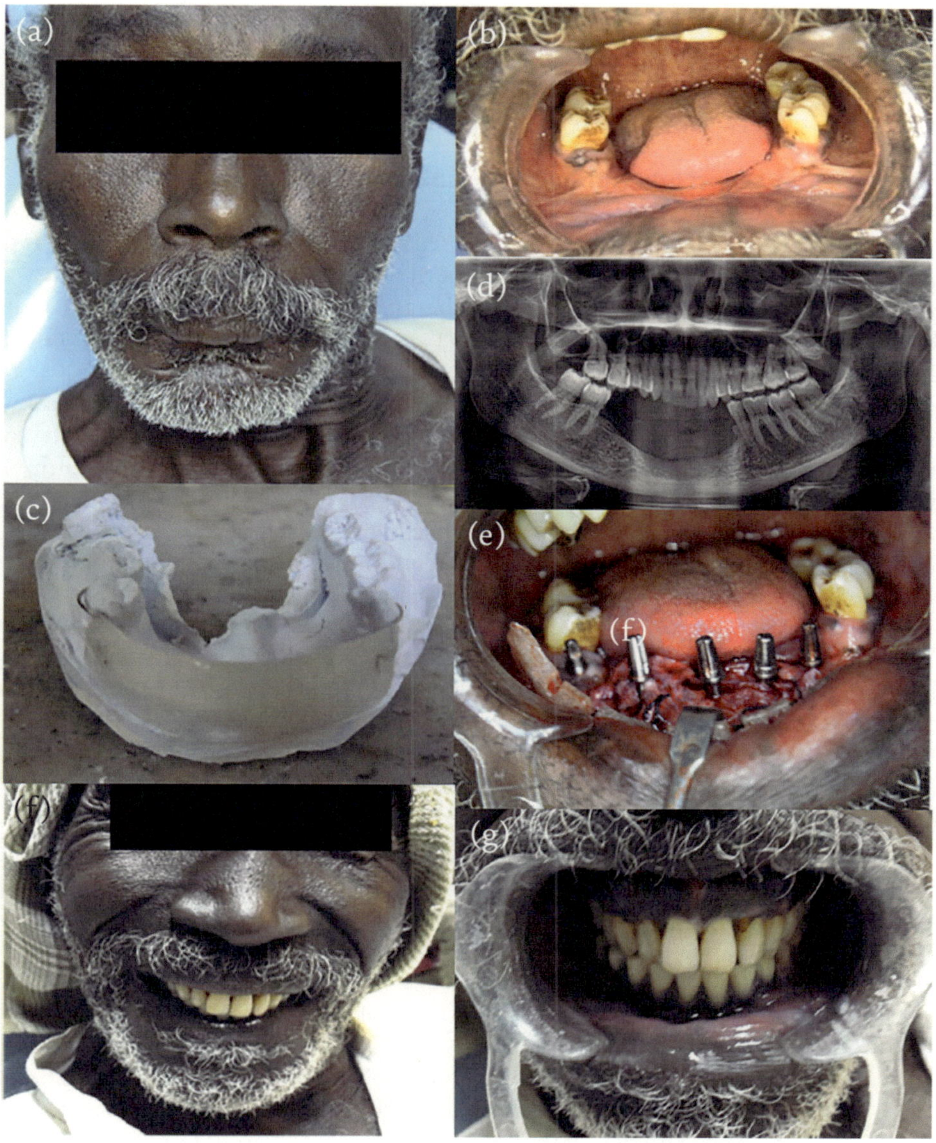

Figure 13.
(a) Extra-oral frontal view of a patient presenting with anterior marginal mandibular resection. (b) Intra-oral view of the patient showing reduced ridge height after marginal mandibulectomy and obliterated mandibular sulci anteriorly. (c) Dental panoramic view showing anterior marginal resection. (d) Vestibuloplasty acrylic stent o cast. (e) Clinical intra-oral view of the patient showing the Corticobasal® implant distribution and stent insertion using the flap technique (Corticobasal® implant, BCS® implant design, Dr. Ihde Dental AG, Switzerland). (f) Extra-oral view of the patient showing mandibular implant reconstructive prosthesis insertion. (g) Intra-oral view of the patient at 2 weeks follow-up visit.

7. Timing of dental implantation

Historically, dental implants were placed using a delayed setting in mandibulectomy cases but have more recently been placed immediately into a bony flap freehand without any form of guidance or referencing. This approach yielded satisfactory, functional outcomes [169–172].

With the introduction of Computer-Aided Design/Manufacturing (CAD/CAM), surgeons now have the capability to virtually plan cases with personalized models and guides that minimize operative time and maximize precision outcomes [142, 169, 170].

8. Mandibular resection and patient quality of life

Mandibular resection had adversely affected the patient's esthetic, function, and quality of life (QOL). Several factors can govern this effect, including the patients' age, tumor stage, tumor location, and radiotherapy [171, 172]. Female patients with advanced stage and treated with radiotherapy or chemotherapy showed lower rates of quality of life [172, 173].

In a study by Karayazgan et al. [144] comparing segmental and marginal mandibulectomy patients, the marginal mandibulectomy group documented acceptable levels of function, phonation, and esthetics, as well as improvement in the health quality of life.

Aimaijang et al. [174] reported no difference in patients' quality of life after rehabilitation among patients with marginal mandibulectomy, segmental mandibulectomy, and glossectomy; however, the glossectomy group showed lower food mixing ability.

Resections involving the mandibular angle and parasymphysis have the most adverse effects on appearance and overall QOL. In a study conducted by Warshavsky et al. [95, 175, 176], patients who underwent a segmental mandibulectomy that included the symphysis had worse outcomes in chewing, recreation, health-related, and social QOL domains compared to those whose mandibulectomy did not involve the symphysis. Increased time intervals from the initial resection and the stage of reconstruction were associated with better QOL [11].

Landstrom et al. [176] documented a significant decrease in all the functional outcomes after 1 year of tumor treatment with reported problems associated with taste and smell, talking, mouth opening, and dry mouth with better-reported overall function following reconstruction [177].

Terrell et al. [177] described 13 factors in relation to the deterioration of the head and neck cancer patient's quality of life, including the presence of a feeding tube, comorbid medical conditions, tracheotomy, chemotherapy, and neck dissection. Moreover, a history of radiation exposure exacerbates the condition. Furthermore, male patients reported a higher quality of life (QOL) compared to female patients, likely due to their higher esthetic concerns.

Mandibular reconstruction with reconstruction plates tended to have a lower QOL and is subject to plate fracture eventually [177]. Davudov et al. [173] compared the health-related quality of life in patients who received free fibula flaps versus reconstruction plates following the segmental resection of the lateral mandible, despite the fact that a non-significant difference was reported among the three groups. Patients receiving free fibula flaps reported better function and fewer complications, while those with no reconstruction showed the worse state.

On the other hand, the history of radiation is a delineating factor affecting QOL [178, 179]. Men have better QOL compared to women, as females are more concerned with esthetics [180, 181]. Patients with an implant-supported prosthodontic reconstruction achieved a higher overall QOL [182].

Garrett et al. [183] studied the effectiveness of conventional and implant-supported prostheses following surgical reconstruction; they recommended the use of implant prostheses after 1 year of resection to avoid recurrence risk and to reduce the patient complication turnover in comparison to conventional prostheses.

Moreover, Karayazgan et al. [144] compare the patient satisfaction and oral health quality of life in patients with marginal mandibulectomy rehabilitated with implant-retained overdentures and fixed metal acrylic resin prostheses; the overdenture prosthesis revealed a higher improvement.

A recent review conducted by Shankar et al. [184] found that restoration of the function, psychological comfort, and improvement in esthetics were significantly improved in patients who underwent prosthetic rehabilitation. Similar QoL was reported between conventional and implant prostheses. Despite the fact that the number of implants does not affect the quality and denture satisfaction, it improves their chewing ability. Additionally, the quality and quantity of the remaining hard and soft tissue structures have a major influence on patient comfort, emphasizing the influence of the extent of surgical excision.

9. Conclusion

Management of mandibular resection cases necessitates the interaction between the different oral and maxillofacial team members for successful treatment outcomes.

Rehabilitation of a patient with mandibular resection can be performed using several surgical reconstruction techniques based on the extension of the resection; however, to retain the patient's normal functions, a prosthetic rehabilitation is mandatory.

In a complete edentulous marginal mandibulectomy patients with favorable bony support, removable reconstructive appliance can be used with high success rate.

For partial edentulous patients, implant-supported prostheses are advantageous in cases with favorable bony support, while tooth-supported removable and telescopic removable prostheses can be used in posterior and anterior defects with sufficient remaining teeth.

Basal implant reconstructive prostheses can be considered a treatment modality offering the advantage of eliminating the need for bone grafting and ensuring a predictable success rate.

For segmental mandibulectomy patients, both removable and fixed implant reconstructive prostheses can be considered after providing the hard and soft tissue-supported foundation through surgical reconstruction, with priority given to the free fibula flap in large defects.

In cases of deviated mandible, the use of a guidance appliance is mandatory to improve the final treatment outcome.

Surgical and prosthetic rehabilitations following mandibular resection significantly improve the patient's esthetic, function, satisfaction, and hence quality of life.

Acknowledgements

There are no acknowledgments to declare.

Conflict of interest

There are no conflicts of interest to declare.

Ethical approval

Institutional approval was not required.

Author details

Fadia Awadalkreem[1*] and Haifa Kamal[2]

1 Department of Prosthodontics, RAK College of Dental Sciences, RAK Medical and Health Sciences University, Ras Al Khaimah, United Arab Emirates

2 Student counselor and lecturer Psychology, RAK Medical and Health Sciences University, Ras Al Khaimah, United Arab Emirates

*Address all correspondence to: fadia.alfateh@rakmhsu.ac.ae

References

[1] Rana M, Warraich R, Kokemuller H, Lemound J, Essig H, Tavassol F, et al. Reconstruction of mandibular defects - clinical retrospective research over a 10-year period. Head & Neck Oncology. 2011;**3**:23. DOI: 10.1186/1758-3284-3-23

[2] Torroni A, Marianetti TM, Romandini M, Gasparini G, Cervelli D, Pelo S. Mandibular reconstruction with different techniques. Journal of Craniofacial Surgery. 2015;**26**(3):885-890. DOI: 10.1097/SCS.0000000000001411

[3] Awadalkreem F, Khalifa N, Ahmad AG, Suliman AM, Osman M. Rehabilitation of an irradiated marginal mandibulectomy patient using immediately loaded basal implant-supported fixed prostheses and hyperbaric oxygen therapy: A 2-year follow-up. International Journal of Surgery Case Reports. 2020;**71**:297-302. DOI: 10.1016/j.ijscr.2020.05.018

[4] Takaoka K, Segawa E, Yamamura M, Zushi Y, Urade M, Kishimoto H. Dental implant treatment in a young woman after marginal mandibulectomy for treatment of mandibular gingival carcinoma: A case report. International Journal of Implant Dentistry. 2015;**1**:1-7. DOI: 10.1186/s40729-015-0022-2

[5] Awadalkreem F, Khalifa N, Satti A, Suliman AM. Rehabilitation of marginal mandibulectomy patients using immediately loaded basal implant-supported prostheses. Journal of Oral and Maxillofacial Surgery, Medicine, and Pathology. 2022;**34**(1):24-35. DOI: 10.1016/j.ajoms.2021.07.002

[6] Petrovic I, Rosen EB, Matros E, Huryn JM, Shah JP. Oral rehabilitation of the cancer patient: A formidable challenge. Journal of Surgical Oncology. 2018;**117**(8):1729-1735. DOI: 10.1002/jso.25075

[7] Petrovic I, Ahmed ZU, Huryn JM, Nelson J, Allen RJ Jr, Matros E, et al. Oral rehabilitation for patients with marginal and segmental mandibulectomy: A retrospective review of 111 mandibular resection prostheses. The Journal of Prosthetic Dentistry. 2019;**122**(1):82-87. DOI: 10.1016/j.prosdent.2018.09.020

[8] Beumer JB III, CT, Marunick MT. Maxillofacial Rehabilitation: Prosthodontic and Surgical Considerations. 2nd ed. St. Louis: Ishiyaku Euromerica; 1996

[9] Castagnola R, Rupe C, Gioco G, Almadori G, Galli J, Tagliaferri L, et al. Clinical outcomes of teeth adjacent to the site of mandibulotomy or mandibulectomy in patients with head and neck cancer: Results from a multidisciplinary mono-institutional head and neck tumor board. BMC Oral Health. 2023;**23**(1):357. DOI: 10.1186/s12903-023-03050-7

[10] Sung H, Ferlay J, Siegel RL, Laversanne M, Soerjomataram I, Jemal A, et al. Global cancer statistics 2020: GLOBOCAN estimates of incidence and mortality worldwide for 36 cancers in 185 countries. CA: a Cancer Journal for Clinicians. 2021;**71**(3):209-249. DOI: 10.3322/caac.21660

[11] Conway DI, Purkayastha M, Chestnutt I. The changing epidemiology of oral cancer: Definitions, trends, and risk factors. British Dental Journal. 2018;**225**(9):867-873. DOI: 10.1038/sj.bdj.2018.922

[12] Sproll CK, Holtmann H, Schorn LK, Jansen TM, Reifenberger J, Boeck I,

et al. Mandible handling in the surgical treatment of oral squamous cell carcinoma: Lessons from clinical results after marginal and segmental mandibulectomy. Oral Surgery, Oral Medicine, Oral Pathology, Oral Radiology. 2020;**129**(6):556-564. DOI: 10.1016/j.oooo.2019.11.011

[13] Salvatori P, Paradisi S, Calabrese L, Zani A, Cantu G, Cappiello J, et al. Patients' survival after free flap reconstructive surgery of head and neck squamous cell carcinoma: A retrospective multicentre study. Acta Otorhinolaryngologica Italica. 2014;**34**(2):99-104

[14] The glossary of prosthodontic terms 2023: Tenth edition. The Journal of Prosthetic Dentistry. 2023;**130**(e1-e3):e1-e3. DOI: 10.1016/j.prosdent.2023.03.003

[15] Kumar BP, Venkatesh V, Kumar KJ, Yadav BY, Mohan SR. Mandibular reconstruction: Overview. Journal of Maxillofacial and Oral Surgery. 2016;**15**:425-441. DOI: 10.1007/s12663-015-0766-5

[16] Lin P-Y, Lin KC, Jeng S-F. Oromandibular reconstruction: The history, operative options and strategies, and our experience. International Scholarly Research Notices. 2011;**2011**(1):824251. DOI: 10.5402/2011/824251

[17] Konstantinovic VS, Todorovic VS, Lazic VM. Possibilities of reconstruction and implant-prosthetic rehabilitation following mandible resection. Vojnosanitetski Pregled. 2013;**70**(1):80-85. DOI: 10.2298/vsp1301080k

[18] Awadalkreem F, Khalifa N, Ahmad AG, Osman M, Suliman AM. Rehabilitation of mandibular resected patients using fixed immediately loaded corticobasal implant -supported prostheses. A case series. International Journal of Surgery Case Reports. 2024;**119**:109707. DOI: 10.1016/j.ijscr.2024.109707

[19] Karandikar S, Bhawsar S, Varsha Murthy J, Pawar P, Yuvaraj V, Dalsingh V. Bhawsar-karandikar stent: an aid to vestibuloplasty. Journal of Oral and Maxillofacial Surgery. 2013;**12**(2):237-239. DOI: 10.1007/s12663-012-0344-z

[20] Hanasono MM. Reconstructive surgery for head and neck cancer patients. Advances in Medicine. 2014;**2014**(1):795483. DOI: 10.1155/2014/795483

[21] Petrovic I, Shah JP, Huryn JM, Ahmed ZU, Rosen EB. Intraoral rehabilitation after marginal mandibulectomy. The International Journal of Prosthodontics. 2019;**32**(3):241-247. DOI: 10.11607/ijp.6181

[22] Awadalkreem F, Khalifa N, Satti A, Suleiman AM. The influence of immediately loaded basal implant treatment on patient satisfaction. International Journal of Dentistry. 2020;**2020**:6590202. DOI: 10.1155/2020/6590202

[23] Jewer DD, Boyd JB, Manktelow RT, Zuker RM, Rosen IB, Gullane PJ, et al. Orofacial and mandibular reconstruction with the iliac crest free flap: A review of 60 cases and a new method of classification. Plastic and Reconstructive Surgery. 1989;**84**(3):391-403; discussion 4-5

[24] Maurer P, Eckert AW, Kriwalsky MS, Schubert J. Scope and limitations of methods of mandibular reconstruction: A long-term follow-up. The British Journal of Oral & Maxillofacial Surgery. 2010;**48**(2):100-104. DOI: 10.1016/j.bjoms.2009.07.005

[25] Boyd JB, Mulholland RS, Davidson J, Gullane PJ, Rotstein LE, Brown DH, et al. The free flap and plate in oromandibular reconstruction: Long-term review and indications. Plastic and Reconstructive Surgery. 1995;**95**(6):1018-1028. DOI: 10.1097/00006534-199505000-00010

[26] Urken ML. Composite free flaps in oromandibular reconstruction. Review of the literature. Archives of Otolaryngology – Head & Neck Surgery. 1991;**117**(7):724-732. DOI: 10.1001/archotol.1991.01870190036009

[27] Schusterman MA, Harris SW, Raymond AK, Goepfert H. Immediate free flap mandibular reconstruction: Significance of adequate surgical margins. Head & Neck. 1993;**15**(3):204-207. DOI: 10.1002/hed.2880150305

[28] Cordeiro PG, Hidalgo DA. Conceptual considerations in mandibular reconstruction. Clinics in Plastic Surgery. 1995;**22**(1):61-69

[29] Baker A, McMahon J, Parmar S. Immediate reconstruction of continuity defects of the mandible after tumor surgery. Journal of Oral and Maxillofacial Surgery. 2001;**59**(11):1333-1339. DOI: 10.1053/joms.2001.27825

[30] Li X, Zhu K, Liu F, Li H. Assessment of quality of life in giant ameloblastoma adolescent patients who have had mandible defects reconstructed with a free fibula flap. World Journal of Surgical Oncology. 2014;**12**:1-6. DOI: 10.1186/1477-7819-12-201

[31] Netscher DT, Meade RA, Goodman CM, Alford EL, Stewart MG. Quality of life and disease-specific functional status following microvascular reconstruction for advanced (T3 and T4) oropharyngeal cancers. Plastic and Reconstructive Surgery. 2000;**105**(5):1628-1634. DOI: 10.1097/00006534-200004050-00005

[32] Weymuller EA, Yueh B, Deleyiannis FW, Kuntz AL, Alsarraf R, Coltrera MD. Quality of life in patients with head and neck cancer: Lessons learned from 549 prospectively evaluated patients. Archives of Otolaryngology – Head & Neck Surgery. 2000;**126**(3):329-335; discussion 35-6. DOI: 10.1001/archotol.126.3.329

[33] Petrovic I, Montero PH, Migliacci JC, Palmer FL, Ganly I, Patel SG, et al. Influence of bone invasion on outcomes after marginal mandibulectomy in squamous cell carcinoma of the oral cavity. Journal of Cranio-Maxillo-Facial Surgery. 2017;**45**(2):252-257. DOI: 10.1016/j.jcms.2016.11.017

[34] Chen YL, Kuo SW, Fang KH, Hao SP. Prognostic impact of marginal mandibulectomy in the presence of superficial bone invasion and the nononcologic outcome. Head & Neck. 2011;**33**(5):708-713. DOI: 10.1002/hed.21530

[35] Seok H. Role of oral and maxillofacial surgeons in treating oral cancer. Journal of the Korean Association of Oral and Maxillofacial Surgeons. 2022;**48**(6):329-330. DOI: 10.5125/jkaoms.2022.48.6.329

[36] Wang YH, Kung PT, Tsai WC, Tai CJ, Liu SA, Tsai MH. Effects of multidisciplinary care on the survival of patients with oral cavity cancer in Taiwan. Oral Oncology. 2012;**48**(9):803-810. DOI: 10.1016/j.oraloncology.2012.03.023

[37] de Boutray M, Cuau L, Ohayon M, Garrel R, Poignet P, Zemiti N. Robot-guided osteotomy in fibula free flap mandibular reconstruction: A preclinical study. International Journal of Oral and

Maxillofacial Surgery. 2024;**53**(4):343-346. DOI: 10.1016/j.ijom.2023.07.010

[38] Kutuk T, Atak E, Villa A, Kalman NS, Kaiser A. Interdisciplinary collaboration in head and neck cancer care: Optimizing oral health management for patients undergoing radiation therapy. Current Oncology. 2024;**31**(4):2092-2108. DOI: 10.3390/curroncol31040155

[39] Ahmed S, Awadalkreem F, Baroudi K. Knowledge and practice of the different maxillofacial prostheses among Sudanese dental practitioners: A cross-sectional study. The Open Dentistry Journal. 2024;**18**(1):e18742106319214. DOI: 10.2174/01187421 06319214240705113136

[40] Shah JP. The role of marginal mandibulectomy in the surgical management of oral cancer. Archives of Otolaryngology – Head & Neck Surgery. 2002;**128**(5):604-605. DOI: 10.1001/archotol.128.5.604

[41] Suliman RM, Awadalkreem F. Knowledge and practice of radiation stents for oral cancer patients among the Sudanese's maxillofacial surgeons, prosthodontists, oncologists, and radiotherapists. The Journal of Contemporary Dental Practice. 2023;**24**(3):168-175. DOI: 10.5005/jp-journals-10024-3491

[42] Turco C, Nisio A, Lofano B. I tumori benigni della mandibola. Esperienza di ricostruzione mediante innesti ossei immediati [benign tumors of the mandible. The experience of reconstruction using immediate bone grafts]. Minerva Stomatologica. 1990;**39**(2):101-108. Italian

[43] Losapio P, Faldi F. Reconstruction of extensive mandibular defects with the use of osteo-mesh and a bone graft. A preliminary report. Minerva Stomatologica. 1989;**38**(10):1059-1063

[44] Harsha BC, Turvey TA, Powers SK. Use of autogenous cranial bone grafts in maxillofacial surgery: A preliminary report. Journal of Oral and Maxillofacial Surgery. 1986;**44**(1):11-15. DOI: 10.1016/0278-2391(86)90008-x

[45] Petroff MA, Burgess LP, Anonsen CK, Lau P, Goode RL. Cranial bone grafts for post-traumatic facial defects. The Laryngoscope. 1987;**97**(11):1249-1253. DOI: 10.1288/00005537-198711000-00001

[46] Carlson ER, Marx RE. Part II. Mandibular reconstruction using cancellous cellular bone grafts. Journal of Oral and Maxillofacial Surgery. 1996;**54**(7):889-897. DOI: 10.1016/s0278-2391(96)90543-1

[47] Tidstrom KD, Keller EE. Reconstruction of mandibular discontinuity with autogenous iliac bone graft: Report of 34 consecutive patients. Journal of Oral and Maxillofacial Surgery. 1990;**48**(4):336-346; discussion 47. DOI: 10.1016/0278-2391(90)90427-4

[48] Wersäll J, Bergstedt H, Korlof B, Lind MG. Split-rib graft for reconstruction of the mandible. Otolaryngology and Head and Neck Surgery. 1984;**92**(3):271-276

[49] Conley J. Use of composite flaps containing bone for major repairs in the head and neck. Plastic and Reconstructive Surgery. 1972;**49**(5):522-526. DOI: 10.1097/00006534-197205000-00008

[50] Siemssen SO, Kirkby B, O'Connor TP. Immediate reconstruction of a resected segment of the lower jaw, using a compound flap of clavicle and sternomastoid muscle. Plastic and

Reconstructive Surgery. 1978;**61**(5):724-735. DOI: 10.1097/00006534-197805000-00011

[51] Panje W, Cutting C. Trapezius osteomyocutaneous island flap for reconstruction of the anterior floor of the mouth and the mandible. Head & Neck Surgery. 1980;**3**(1):66-71. DOI: 10.1002/hed.2890030112

[52] Green MF, Gibson JR, Bryson JR, Thomson E. A one-stage correction of mandibular defects using a split sternum pectoralis major osteo-musculocutaneous transfer. British Journal of Plastic Surgery. 1981;**34**(1):11-16. DOI: 10.1016/0007-1226(81)90087-4

[53] Judd RT, McCrary HC, Farlow JL, Li M, Godsell J, Kneuertz PJ, et al. Pedicled osteomyocutaneous pectoralis major flap with osseous rib harvest for salvage mandibular reconstruction: Case and technique. Head & Neck. 2024;**46**(2):447-451. DOI: 10.1002/hed.27586

[54] Maruyama Y, Urita Y, Ohnishi K. Rib-latissimus dorsi osteomyocutaneous flap in reconstruction of a mandibular defect. British Journal of Plastic Surgery. 1985;**38**(2):234-237. DOI: 10.1016/0007-1226(85)90055-4

[55] Pai D, Wodeyar A, Raja P, Nishad M, Martis E, Kumar K. Evolution of mandibular defects reconstruction procedures: From older principles to newer techniques and technology. Acta Scientific Dental Sciences. 2019;**3**(5):08-18. Available from: https://actascientific.com/ASDS/pdf/ASDS-03-0510.pdf

[56] Schusterman MA, Reece GP, Kroll SS, Weldon ME. Use of the AO plate for immediate mandibular reconstruction in cancer patients. Plastic and Reconstructive Surgery. 1991;**88**(4):588-593

[57] Chow JM, Hill JH. Primary mandibular reconstruction using the AO reconstruction plate. The Laryngoscope. 1986;**96**(7):768-773. DOI: 10.1097/00006534-199110000-00005

[58] Ali MN, Anwar RB, Banik R, Hasan S, Arefin MRU, Uddin MW. Mandibular reconstruction: A review. Update Dental College Journal. 2019;**9**(2):50-54. Available from: https://banglajol.info/index.php/UpDCJ/article/view/43742

[59] Ferreira JJ, Zagalo CM, Oliveira ML, Correia AM, Reis AR. Mandible reconstruction: History, state of the art and persistent problems. Prosthetics and Orthotics International. 2015;**39**(3):182-189. DOI: 10.1177/0309364613520032

[60] Hjørting-Hansen E. Bone grafting to the jaws with special reference to reconstructive preprosthetic surgery. A historical review. Mund-, Kiefer- und Gesichtschirurgie. 2002;**6**(1):6-14. DOI: 10.1007/s10006-001-0343-6

[61] Fang F, Chung KC. An evolutionary perspective on the history of flap reconstruction in the upper extremity. Hand Clinics. 2014;**30**(2):109-122. DOI: 10.1016/j.hcl.2013.12.001

[62] Taylor GI, Townsend P, Corlett R. Superiority of the deep circumflex iliac vessels as the supply for free groin flaps clinical work. Plastic and Reconstructive Surgery. 1979;**64**(6):745-759. DOI: 10.1097/00006534-197912000-00001

[63] Sanders R, Mayou BJ. A new vascularized bone graft transferred by microvascular anastomosis as a free flap. The British Journal of Surgery. 1979;**66**(11):787-788. DOI: 10.1002/bjs.1800661111

[64] Swartz WM, Banis JC, Newton ED, Ramasastry SS, Jones NF, Acland R. The osteocutaneous scapular flap for mandibular and maxillary reconstruction. Plastic and Reconstructive Surgery. 1986;**77**(4):530-545. DOI: 10.1097/00006534-198604000-00003

[65] Brown JS, Jones DC, Summerwill A, Rogers SN, Howell RA, Cawood JI, et al. Vascularized iliac crest with internal oblique muscle for immediate reconstruction after maxillectomy. The British Journal of Oral & Maxillofacial Surgery. 2002;**40**(3):183-190. DOI: 10.1054/bjom.2001.0774

[66] Spiro RH, Strong EW, Shah JP. Maxillectomy and its classification. Head & Neck. 1997;**19**(4):309-314. DOI: 10.1002/(sici)1097-0347(199707)19:4<309::aid-hed9>3.0.co;2-4

[67] Genden EM, Okay D, Stepp MT, Rezaee RP, Mojica JS, Buchbinder D, et al. Comparison of functional and quality-of-life outcomes in patients with and without palatomaxillary reconstruction: A preliminary report. Archives of Otolaryngology–Head & Neck Surgery. 2003;**129**(7):775-780. DOI: 10.1001/archotol.129.7.775

[68] Rogers SN, Lowe D, McNally D, Brown JS, Vaughan ED. Health-related quality of life after maxillectomy: A comparison between prosthetic obturation and free flap. Journal of oral and maxillofacial surgery. 2003;**61**(2):174-181. DOI: 10.1053/joms.2003.50044

[69] Cordeiro PG, Santamaria E. A classification system and algorithm for reconstruction of maxillectomy and midfacial defects. Plastic and Reconstructive Surgery. 2000;**105**(7):2331-2346; discussion 47-8. DOI: 10.1097/00006534-200006000-00004

[70] Rodriguez ED, Martin M, Bluebond-Langner R, Khalifeh M, Singh N, Manson PN. Microsurgical reconstruction of posttraumatic high-energy maxillary defects: Establishing the effectiveness of early reconstruction. Plastic and Reconstructive Surgery. 2007;**120** (7 Suppl. 2):103S-117S. DOI: 10.1097/01.prs.0000260728.60178.de

[71] Hanasono MM, Lee JC, Yang JS, Skoracki RJ, Reece GP, Esmaeli B. An algorithmic approach to reconstructive surgery and prosthetic rehabilitation after orbital exenteration. Plastic and Reconstructive Surgery. 2009;**123**(1):98-105. DOI: 10.1097/PRS.0b013e3181904b95

[72] Hanasono MM, Utley DS, Goode RL. The temporalis muscle flap for reconstruction after head and neck oncologic surgery. The Laryngoscope. 2001;**111**(10):1719-1725. DOI: 10.1097/00005537-200110000-00009

[73] Seikaly H, Chau J, Li F, Driscoll B, Seikaly D, Calhoun J, et al. Bone that best matches the properties of the mandible. Journal of Otolaryngology. 2003;**32**(4):262-265. DOI: 10.2310/7070.2003.41646

[74] Johansson B, Grepe A, Wannfors K, Hirsch JM. A clinical study of changes in the volume of bone grafts in the atrophic maxilla. Dento Maxillo Facial Radiology. 2001;**30**(3):157-161. DOI: 10.1038/sj/dmfr/4600601

[75] Kim RY, Sokoya M, Ducic Y, Williams F. Free-flap reconstruction of the mandible. Seminars in Plastic Surgery. Feb 2019;**33**(1):46-53. DOI: 10.1055/s-0039-1677791

[76] Okay DJ, Genden E, Buchbinder D, Urken M. Prosthodontic guidelines for surgical reconstruction of the maxilla: A classification system of defects. The Journal of Prosthetic Dentistry. 2001;**86**(4):352-363. DOI: 10.1067/mpr.2001.119524

[77] Hurley CM, McConn Walsh R, Shine NP, O'Neill JP, Martin F, O'Sullivan JB. Current trends in craniofacial reconstruction. The Surgeon. 2023;**21**(3):e118-ee25. DOI: 10.1016/j.surge.2022.04.004

[78] Tatti M, Carta F, Bontempi M, Deriu S, Mariani C, Marrosu V, et al. Segmental mandibulectomy and mandibular reconstruction with fibula-free flap using a 3D template. Journal of Personalized Medicine. 2024;**14**(5):512. DOI: 10.3390/jpm14050512

[79] Tahmasebi E, Keykha E, Hajisadeghi S, Moslemi H, Shafiei S, Motamedi MHK, et al. Outcomes and influential factors in functional and dental rehabilitation following microvascular fibula flap reconstruction in the maxillomandibular region: A systematic review and meta-analysis. Maxillofacial Plastic and Reconstructive Surgery. 2023;**45**(1):24. DOI: 10.1016/j.ijscr.2024.110433

[80] van Gemert JTM, Abbink JH, van Es RJJ, Rosenberg A, Koole R, Van Cann EM. Early and late complications in the reconstructed mandible with free fibula flaps. Journal of Surgical Oncology. 2018;**117**(4):773-780. DOI: 10.1186/s40902-023-00392-8

[81] Urken ML, Buchbinder D, Costantino PD, Sinha U, Okay D, Lawson W, et al. Oromandibular reconstruction using microvascular composite flaps: Report of 210 cases. Archives of Otolaryngology – Head & Neck Surgery. 1998;**124**(1):46-55. DOI: 10.1001/archotol.124.1.46

[82] Chim H, Salgado CJ, Mardini S, Chen HC. Reconstruction of mandibular defects. Seminars in Plastic Surgery. 2010;**24**(2):188-197. DOI: 10.1055/s-0030-1255336

[83] Soutar DS, Widdowson WP. Immediate reconstruction of the mandible using a vascularized segment of radius. Head & Neck Surgery. 1986;**8**(4):232-246. DOI: 10.1002/hed.2890080403

[84] Gilbert A, Teot L. The free scapular flap. Plastic and Reconstructive Surgery. 1982;**69**(4):601-604. DOI: 10.1097/00006534-198204000-00002

[85] Marttila E, Salli M, Mesimaki K, Kainulainen S, Snall J, Wilkman T. The combined anterolateral thigh-partial iliac crest minihybrid free flap for mandibular reconstruction. Microsurgery. 2022;**42**(4):312-318. DOI: 10.1002/micr.30854

[86] Akifuddin S, Awadalkreem F. Prosthetic rehabilitation of segmental mandibulectomy patient using a free fibula flap and Corticobasal implant supported prosthesis: A case report. International Journal of Surgery Case Reports. 2024;**124**:110433. DOI: 10.1016/j.ijscr.2024.110433

[87] Takushima A, Harii K, Asato H, Momosawa A, Okazaki M, Nakatsuka T. Choice of osseous and osteocutaneous flaps for mandibular reconstruction. International Journal of Clinical Oncology. 2005;**10**(4):234-242. DOI: 10.1007/s10147-005-0504-y

[88] Al-Namnam NMN, Hariri F, Rahman ZAA. Distraction osteogenesis in the surgical management of syndromic craniosynostosis: A comprehensive review of published papers. The British Journal of Oral & Maxillofacial Surgery.

2018;**56**(5):353-366. DOI: 10.1016/j.bjoms.2018.03.002

[89] Iwai T, Sugiyama S, Hirota M, Mitsudo K. Horizontal alveolar transport distraction osteogenesis to stabilize removable prosthesis after mandibular reconstruction. The Journal of Dental Sciences. 2023;**18**(4):1895-1896. DOI: 10.1016/j.jds.2023.07.022

[90] Wang C, Gao M, Yu Y, Zhang W, Peng X. Clinical analysis of denture rehabilitation after mandibular fibula free-flap reconstruction. Beijing Da Xue Xue Bao Yi Xue Ban. 2024;**56**(1):66-73. DOI: 10.19723/j.issn.1671-167X.2024.01.011

[91] Dibbs RP, Ferry AM, Sarrami SM, Abu-Ghname A, Dempsey RF, Buchanan EP. Distraction osteogenesis: Mandible and maxilla. Facial Plastic Surgery. 2021;**37**(06):751-758. DOI: 10.1055/s-0041-1727248

[92] Cheung LK, Samman N, Chow TW, Clark RK, Tideman H. A bone graft condensing syringe system for maxillofacial reconstructive surgery. The British Journal of Oral & Maxillofacial Surgery. 1997;**35**(4):267-270. DOI: 10.1016/s0266-4356(97)90045-0

[93] Albert TW, Smith JD, Everts EC, Cook TA. Dacron mesh tray and cancellous bone in reconstruction of mandibular defects. Archives of Otolaryngology – Head & Neck Surgery. 1986;**112**(1):53-59. DOI: 10.1001/archotol.1986.03780010055010

[94] Moghadam HG, Urist MR, Sandor GK, Clokie CM. Successful mandibular reconstruction using a BMP bioimplant. The Journal of Craniofacial Surgery. 2001;**12**(2):119-127; discussion 28. DOI: 10.1097/00001665-200103000-00005

[95] Herford AS, Boyne PJ. Reconstruction of mandibular continuity defects with bone morphogenetic protein-2 (rhBMP-2). Journal of Oral and Maxillofacial Surgery. 2008;**66**(4):616-624. DOI: 10.1016/j.joms.2007.11.021

[96] Clokie CM, Sandor GK. Reconstruction of 10 major mandibular defects using bioimplants containing BMP-7. Journal of the Canadian Dental Association. 2008;**74**(1):67-72

[97] Carter TG, Brar PS, Tolas A, Beirne OR. Off-label use of recombinant human bone morphogenetic protein-2 (rhBMP-2) for reconstruction of mandibular bone defects in humans. Journal of Oral and Maxillofacial Surgery. 2008;**66**(7):1417-1425. DOI: 10.1016/j.joms.2008.01.058

[98] Glied AN, Kraut RA. Off-label use of rhBMP-2 for reconstruction of critical-sized mandibular defects. The New York State Dental Journal. 2010;**76**(4):32-35

[99] Herford AS, Cicciu M. Recombinant human bone morphogenetic protein type 2 jaw reconstruction in patients affected by giant cell tumor. The Journal of Craniofacial Surgery. 2010;**21**(6):1970-1975. DOI: 10.1097/SCS.0b013e3181f502fa

[100] Desai SC, Sclaroff A, Nussenbaum B. Use of recombinant human bone morphogenetic protein 2 for mandible reconstruction. JAMA Facial Plastic Surgery. 2013;**15**(3):204-209. DOI: 10.1001/jamafacial.2013.650

[101] Chanchareonsook N, Junker R, Jongpaiboonkit L, Jansen JA. Tissue-engineered mandibular bone reconstruction for continuity defects: A systematic approach to the literature. Tissue Engineering. Part B, Reviews. 2014;**20**(2):147-162. DOI: 10.1089/ten.TEB.2013.0131

[102] Konopnicki S, Troulis MJ. Mandibular tissue engineering: Past, present, future. Journal of Oral and Maxillofacial Surgery. 2015;**73**(Suppl. 12):S136-S146. DOI: 10.1016/j.joms.2015.05.037

[103] Dumbach J, Rodemer H, Spitzer WJ, Steinhauser EW. Mandibular reconstruction with cancellous bone, hydroxylapatite and titanium mesh. Journal of Cranio-Maxillo-Facial Surgery. 1994;**22**(3):151-155. DOI: 10.1016/s1010-5182(05)80381-6

[104] Iino M, Fukuda M, Nagai H, Hamada Y, Yamada H, Nakaoka K, et al. Evaluation of 15 mandibular reconstructions with Dumbach titan mesh-system and particulate cancellous bone and marrow harvested from bilateral posterior ilia. Oral Surgery, Oral Medicine, Oral Pathology, Oral Radiology, and Endodontics. 2009;**107**(4):e1-e8. DOI: 10.1016/j.tripleo.2008.12.018

[105] Miyamoto I, Yamashita Y, Yamamoto N, Nogami S, Yamauchi K, Yoshiga D, et al. Evaluation of mandibular reconstruction with particulate cancellous bone marrow and titanium mesh after mandibular resection due to tumor surgery. Implant Dentistry. 2014;**23**(2):108-115. DOI: 10.1097/ID.0000000000000041

[106] Yamada H, Nakaoka K, Horiuchi T, Kumagai K, Ikawa T, Shigeta Y, et al. Mandibular reconstruction using custom-made titanium mesh tray and particulate cancellous bone and marrow harvested from bilateral posterior ilia. Journal of Plastic Surgery and Hand Surgery. 2014;**48**(3):183-190. DOI: 10.3109/2000656X.2013.848809

[107] Dawood A, Marti BM, Sauret-Jackson V, Darwood A. 3D printing in dentistry. British Dental Journal. 2015;**219**(11):521-529. DOI: 10.1038/sj.bdj.2016.50

[108] Zhou LB, Shang HT, He LS, Bo B, Liu GC, Liu YP, et al. Accurate reconstruction of discontinuous mandible using a reverse engineering/computer-aided design/rapid prototyping technique: A preliminary clinical study. Journal of Oral and Maxillofacial Surgery. 2010;**68**(9):2115-2121. DOI: 10.1016/j.joms.2009.09.033

[109] Yamada H, Nakaoka K, Sonoyama T, Kumagai K, Ikawa T, Shigeta Y, et al. Clinical usefulness of mandibular reconstruction using custom-made titanium mesh tray and autogenous particulate cancellous bone and marrow harvested from tibia and/or Ilia. The Journal of Craniofacial Surgery. 2016;**27**(3):586-592. DOI: 10.1097/SCS.0000000000002472

[110] Khalifa GA, Abd El Moniem NA, Elsayed SA-E, Qadry Y. Segmental mirroring: Does it eliminate the need for intraoperative readjustment of the virtually pre-bent reconstruction plates and is it economically valuable? Journal of Oral and Maxillofacial Surgery. 2016;**74**(3):621-630. DOI: 10.1016/j.joms.2015.09.036

[111] Shen Y, Sun J, Li J, Ji T, Li MM, Huang W, et al. Using computer simulation and stereomodel for accurate mandibular reconstruction with vascularized iliac crest flap. Oral Surgery, Oral Medicine, Oral Pathology, Oral Radiology. 2012;**114**(2):175-182. DOI: 10.1016/j.tripleo.2011.06.030

[112] Ramezanzade S, Aeinehvand M, Ziaei H, Khurshid Z, Keyhan SO, Fallahi HR, et al. Reconstruction of critical sized maxillofacial defects using composite allogeneic tissue engineering: Systematic review of current literature. Biomimetics (Basel). 2023;**8**(2):142. DOI: 10.3390/biomimetics8020142

[113] Quek J, Vizetto-Duarte C, Teoh SH, Choo Y. Towards stem cell therapy for critical-sized segmental bone defects: Current trends and challenges on the path to clinical translation. Journal of Functional Biomaterials. 2024;**15**(6):145. DOI: 10.3390/jfb15060145

[114] Hutmacher DW. Scaffold design and fabrication technologies for engineering tissues--state of the art and future perspectives. Journal of Biomaterials Science. Polymer Edition. 2001;**12**(1):107-124. DOI: 10.1163/156856201744489

[115] Jukes JBS, Post J. In: Potten C, editor. Stem Cells. 1st ed. London: Elsevier; 2008. ISBN: 9780080541761

[116] Zhao J, Zhou YH, Zhao YQ, Gao ZR, Ouyang ZY, Ye Q, et al. Oral cavity-derived stem cells and preclinical models of jaw-bone defects for bone tissue engineering. Stem Cell Research & Therapy. 2023;**14**(1):39. DOI: 10.1186/s13287-023-03265-z

[117] Probst FA, Liokatis P, Mast G, Ehrenfeld M. Virtual planning for mandible resection and reconstruction. Innovative Surgical Sciences. 2023;**8**(3):137-148. DOI: 10.1515/iss-2021-0045

[118] Park HI, Lee JH, Lee SJ. The comprehensive on-demand 3D bio-printing for composite reconstruction of mandibular defects. The Journal of Indian Prosthodontic Society. 2022;**44**(1):31. DOI: 10.1186/s40902-022-00361-7

[119] Onodera K, Miyamoto I, Hoshi I, Kawamata S, Takahashi N, Shimazaki N, et al. Towards optimum mandibular reconstruction for dental occlusal rehabilitation: From preoperative virtual surgery to autogenous particulate cancellous bone and marrow graft with custom-made titanium mesh-A retrospective study. Journal of Clinical Medicine. 2023;**12**(3):112. DOI: 10.3390/jcm12031122

[120] Sedgley CM, Botero TM. Dental stem cells and their sources. Dental Clinics of North America. 2012;**56**(3):549-561. DOI: 10.1016/j.cden.2012.05.004. Epub 2012 Jun 23

[121] Liu A, Lin D, Zhao H, Chen L, Cai B, Lin K, et al. Optimized BMSC-derived osteoinductive exosomes immobilized in hierarchical scaffold via lyophilization for bone repair through Bmpr2/Acvr2b competitive receptor-activated Smad pathway. Biomaterials. 2021;**272**:120718. DOI: 10.1016/j.biomaterials.2021.120718

[122] Dholaria B, Labopin M, Sanz J, Ruggeri A, Cornelissen J, Labussiere-Wallet H, et al. Allogeneic hematopoietic cell transplantation with cord blood versus mismatched unrelated donor with post-transplant cyclophosphamide in acute myeloid leukemia. Journal of Hematology & Oncology. 2021;**14**(1):76. DOI: 10.1186/s13045-021-01086-2

[123] Corvera S. Cellular heterogeneity in adipose tissues. Annual Review of Physiology. 2021;**83**:257-278. DOI: 10.1146/annurev-physiol-031620-095446

[124] Arora S, Srinivasan A, Leung CM, Toh YC. Bio-mimicking shear stress environments for enhancing mesenchymal stem cell differentiation. Current Stem Cell Research & Therapy. 2020;**15**(5):414-427. DOI: 10.2174/1574888X15666200408113630

[125] Wu V, Helder MN, Bravenboer N, Ten Bruggenkate CM, Jin J, Klein-Nulend J, et al. Bone tissue regeneration in the oral and maxillofacial region:

A review on the application of stem cells and new strategies to improve vascularization. Stem Cells International. 2019;**2019**:6279721. DOI: 10.1155/2019/6279721

[126] Takahashi D, Suzuki H, Komori T. A clinical study of 103 dental implants in oral cancer patients after jaw resection. Journal of Oral and Maxillofacial Surgery, Medicine, and Pathology. 2018;**30**(3):206-211. DOI: 10.1016/j.ajoms.2017.12.006

[127] Deleyiannis FW, Dunklebarger J, Lee E, Gastman B, Lai S, Ferris R, et al. Reconstruction of the marginal mandibulectomy defect: An update. American Journal of Otolaryngology. 2007;**28**(6):363-366. DOI: 10.1016/j.amjoto.2006.10.017

[128] Mosahebi A, Chaudhry A, McCarthy CM, Disa JJ, Mehrara BJ, Pusic AL, et al. Reconstruction of extensive composite posterolateral mandibular defects using nonosseous free tissue transfer. Plastic and Reconstructive Surgery. 2009;**124**(5):1571-1577. DOI: 10.1097/PRS.0b013e3181b98b78

[129] Hanasono MM, Zevallos JP, Skoracki RJ, Yu P. A prospective analysis of bony versus soft-tissue reconstruction for posterior mandibular defects. Plastic and Reconstructive Surgery. 2010;**125**(5):1413-1421. DOI: 10.1097/PRS.0b013e3181d62aef

[130] Hutmacher DW, Tandon B, Dalton PD. Scaffold design and fabrication. In: Tissue Engineering. Amsterdam, Netherlands: Elsevier; 2023. pp. 355-385. DOI: 10.1016/B978-0-12-824459-3.00011-1

[131] Hadad H, Boos Lima FB, Shirinbak I, Porto TS, Chen JE. The impact of 3D printing on oral and maxillofacial surgery. Journal of 3D Printing in Medicine. 2023;7(2). DOI: 10.2217/3dp-2022-0025

[132] Wang X, Mu M, Yan J, Han B, Ye R, Guo G. 3D printing materials and 3D printed surgical devices in oral and maxillofacial surgery: Design, workflow and effectiveness. Regenerative Biomaterials. 2024;**27**(11):rbae066. DOI: 10.1093/rb/rbae066

[133] Bartier S, Mazzaschi O, Benichou L, Sauvaget E. Computer-assisted versus traditional technique in fibular free-flap mandibular reconstruction: A CT symmetry study. European Annals of Otorhinolaryngology, Head and Neck Diseases. 2021;**138**(1):23-27. DOI: 10.1016/j.anorl.2020.06.011

[134] Ren W, Gao L, Li S, Chen C, Li F, Wang Q, et al. Virtual planning and 3D printing modeling for mandibular reconstruction with fibula free flap. Medicina Oral, Patología Oral y Cirugía Bucal. 2018;**23**(3):e359-ee66. DOI: 10.4317/medoral.22295

[135] Liu R, Su Y, Pu J, Zhang C, Yang W. Cutting-edge patient-specific surgical plates for computer-assisted mandibular reconstruction: The art of matching structures and holes in precise surgery. Frontiers in Surgery. 2023;**9**(10):1132669. DOI: 10.3389/fsurg.2023.1132669

[136] Bolzoni AR, Pollice A, Nuti M, Baj A, Rossi DS, Beltramini GA. Clinical and functional outcomes of cad/cam mandibular reconstruction with free fibular flap comparing traditional versus micro-invasive intraoral surgical approaches. Journal of Biological Regulators and Homeostatic Agents. 2020;**34**(5 Suppl. 3):175-184

[137] Zoabi A, Redenski I, Oren D, Kasem A, Zigron A, Daoud S, et al. 3D printing and virtual surgical planning in

oral and maxillofacial surgery. Journal of Clinical Medicine. 2022;**11**(9):2385. DOI: 10.3390/jcm11092385

[138] Lin Q-q, Wang F, Sun J-l, Zhang H-z, Xi Q. Accurate mandible reconstruction by mixed reality, 3D printing, and robotic-assisted navigation integration. Journal of Craniofacial Surgery. 2022;**33**(6):1720-1724. DOI: 10.1097/SCS.0000000000008603

[139] Guo Y, Zhang C, Liu J, Chen X. Accuracy and safe strategies for robotic-assisted mandible reconstruction with fibula free flap. In: 2024 IEEE International Conference on Real- Time Computing and Robotics (RCAR). New York, USA: IEEE; 2024. DOI: 10.1109/RCAR61438.2024.10670945

[140] Ni Y, Zhang X, Meng Z, Li Z, Li S, Xu ZF, et al. Digital navigation and 3D model technology in mandibular reconstruction with fibular free flap: A comparative study. Journal of Stomatology, Oral and Maxillofacial Surgery. 2021;**122**(4):e59-e64. DOI: 10.1016/j.jormas.2020.11.002

[141] Shao L, Li X, Fu T, Meng F, Zhu Z, Zhao R, et al. Robot-assisted augmented reality surgical navigation based on optical tracking for mandibular reconstruction surgery. Medical Physics. 2024;**51**(1):363-377. DOI: 10.1002/mp.16598. Epub 2023 Jul 11

[142] Nakayama Y, Yamashita Y, Shimohira D, Aijima R, Danjo A. A long-term clinical statistical analysis of machined-surface Brånemark implants used in patients undergoing oral and maxillofacial surgery. Journal of Oral and Maxillofacial Surgery, Medicine, and Pathology. 2019;**31**(4):237-240. DOI: 10.1016/j.ajoms.2019.01.001

[143] Oliveira MT, Rocha FS, de Paulo LF, Rodrigues AR, Zanetta-Barbosa D. The approach of ameloblastoma of the mandible: A case treated by hyperbaric oxygen therapy and bone graft reconstruction. Oral and Maxillofacial Surgery. 2013;**17**(4):311-314. DOI: 10.1007/s10006-013-0390-9

[144] Karayazgan-Saracoglu B, Atay A, Korkmaz C, Gunay Y. Quality of life assessment of implant-retained overdentures and fixed metal-acrylic resin prostheses in patients with marginal mandibulectomy. The Journal of Prosthetic Dentistry. 2017;**118**(4):551-560. DOI: 10.1016/j.prosdent.2017.01.025

[145] Kumthekar MS, Sanyal PK, Tewary S. Anchored guided rehabilitation. Journal of Indian Prosthodontic Society. 2020;**20**(3):321-325. DOI: 10.4103/jips.jips_311_19. Epub 2020 Jul 17

[146] Gupta S, Bhargava A, Mehra P. A bar and ball attachment prosthesis over osseointegrated implants post mandibular resection. The Journal of Indian Prosthodontic Society. 2016;**16**(4):395-399. DOI: 10.4103/0972-4052.176523

[147] Singh D, Kumari S. Twin occlusion: A solution to rehabilitate hemimandibulectomy patient: A case report. Journal of Applied Dental and Medical Sciences. 2019;**5**:31-34. ISSN:2454-2288

[148] Marathe AS, Kshirsagar PS. A systematic approach in rehabilitation of hemimandibulectomy: A case report. The Journal of Indian Prosthodontic Society. 2016;**16**(2):208-212. DOI: 10.4103/0972-4052.164914

[149] Singh B, Sinha N, Sharma R, Parekh N. Non surgical correction of mandibular deviation and neuromuscular coordination after two

years of mandibular guidance therapy: A case report. Journal of Clinical and Diagnostic Research. 2015;**9**(11):ZD07-9. DOI: 10.7860/JCDR/2015/16309.6730

[150] Choudhary S, Ram S, Kumar A. Prosthetic management of a hemi-mandibulectomy patient. Indian Journal of Dental Sciences. 2018;**10**(2):118-120. DOI: 10.4103/IJDS.IJDS_122_17

[151] Madan S, Rani S, Jainer R, Kumar S, Kumar M, Varshney N. Guide flange prosthesis for deviation in mandibulectomy patients: A case report. International Journal of Research and Reports in Dentistry. 2018;**1**:64-69. Available from: https://journalijrrd.com/index.php/IJRRD/article/view/4

[152] Mohapatra A. Rehabilitating occlusion with a guiding flange prosthesis in a patient with mandibular resection: A case report. Indian Journal of Forensic Medicine & Toxicology. 2020;**14**(4):8897-8901. DOI: 10.37506/ijfmt.v14i4.13118

[153] Kumar S, Dwivedi H, Singh B, Jha AK, Jain R, Singh S. A systematic review on prosthodontic rehabilitation of hemimandibulectomy defects. Cureus. 2023;**15**(9):e44647. DOI: 10.7759/cureus.44647

[154] Singh M, Mattoo K, Yadav L. Clinical variables associated with the rehabilitation of a hemimandibulectomy patient. Medico Research Chronicles. 2015;**2**(1):14-18. Available from: https://medrech.com/index.php/medrech/article/view/42

[155] Rathee M, Tamrakar A, Bhoria M, Boora P. Prosthetic rehabilitation of surgically treated case of squamous cell carcinoma of retromolar trigone: A case report. Research and Reviews: Journal of Medical and Health Sciences. 2014;**3**:26-32. e-ISSN: 2319-9865

[156] Kumar CD, Zankari V, Harichandan S, Yuvaraja G. Prosthodontic rehabilitation of the patient with acquired maxillo-mandibular defect. Kerala Dental Journal. 2013;**36**:146-148. Available from: https://www.idakerala.com/publications/KDJVol36No2_KeralaDentalJournal.pdf

[157] Aggarwal H, Jurel SK, Kumar P, Chand P. Rehabilitating mandibular resection with guide flange prosthesis. Journal of the College of Physicians and Surgeons–Pakistan. 2014;**24**(Suppl 2):S135-S137

[158] Hazra R, Srivastava A, Kumar D. Mandibular guidance prosthesis: Conventional and innovative approach: A case series. The Journal of Indian Prosthodontic Society. 2021;**21**(2):208-214. DOI: 10.4103/jips.jips_12_21

[159] Kar S, Tripathi A, Madhok R. Treatment outcome with guiding flange prosthesis in hemimandibulectomy patients: Case series of three patients. Annals of Maxillofacial Surgery. 2015;**5**(2):266-270. DOI: 10.4103/2231-0746.175750

[160] Lingeshwar D, Appadurai R, Sswedheni U, Padmaja C. Prosthodontic management of hemimandibulectomy patients to restore form and function - a case series. World Journal of Clinical Cases. 2017;**5**(10):384-389. DOI: 10.12998/wjcc.v5.i10.384

[161] Jain V, Pruthi G, Mundhe K. Clinical considerations for prosthodontic rehabilitation of intermediate form of osteopetrosis: A report of two cases. Journal of Oral Biology and Craniofacial Research. 2012;**2**(2):126-130. DOI: 10.1016/j.jobcr.2012.05.008

[162] Gupta SG, Sandhu D, Arora A, Pasam N. The use of mandibular guidance prosthesis to correct

mandibular deviation following hemimandibulectomy: Case reports. Indian Journal of Dental Research. April-Sep 2012:71-73

[163] Hindocha AD, Dudani MT. Detachable palatal ramp of teeth to improve comfort in a completely edentulous patient with a segmentally resected mandible. Journal of Prosthodontics. 2017;**26**(5):474-480. DOI: 10.1111/jopr.12427

[164] Coutinho CA, Hegde D, Vijayalakshmi CR, Iyer R, Priya A. Twin-occlusion prosthesis in a class III hemimandibulectomy patient. International Journal of Prosthodontics and Restorative Dentistry. 2020;**10**:35-38. DOI: 10.5005/jp-journals-10019-1257

[165] Shashidhara HS, Thippanna RK, Dang K, Hajira N, Sharma A. Modified occlusal table - an aid to enhance function of hemimandibulectomy patient: A case report. Journal of Clinical and Diagnostic Research. 2015;**9**(9):ZD01-3. DOI: 10.7860/JCDR/2015/13267.6414

[166] Talukder D, Datta P, Raheja A, Dua B. Twin occlusion prosthesis: Management of hemimandibulectomy patient. Indian Journal of Dental Education. 2017;**10**:235-238

[167] Koralakunte PR, Shamnur SN, Iynalli RV, Shivmurthy S. Prosthetic management of hemimandibulectomy patient with guiding plane and twin occlusion prosthesis. Journal of Natural Science, Biology and Medicine. 2015;**6**(2):449-453. DOI: 10.4103/0976-9668.160036

[168] Sahu SK, Motwani BK, Dani A. Prosthetic rehabilitation of edentulous hemimandibulectomy patient: A clinical report. Clinical Case Reports. 2017;**5**(11):1739-1742. DOI: 10.1002/ccr3.1125

[169] Matros E, Albornoz CR, Rensberger M, Weimer K, Garfein ES. Computer-assisted design and computer-assisted modeling technique optimization and advantages over traditional methods of osseous flap reconstruction. Journal of Reconstructive Microsurgery. 2014;**30**(5):289-296. DOI: 10.1055/s-0033-1358789

[170] Okay DJ, Buchbinder D, Urken M, Jacobson A, Lazarus C, Persky M. Computer-assisted implant rehabilitation of maxillomandibular defects reconstructed with vascularized bone free flaps. JAMA Otolaryngology. Head & Neck Surgery. 2013;**139**(4):371-381. DOI: 10.1001/jamaoto.2013.83

[171] Pierre CS, Dassonville O, Chamorey E, Poissonnet G, Riss JC, Ettaiche M, et al. Long-term functional outcomes and quality of life after oncologic surgery and microvascular reconstruction in patients with oral or oropharyngeal cancer. Acta Oto-Laryngologica. 2014;**134**(10):1086-1093. DOI: 10.3109/00016489.2014.913809

[172] de Melo NB, Bernardino IM, de Melo DP, Gomes DQC, Bento PM. Head and neck cancer, quality of life, and determinant factors: A novel approach using decision tree analysis. Oral Surgery, Oral Medicine, Oral Pathology, Oral Radiology. 2018;**126**(6):486-493. DOI: 10.1016/j.oooo.2018.07.055

[173] Davudov MM, Harirchi I, Arabkheradmand A, Garajei A, Mahmudzadeh H, Shirkhoda M, et al. Evaluation of quality of life in patients with oral cancer after mandibular resection: Comparing no reconstruction, reconstruction with plate, and reconstruction with flap. Medicine. 2019;**98**(41):e17431. DOI: 10.1097/MD.0000000000017431

[174] Aimaijiang Y, Otomaru T, Taniguchi H. Relationships between

perceived chewing ability, objective masticatory function and oral health-related quality of life in mandibulectomy or glossectomy patients with a dento-maxillary prosthesis. Journal of Prosthodontic Research. 2016;**60**(2):92-97. DOI: 10.1016/j.jpor.2015.07.005

[175] Warshavsky A, Fliss DM, Frenkel G, Kupershmidt A, Moav N, Rosen R, et al. Quality of life after mandibulectomy: The impact of the resected subsite. International Journal of Oral and Maxillofacial Surgery. 2019;**48**(10):1273-1278. DOI: 10.1016/j.ijom.2019.02.013

[176] Landström FJ, Reizenstein JA, Nilsson CO, Beckerath MV, Löfgren AL, Adamsson GB, et al. Electrochemotherapy - possible benefits and limitations to its use in the head and neck region. Acta Oto-Laryngologica. 2015;**135**(1):90-95. DOI: 10.3109/00016489.2014.947655

[177] Terrell JE, Ronis DL, Fowler KE, Bradford CR, Chepeha DB, Prince ME, et al. Clinical predictors of quality of life in patients with head and neck cancer. Archives of Otolaryngology – Head & Neck Surgery. 2004;**130**(4):401-408. DOI: 10.1001/archotol.130.4.401

[178] Vu DD, Schmidt BL. Quality of life evaluation for patients receiving vascularized versus nonvascularized bone graft reconstruction of segmental mandibular defects. Journal of Oral and Maxillofacial Surgery. 2008;**66**(9):1856-1863. DOI: 10.1016/j.joms.2008.04.021

[179] Clemente JT, Parada CA, Veiga MC, Gear RW, Tambeli CH. Sexual dimorphism in the antinociception mediated by kappa opioid receptors in the rat temporomandibular joint. Neuroscience Letters. 2004;**372**(3):250-255. DOI: 10.1016/j.neulet.2004.09.048

[180] de Coupade C, Gear RW, Dazin PF, Sroussi HY, Green PG, Levine JD. β2-adrenergic receptor regulation of human neutrophil function is sexually dimorphic. British Journal of Pharmacology. 2004;**143**(8):1033-1041. DOI: 10.1038/sj.bjp.0705972

[181] Fillingim RB, Gear RW. Sex differences in opioid analgesia: Clinical and experimental findings. European Journal of Pain. 2004;**8**(5):413-425. DOI: 10.1016/j.ejpain.2004.01.007

[182] Jacobsen HC, Wahnschaff F, Trenkle T, Sieg P, Hakim SG. Oral rehabilitation with dental implants and quality of life following mandibular reconstruction with free fibular flap. Clinical Oral Investigations. 2016;**20**(1):187-192. DOI: 10.1007/s00784-015-1487-3

[183] Garrett N, Roumanas ED, Blackwell KE, Freymiller E, Abemayor E, Wong WK, et al. Efficacy of conventional and implant-supported mandibular resection prostheses: Study overview and treatment outcomes. The Journal of Prosthetic Dentistry. 2006;**96**(1):13-24. DOI: 10.1016/j.prosdent.2006.05.010

[184] Shankar RK, Raza FB, Kumar VA. Quality of life with the rehabilitation after partial mandibulectomy: A systematic review. Indian Journal of Surgical Oncology. 2023;**14**(2):292-300. DOI: 10.1007/s13193-022-01664-x. Epub 2022 Oct 12

Chapter 5

Long-Lasting and Natural-Looking Face with Optimal Hyaluronic Acid Filler Injection

Devin Su

Abstract

Since the approval of the U.S. Food and Drug Administration (FDA) in 2003, the first hyaluronic acid filler (HAF), Restylane, has opened up a new era of nonsurgical soft tissue augmentation without the requirement of a skin test. Although other dermal fillers, such as collagen stimulators and some composite fillers, have emerged over the past few years, the HAF remains the most widely used material today for esthetic use due to its safety, reliability, and favorable duration of action. The past two decades have not only brought an expansion of available HAF products, but also evolving concepts of how HAF can be incorporated into human faces. However, facial overfilled syndrome (FOS) is an emerging esthetic problem resulting from various types of filler injection. In this chapter, the author would like to introduce an injecting technique for HAF into the deep pyriform space under the nasolabial fold (NLF) for opening a door to a long-lasting and natural-looking face.

Keywords: hyaluronic acid, nonsurgical, overfilled, nasolabial fold, natural-looking

1. Introduction

Facial overfilled syndrome (FOS) is an arising esthetic problem due to multiple sessions of incorrectly placed dermal fillers [1, 2]. Over the past decade, we have experienced a massive approach in dermal fillers for esthetic medicine. In that process, we some success in restoring youth and beauty in people, but in some instances, we might have done worse outcomes for our customers. The most commonly used dermal fillers include HAF, collagen stimulators, and composite fillers. These dermal fillers were considered safe. For those people who had undergone dermal fillers, some might be aware that he or she was overfilled, but others might be satisfied with his or her weird face and regard it as normal. Distorted appearance due to FOS might occur after multiple sessions of filler injection, one single modality of large amounts of volume overload, or even one outrageous placement of small amounts of dermal filler. Eventually, a conscientious and well-experienced physician would do his best to prevent FOS. Facial aging was a process that resulted from a combination of bone resorption, degeneration and weakening of supportive osseocutaneous ligaments, and volume change of superficial subcutaneous fat or deep fat pads. A physician without

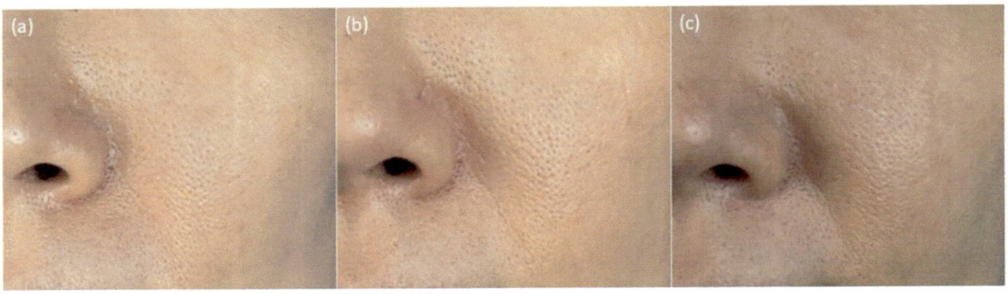

Figure 1.
(a) A 47-year-old woman underwent two sessions of collagen stimulator injection for her mid- and lower-face rejuvenation within 2 months. (b) 4 months later, she underwent another session of collagen stimulator injection. (c) 9 months later, the NLF became even deeper than the original state, consistent with FOS.

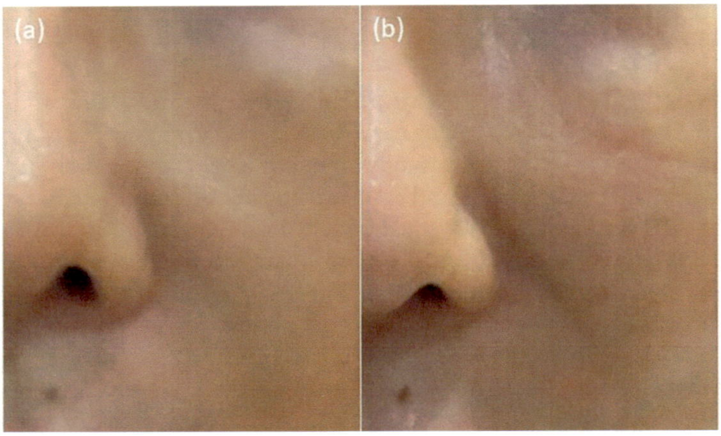

Figure 2.
(a) A 50-year-old woman underwent unknown sessions of dermal filler injection into her face. (b) 2 years later, the NLF became deeper, resulting from compression of the above superficial NLF fat. Note the nostril also being compressed. Her face was consistent with FOS.

adequate training or certification might inject some dermal fillers into customers' faces just based on a traditional theory that volume loss contributes to human facial aging. However, these operations sometimes worked, but they sometimes did not achieve the anti-aging function and instead increased the load on the face. Moreover, there was no knowing exactly when any kind of dermal fillers would completely go away, and hence, these operations, in turn, expedited the aging process (**Figures 1** and **2**). Almost all of the indications of the dermal filler included NLF, so the most important risk factor contributing to FOS might be NLF.

2. Discussion

Methods to correct NLF include surgical implants, face lifts with surgery or threads, and filler injection. Filler injection is the most common method and hence easily contributes to FOS. Filler is not well-maintained at NLF. A detailed understanding of the anatomy of NLF helps us to prevent ineffective treatments [3–10]. A Micro-Computed Tomography Study revealed that the medial part of NLF has dense connective tissue with interlacing muscle fibers, and the lateral part of NLF has loose adipose tissue [3]. Superficial mimetic muscle, including levator labii superioris alaeque nasi, levator labii superioris, and zygomaticus minor, tightly tethers to the dermis of the medial part of NLF. The lateral border of the above muscle attachment corresponds to NLF. The musculodermal theory offers an insight into the fact that NLF corresponds to a groove along the lateral margin of these mimetic muscle attachments. Senescence-related distribution change of the fat-rich part lateral to the NLF, sunken from pyriform resorption, or both, makes the fold deeper [11–14].

The author would like to present a detailed operating process on how to inject HAF into a potential deep space under NLF. The concept of "deep pyriform space" was first proposed by Christopher in 2016 [15]. This potential deep space can be "weaker" with bony resorption of pyriform aperture, lipoatrophy of medial deep fat pad, and aging-associated loosening of perioral superficial fibromuscular layer.

Place the patient in the supine position. A 27-gauge short needle is preferred for this technique. The NLF is anesthetized with the infraorbital nerve block using 2% lidocaine, 1-c.c. for either side. Press the innermost NLF toward the pyriform aperture with the index finger. After the removal of the index finger, an obtuse-angle L-shape dent would appear before it totally rebounds. After sterilization of the nose, NLF, and medial cheeks, check the bevel of the needle parallel to the NLF. An entry point about 5-mm above the vertex of the angle is punctured using a 27-gauge unprimed needle. On the first step, the needle is directed at a 45- to 60-degree angle to the vertical line in the sagittal plane. The needle is guided smoothly along the downward slope of the pyriform aperture, and any resistance should not be felt while advancing the needle through the soft tissue. Hold the syringe with the bevel toward the bone, and eventually into the supraperiosteum of the deep pyriform space. At this point, the needle should not be pushed hard toward the bone. On the second step, the needle is turned at a 45-degree angle directed inferiorly and medially. Advance the needle to a depth of about three-fourths of its total length until tight contact with the bone is reached. Before injecting, aspiration should be made to avoid accidental injection into the angular artery. After a negative aspiration, the filler should be injected without obvious resistance. Keep the needle in a steady position. Slight squeezing of the area of entry helps tenting the skin and preventing retrograde spread of the filler. Always be aware of any response from the patient. Neither linear threading nor fanning technique is utilized. Instead, if the needle moves, re-aspirate before keeping going. If positive aspiration occurs, slowly retract the needle and change to a new one. Gauze compression should be made before re-entry. A successful injection technique results in the sunken groove of the NLF being naturally lifted and smoothened. No superficial fatty layer or subdermal layer was injected. When HAF is attached to the pyriform aperture instead of the inner superficial fibromuscular subcutaneous layer of NLF, which allows it to restore and support this potential deep space. A highly cohesive and highly elastic HAF would be preferred because this type of HAF could fix well regardless of the strength of the above mimetic muscle. After all, a combination of downward pushing using one index finger on the NLF skin and medial pushing using another one on the oral mucosa, molds the HAF into a pyramid-like shape firmly fit to the pyriform aperture. The interference of facial expression involving the mimetic muscle would be minimal. More importantly, inevitable displacement of any type of fillers from inner dense nasolabial fat to upper-outward loose area could be well prevented with this technique. In brief, the illustration depicts an insight of the needle in position under the roof of the mimetic muscle (**Figure 3**). In general, the injected amount of HAF from this technique is about 1.0 to 1.5-c.c. for either side.

Some practitioners inject directly at a 45- to 90-degree angle, placing the bevel of the needle close to the bone. Disadvantages of this one-step technique include hitting

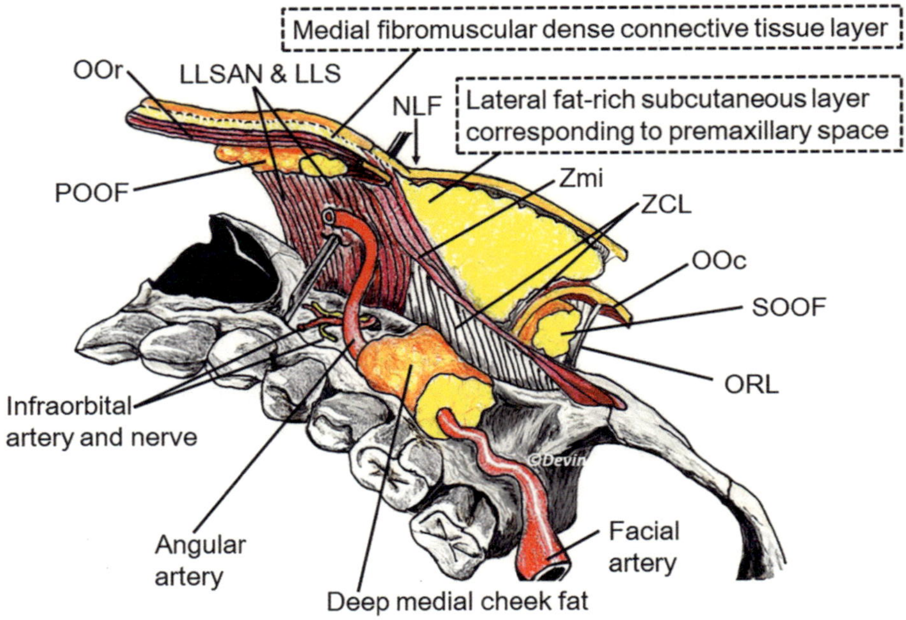

Figure 3.
The illustration briefly demonstrates the needle approaching the pyriform aperture. The overlying mimetic muscle comprises the roof of this space. The distinct difference between the medial fibromuscular dense connective tissue layer and the lateral fat-rich superficial nasolabial fat is depicted. The lateral border of the mimetic muscle attachment corresponds to a distinct cutaneous furrow named NLF. (LLS, levator labii superioris; LLSAN, Levator labii superioris alaeque nasi; OOr, orbicularis oris muscle; OOc, orbicularis oculi muscle; ORL, orbicularis retaining ligament; POOF, post-orbicularis oris fat; SOOF, sub-orbicularis oculi fat; ZCL, zygomatic cutaneous ligament; Zmi, zygomaticus minor muscle.)

the superficial wall, probably the depressor septi nasi, before entering the deep pyriform space and a higher risk of accidentally tearing the angular artery, resulting in a false deep pyriform space injection. Some practitioners get deep pyriform space injection with a cannula. The entry was usually lateral to the NLF and the cannula was inserted deep under the NLF and slid toward the alar base. Disadvantages of this injection method include unexpected breakthrough of the oral mucosa, unworkable or unreliable aspiration with a cannula before a bolus injection, easily dispersed spreading of the filler material from the side hole of the cannula, and unsteady sliding of the cannula while injecting a bolus in such a deep plane. However, if one can manipulate well with an ultrasound guide, it could be feasible.

It is a controversial issue how to inject appropriately and to prevent potential risk of vascular complications. In most circumstances, physicians correct nasolabial folds with a variety of dermal fillers. Injecting techniques include anterograde or retrograde linear threading, fanning, or a combination in multiple layers [16]. Although a mainstream consensus about minimizing the chance of vascular complications includes slow injection, small aliquots, low extrusion pressure, preferring cannula, and deeply understanding anatomical plane and vessel distribution [17, 18]. These theories are very general and might be unworkable for some value areas, such as deep pyriform space. In addition, the main trunk and its branches of the facial artery are distributed in the vicinity of NLF in more than 90% of cases [19]. Therefore, even taking the above injection consensus could not assure preventing vascular compromise. The course of the angular artery was described as running superficially in the roof of the pyriform space, which allowed a deep injection on the bone safer [15]. Nevertheless, the recent research demonstrated that the angular artery ran <1 mm from the bone of the pyriform space in 3% of the cases [20]. The variations of the angular artery could not ensure a totally safe procedure, but it is still looking quite promising for operating in this potential space. In the author's opinion, it might not be safer to continue moving even with a cannula when operating toward deep pyriform space. The continuous moving in this space might make the angular artery easily injured or cause an unexpected breakthrough of the oral mucosa. On the contrary, for example, if a healthy provider needs to set an intravenous route, instead, he or she must assure cannulating the vessel. In this situation, continuous dripping cannot be feasible if a healthy provider does not see a blood withdrawal in the needle hub and set the cannula well. The general guideline for intravenous or intra-arterial route insertion is never questioned. At present, the 27-gauge or 30-gauge thin-walled needles included in the product boxes are still standard instead of a cannula. Available studies demonstrated that aspiration alone does not assure safety. An expert physician would notice many aspects of abnormal signs except a positive aspiration, including abnormal stabbing pain, unsteady bevel position, feeling of an elastic touch from the needle, and abrupt increased injection resistance, all of which might indicate false-negative aspiration. Ultrasound might provide a reliable insight to operate the pyriform space injection [20]. The choice of injection tool, either needle or cannula, would not guarantee safety. Accordingly, aspiration should still be a basic and standard step that should not be easily abandoned. Always remember to notice any sign and response from your patient during the injection.

With regard to the choice of HAF for the purpose of offering a well-maintained support for the deep pyriform aperture, a HAF capable of providing both adequate support and high flexibility, such as Restylane® DEFYNE™ (HADEF), is preferred [21]. HADEF has been approved in the United States since 2016 for the correction of moderate to severe, deep facial wrinkles and folds, such as the NLF, or for the augmentation of mild to moderate chin retrusion in patients over the age of 21 [22]. HADEF is designed with OBT™/XpresHAn™ technology, capable of providing both adequate firmness (higher G′), high flexibility, and high tissue integration [21, 23]. HADEF has been proven effective for lower-face contouring and structural reshaping while maintaining natural facial expression [24, 25]. More importantly, unlike surgical implants, which are difficult to carve in

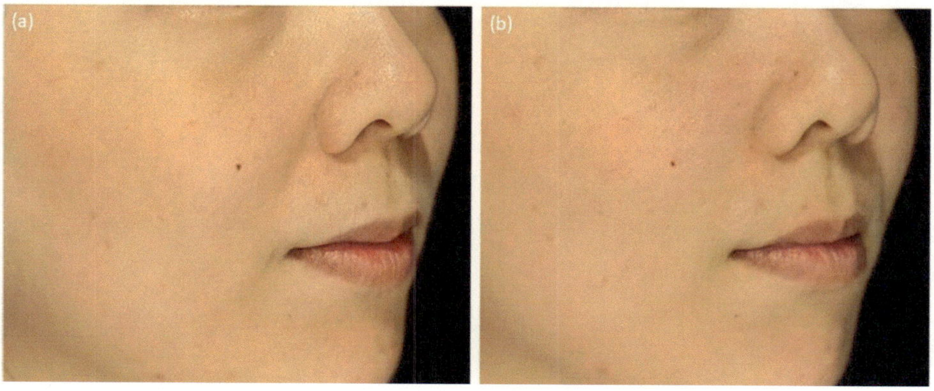

Figure 4.
(a) A 38-year-old woman underwent 2-c.c. HADEF injection (1-c.c. for either side) with the author's injection technique for correction of her NLF. No superficial injection was given. (b) Right after the HA augmentation on the pyriform aperture area, the lower midface profile changed from concavity to relative convexity. The NLF smoothened naturally. In addition, the alar lobule and the marionette line of the mouth corner profited from the support of the potential deep space.

place, HADEF can be easily contoured right after a bolus injection and would be hard to be displaced while sitting well in the pyriform space.

This 2-step method pronounced by the author was performed in hundreds of patients during the past decade, and there were no significant vascular complications. Some patients benefited soon after the procedure (**Figure 4**). Dynamic facial expression involving the mimetic muscle was usually not interfered with (**Figure 5**). Even some cases consistent with FOS might benefit from this augmentation method (**Figure 6**). The longest duration of this injection method from the author lasted more than 3 years (**Figure 7**). The long-lasting maintenance of HAF has been reported previously and this phenomenon may explain why some cases last so long from the injection [26, 27]. Most common complications included slightly erythematous swelling or ecchymosis, and all of these signs went away within 1–2 weeks. The risk of vascular compromise always exists. Therefore, it is still necessary to inject fillers

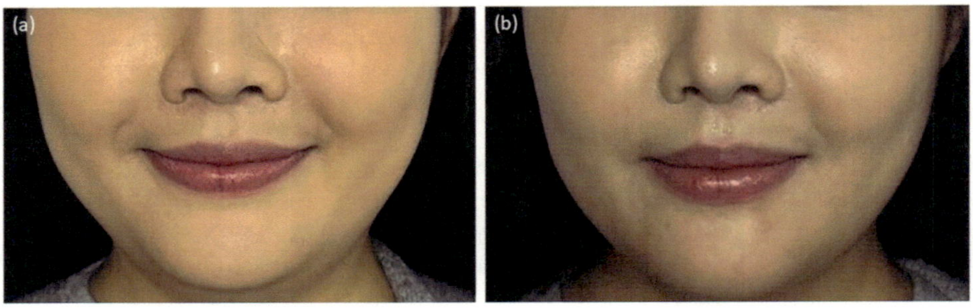

Figure 5.
(a) A 31-year-old woman underwent 5-c.c. HAF injection for correction of her NLF and chin contouring, including 2-c.c. for NLF (1-c.c. for either side) with the author's injection technique on the pyriform aperture area. No superficial-layer injection was given. (b) 1 week after the procedure, the dynamic smile expression looked smooth and natural without signs of FOS.

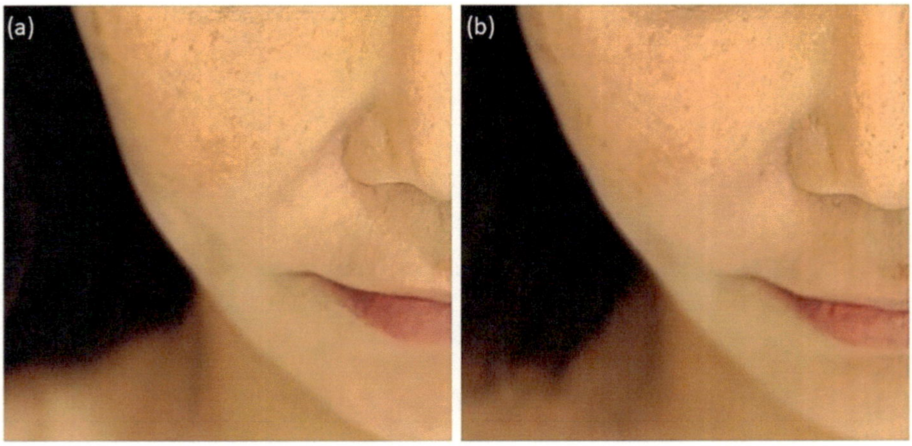

Figure 6.
(a) A 52-year-old woman whose face was consistent with FOS resulting from previous unknown sessions of filler injection, underwent 8-c.c. HADEF injection in total for whole-face rejuvenation, including 0.8-c.c. for the NLF (0.5-c.c. for the right side and 0.3-c.c. for the left side) with the author's injection technique. No superficial injection was given. A combination of whole-face Ultherapy was given before the HADEF injection on the same day. (b) Right after the whole-face procedure, the lower midface profile changed from drooping concavity to relatively smooth convexity. The sharp NLF smoothened naturally.

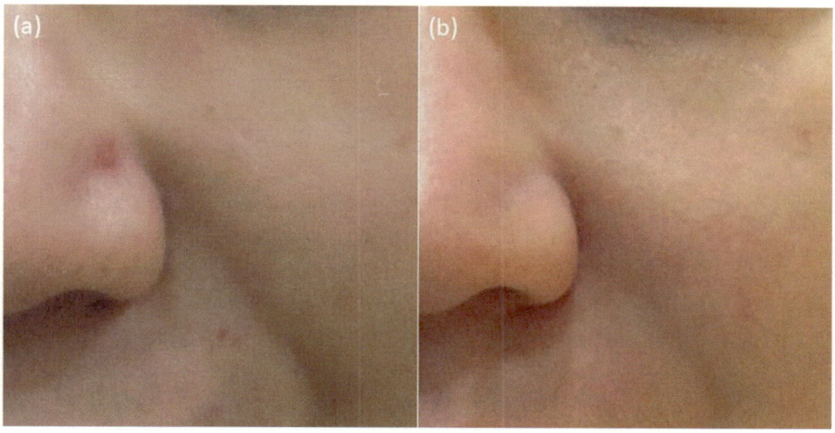

Figure 7.
(a) A 30-year-old woman underwent a session of Ultherapy and 2-c.c. HAF injection (1-c.c. for either side) with the author's injection technique for correction of her NLF. No superficial injection was given. (b) About 3.6 years after the procedure, the naturally smoothened NLF still maintained well.

gently and slowly with a lot of care. The author prefers the injection technique so that the change of NLF would not merely be superficial or temporary. Most importantly, the filler was able to support more than just the depressed NLF for a long time instead of being a risk factor for FOS. There were still limitations to this injection technique. One was a history of paranasal (pyriform aperture) implants, which usually sit on the bone. Another is severe fibrosis resulting from multiple sessions of collagen stimulators in NLF. Both of them would restrict the space for further operation.

3. Conclusion

Widely used injection techniques to correct the NLF include fanning or linear threading across the NLF. However, these outcomes inevitably lasted for a short or evenly became worse resulting from the traction of the mimetic muscle. The author hereby proposes an innovative 2-step injection technique using a 27-gauge needle with the bevel closed, appressed to the slope bottom of the pyriform aperture. It is worth noting that a single bolus injection of HAF at the base of the pyriform aperture did not result in any safety compromise during the author's past decade of clinical practice with hundreds of patients. It might be challenging for operators to continuously inject a relatively large amount of HA bolus with a needle. Furthermore, this technique might be considered controversial. Eventually, expertise in anatomy, confidence from cumulative clinical experience, and exquisite injection skills are still necessary to provide exact effectiveness, safety, and a good first step to prevent FOS.

Conflict of interest

The authors declare no conflict of interest.

Author details

Devin Su
Ultimate Beauty Clinic, Taipei, Taiwan

*Address all correspondence to: beauty.in.nature.21@gmail.com

References

[1] Lim T. Facial overfilled syndrome. Dermatologic Clinics. 2024;**42**(1):121-128. DOI: 10.1016/j.det.2023.06.007. Epub 2023 Jul 26

[2] Lim TS, Wanitphakdeedecha R, Yi KH. Exploring facial overfilled syndrome from the perspective of anatomy and the mismatched delivery of fillers. Journal of Cosmetic Dermatology. 2024;**23**(6):1964-1968. DOI: 10.1111/jocd.16244. Epub 2024 Feb 18

[3] Kwon HJ, Cho TH, Choi YJ, Yang HM. The nasolabial fold: A micro-computed tomography study. Plastic and Reconstructive Surgery. 2020;**145**(1):71-79. DOI: 10.1097/PRS.0000000000006328

[4] Pessa JE, Brown F. Independent effect of various facial mimetic muscles on the nasolabial fold. Aesthetic Plastic Surgery. 1992;**16**:167-171

[5] Beer GM, Manestar M, Mihic-Probst D. The causes of the nasolabial crease: A histomorphological study. Clinical Anatomy. 2013;**26**:196-203

[6] Sandulescu T, Spilker L, Rauscher D, Naumova EA, Arnold WH. Morphological analysis and three-dimensional reconstruction of the SMAS surrounding the nasolabial fold. Annals of Anatomy. 2018;**217**:111-117

[7] Barton FE Jr, Gyimesi IM. Anatomy of the nasolabial fold. Plastic and Reconstructive Surgery. 1997;**100**:1276-1280

[8] Rubin LR, Mishriki Y, Lee G. Anatomy of the nasolabial fold: The keystone of the smiling mechanism. Plastic and Reconstructive Surgery. 1989;**83**:1-10

[9] Pogrel MA, Shariati S, Schmidt B, Faal ZH, Regezi J. The surgical anatomy of the nasolabial fold. Oral Surgery, Oral Medicine, Oral Pathology, Oral Radiology, and Endodontics. 1998;**86**:410-415

[10] Zufferey J. Anatomic variations of the nasolabial fold. Plastic and Reconstructive Surgery. 1992;**89**:225-231; discussion 232-233

[11] Rohrich RJ, Pessa JE, Ristow B. The youthful cheek and the deep medial fat compartment. Plastic and Reconstructive Surgery. 2008;**121**(6):2107-2112. DOI: 10.1097/PRS.0b013e31817123c6

[12] Donofrio LM. Fat distribution: A morphologic study of the aging face. Dermatologic Surgery. 2000;**26**(12):1107-1112

[13] Mendelson B, Wong CH. Changes in the facial skeleton with aging: Implications and clinical applications in facial rejuvenation. Aesthetic Plastic Surgery. 2012;**36**(4):753-760. DOI: 10.1007/s00266-012-9904-3. Epub 2012 May 12

[14] Shaw RB Jr, Kahn DM. Aging of the midface bony elements: A three-dimensional computed tomographic study. Plastic and Reconstructive Surgery. 2007;**119**(2):675-681; discussion 682-3. DOI: 10.1097/01.prs.0000246596.79795.a8

[15] Surek CK, Vargo J, Lamb J. Deep pyriform space: Anatomical clarifications and clinical implications. Plastic and Reconstructive Surgery. 2016;**138**(1):59-64. DOI: 10.1097/PRS.0000000000002262

[16] Jung GS. Hyaluronic acid filler injection technique in multiple layers

of the nasolabial fold. Plastic and Reconstructive Surgery. Global Open. 2020;**8**(12):e3318. DOI: 10.1097/GOX.0000000000003318

[17] Goodman GJ, Magnusson MR, Callan P, et al. A consensus on minimizing the risk of hyaluronic acid embolic visual loss and suggestions for immediate bedside management. Aesthetic Surgery Journal. 2020;**40**(9):1009-1021

[18] Cotofana S, Alfertshofer M, Schenck TL, et al. Anatomy of the superior and inferior labial arteries revised: An ultrasound investigation and implication for lip volumization. Aesthetic Surgery Journal. 2020;**40**(12):1327-1335

[19] Yang HM, Lee JG, Hu KS, et al. New anatomical insights on the course and branching patterns of the facial artery: Clinical implications of injectable treatments to the nasolabial fold and nasojugal groove. Plastic and Reconstructive Surgery. 2014;**133**:1077-1082

[20] Franceschelli A, Cazzulani M, Urso S, Molinari P, Piludu M, Zuccaro M, et al. In vivo ultrasound study of the angular artery anatomy: Practical indications for the treatment of the deep pyriform space. Aesthetic Surgery Journal Open Forum. 2024;**6**:ojae113. DOI: 10.1093/asjof/ojae113

[21] Öhrlund Å. Evaluation of rheometry amplitude sweep cross-over point as an index of flexibility for HA fillers. Journal of Cosmetics, Dermatological Sciences and Applications. 2018;**8**:47-54

[22] FDA. Directions for Use: Restylane Defyne [package insert]. Available from: https://www.accessdata.fda.gov/cdrh_docs/pdf14/P140029S027C.pdf [Accessed: May 5, 2023]

[23] Lundgren B, Sandkvist U, Bordier N, Gauthier B. Using a new photo scale to compare product integration of different hyaluronan-based fillers after injection in human ex vivo skin. Journal of Drugs in Dermatology. 2018;**17**:982-986

[24] Philipp-Dormston WG, Wong C, Schuster B, Larsson MK, Podda M. Evaluating perceived naturalness of facial expression after fillers to the nasolabial folds and lower face with standardized video and photography. Dermatologic Surgery. 2018;**44**:826-832

[25] Solish N, Bertucci V, Percec I, Wagner T, Nogueira A, Mashburn J. Dynamics of hyaluronic acid fillers formulated to maintain natural facial expression. Journal of Cosmetic Dermatology. 2019;**18**:738-746

[26] Chow KV, Urman DS, Cabral ES, Shim EK, Bennett RG. Hyaluronic acid filler incidentally found during Mohs micrographic surgery: Observations in 36 patients regarding skin depth, degradation size, and estimated persistence time. Dermatologic Surgery. 2022;**48**(4):401-405. DOI: 10.1097/DSS.0000000000003380

[27] Bennett R, Taher M. Restylane persistent for 23 months found during Mohs micrographic surgery: A source of confusion with hyaluronic acid surrounding basal cell carcinoma. Dermatologic Surgery. 2005;**31**(10):1366-1369. DOI: 10.1111/j.1524-4725.2005.31223

Chapter 6

Temporomandibular Joint (TMJ) Dilemma: How to Resolve?

Hossam Barghash

Abstract

Temporomandibular joint (TMJ) dysfunction is one of the most debatable subjects in the field of oral maxillofacial surgery. Debating starts with identifying the problems up to the managing them. The cause for this debate is the confusion and unclear understanding of the dysfunction pathogenesis. Surgical intervention was one of the oldest methods for the management of such conditions, but nowadays, surgery is considered an invasive method with unsatisfactory results, which led to a shift to noninvasive methods. Literature provides different ways of explaining the problem with many different suggestions to manage it. In this chapter, the author explains the cause of confusion and how to solve it.

Keywords: TMJ dysfunction, orofacial pain, myofascial pain syndrome, chronic pain pathogenesis, masticatory system biomechanics

1. Introduction

One of the most debatable subjects in dentistry and in the field of oral and maxillofacial surgery is the management of temporomandibular dysfunction/disorders (TMD). This debate reflects the lack of knowledge regarding the pathology that shows the symptoms of pain and restriction of mouth opening and clicking, resulting in the dysfunction of masticatory system such as difficulty in masticating, swallowing, and speaking. The pathology of this disease in general includes the etiological factors and pathogenesis that lead to structural and functional deviations from normal with the resulting symptoms and signs that help the clinician to make a diagnosis. Another important point regarding the pathology of a disease is the prognosis that is essential in decision-making for management. Without this knowledge of disease pathology, the right diagnosis and hence the selection of the method of management would go wrong.

The first part of this chapter will explain the development of dilemma starting from its historical roots of misconceptions until now. The second part will deal with how to resolve the debate by filling in missing knowledge of pathology that will affect the selection of management methods.

2. The development of TMD dilemma

The history of trying to understand the cause of pain and clicking sound at the TMJ with many explanations and methods of treatments starts many years ago.

For better understanding the TMD dilemma, we can divide this period into:

i. TMD dilemma before the development of MRI.

ii. TMD dilemma after the development of MRI.

2.1 The TMD dilemma before the development of MRI

In 1837, Brodie Benjamine described in his book (Lectures Illustrative of Certain Local Nervous Affections) some cases of pain in different joints of the body have no apparent pathology, the common finding was that they are females, and the condition does not need medical treatment. He described it as hysteria, which meant at that time unhealthy emotions [1].

Surgical intervention began to be performed after the publication by Annandale T. 1887 [2]. The operation he did was based on the same principle for correction of displacement of semilunar cartilage of the knee joint. During the operation, he described how he used catgut suture to fix the interarticular cartilage disc to periosteum of the outer margin of the articulating bone. Although both knee joint and TMJ are synovial joints, their embryological development [3], histological structure of the disc [4], and biomechanics [5, 6] are different. These differences make the TMJ stand out from other joints in the body, and the way it can be affected by diseases is different. TMJ has a unique potential for adaptability, and it is the only joint with hard end point (teeth) during loading (the biting force).

In 1918, Pringle [7] described the attachment of lateral pterygoid muscle to the TMJ disc. And first to suppose the cause of disc displacement is due to hyperactivity of this muscle. He tried to reduce the disc into place using manual manipulation. He also described surgical removal of a loose interarticular disc, noticing that the joint bone surface was free from any abnormality seen in osteoarthritis. This observation was the first description of anterior disc dislocation without any osteoarthritic change in TMJ.

The first description to relate the symptoms of hearing affection and other ENT symptoms due to loss of vertical dimension of the face and occlusion was not Costen as always mentioned, but Monson 1928 [8]. He explained that bringing the mandible close to maxilla will impair the muscle function due to bringing the muscle insertion close to origin and cause backward movement of the condyle impinging on the external auditory meatus. Also, the inadequate space for the tongue will cause difficulty in swallowing and Eustachian tube function. In this chapter, he showed a method for determining the vertical dimension and condylar position by placing his finger in the ear and asking the patient to close his mouth until he first feels the condyle touching his finger after which the patient can stop closing. The severity of symptoms will be related to the degree of vertical loss.

Focusing on TMJ as the cause of dysfunction was obvious in a publication by David J. Goodfriend 1934 [9]. The problem was approached from the anatomical, radiological, psychological, and histopathological aspects. The psychological part consisted of speech and personality disturbance. He was the first to describe the relation of the mandibular condyle to the lower part of the posterior wall of the articular eminence.

Classification for articular problems was described as follows:

1. Mandubular subarthrosis: a degenerative condition of the joint disc and relaxation of articular ligaments associated with either limited or excessive movement of the joint.

2. Mandibular disarthrosis: characterized by chronic and recurrent joint disarticulation as a sequel of mandibular subarthrosis.

3. Mandibular luxation or dislocation: complete disarticulation of the joint.

4. Mandibular ankylosis: limitation of the movement of the mandibular articulation as a result of intra-articular causes.

5. Trismus: limitation of movement of mandibular articulation due to extra-articular causes.

Loss of vertical dimension was mentioned as an etiological factor, and symptoms result from pressure of condyle and articular disc against abnormal articular surface. The most recommended in this chapter is to adjust the occlusal problem by constructing temporary bite plan to release the stress on joint articulating surface.

From 1934 to 1939, Costen published many papers [10–13]. Costen was not the first to make a link between the TMJ and ENT symptoms, but what he did was he called it a syndrome [10], which carried his name Costen's syndrome. Headache, deafness, vertigo, and even sinus problems were all correlated to loss of vertical dimension, due to posterior teeth loss, that caused muscles and TMJ dysfunction. He also pointed out that this loss of vertical dimension will cause pressure on the chorda tympani and auriculotemporal nerves causing pain and affecting saliva production. His recommendation was to correct the vertical dimension, and replacement of the missing molar teeth will result in immediate relief of the symptoms. In 1939, he confirmed that the source of pain around the ear is the irregular movements of the condyle in TMJ with the x-ray confirmation of that (not mentioning what kind of radiological examination), but he stated that the deviation of TMJ from normal with associated symptoms is seen in cases where occlusion is totally normal [13].

In 1947, Block agreed totally with Costen that the loss of vertical dimension is the main cause of the TMJ dysfunction [14]. He asked all the dentists to be aware of TMJ problems as the diagnosis and treatment of such cases are within the limits of the dental specialists and not with ENT doctors. The problem is that the patient goes first to an ENT specialist and even from one dentist to the other, which is due to lack of knowledge about TMJ. He divided the anatomical variations that cause pain into:

1. Loss of vertical dimension due to molar loss or teeth wear led to overclosure and pressure on the auriculotemporal nerve.

2. The backward pressure of the mandibular condyle overeroded the tympanic bone exposing the chorda tympani nerve.

3. Deep erosion of glenoid cavity with exposure of dura, with impact effect of jaw closure on the dura, which is full of sensory innervation.

He introduced the concept of trial dental occlusal appliance to raise the vertical dimension, and if the patient symptoms improved, then permeant restoration was done.

In 1948, Sicher [15] denied the anatomic explanation of pain provided by Block. With his experience in anatomy, Sicher described the auriculotemporal nerve position and the relation of the condyle to glenoid fossa excluding the pressure on nerves as a cause for pain. He described the pain in the ear as referred one, and joint symptoms are caused by arthritis, which is mostly due to trauma. He also mentioned that the deficiency in tympanic plate is a genetic defect, and the thinnest and deepest portion of the glenoid fossa is protected from pressure by the protracting action of external pterygoid muscle during the forced closure.

Ireland in 1951 excluded that the auditory symptoms are due to TMJ problem, and he focused on the clicking jaw problem [16]. He grouped the patients according to the presenting symptoms, which are as follows:

1. Painless clicking during opening
2. Intermittent locking with limitation of mouth opening to finger breadth and accompanied by pain
3. Limitation of opening with pain with history of the previous symptoms
4. Limitation of the mouth opening without history of previous symptoms
5. Clicking at the end of opening and the beginning of closure

Most of the cases, he said, have deep bite. So instead of talking about vertical dimension, the horizontal relation is accused as a cause of joint problem mainly clicking because of backward displacement of the condyle due to either genetic cause or loss of posterior molar stopper that allows mandibular overclosure. Management was described according to presented symptoms, so if the patient is seen immediately after painful locking, the Pringle method for reduction is used [7].

Ireland noticed that when he asked the patients not totally close their mouth, the clicking disappeared. For that reason, he described a bite plane splint that prevented the mandibular closure more than the rest position of the mandible. Description of the construction of such splint is also parented [16]. Surgical interventions are used for advanced cases with the advocation of injection of sclerosing agents to limit the forward sliding of the mandibular condyle.

In 1952, Travell and Rinzler published a unique paper under the title the myofascial genesis of pain [17]. Although this paper did not focus on TMJ dysfunction, by collecting the data from over 1000 patients suffering from chronic pain related to musculoskeletal structure, they came up with the concept of trigger area. Pain is set whenever this trigger area is stimulated by different stimulus like heat extremes, pressure, or motion that stretches the structure containing trigger area. Whenever this area is stimulated, it will cause pain with constant pattern between different individuals, which is traced also for head and neck muscles like masseter, temporalis, and sternocleidomastoid muscles. One crucial point to know is that trigger point will cause the affected muscle to resist stretching, which will shorten the muscle and decrease the range of motion. The initiating factors are claimed to be trauma, muscle strain, myositis, and arthritis. The pain cycle will continue even after the removal of the initiating factors, and to terminate, blocking this point through injection of local anesthetic agents is required.

Directing the attention to the muscles as a source of pain in temporomandibular dysfunction was noticed after the explanation of myofascial pain mechanism. In his publication, Laszlo Schwartz claimed that the main reason for pain in temporomandibular dysfunction is due to muscular causes, and parafunctional habits, as well as malocclusion, were mentioned as a contributing factor [18]. The temporomandibular joint pain dysfunction syndrome was divided into three phases:

1. The incoordination phase, incoordination of mandibular muscles

2. The pain-limitation phase, painful spasm of the masticatory muscles

3. The limitation phase, contracture of the masticatory muscles with painless limitation of mandibular movement

Considering the muscles as the main contributing factor for temporomandibular pain dysfunction, therapeutic exercises for masticatory and neck muscles were the recommended method of treatment.

Dolowitz et al. [19] confirmed the role of muscular incoordination in the pathogenesis of temporomandibular joint syndrome, especially the lateral pterygoid muscle spasm and bruxism in the development of such a dysfunction. The spasm of lateral pterygoid muscles was blamed to prevent the translation movement of the condyle with resultant limitation of mouth opening to the limit of hinge movement. The treatment policy was mainly muscle stretching exercises that should be tailored according to every individual. No recommendation for dental treatment or alteration for bite was advised in the mentioned cases even though some of them were suffering from mild bite deformity.

Laskin [20] proposed the name "myofascial pain dysfunction (MPD) syndrome" for the muscle spasm as the main etiological factor responsible for symptoms and signs of mandibular joint dysfunction. The change in occlusion was explained secondary to muscle spasm. If the abnormal jaw closing movement persists, this will lead to shift in teeth position and changes in occlusion. According to this theory, he explained why some patients complain of occlusal disharmony even after the muscle spasm problem is resolved. The muscle spasm problem is usually associated with psychological disturbance; for that reason, the pathogenesis theory for MPD is known as the psychophysiologic theory. This theory claims that the emotional problem preceded the physiological one, and it must be first targeted in management of such cases.

So, the outcome of TMD dilemma before MRI is that psychophysiological theory is the main accepted theory behind the symptoms of TMD dysfunction with no clear evidence of the role of occlusion and dimensional changes mainly vertical and anteroposterior. The physiological changes tend toward muscular problems as the main factor of dysfunction that can lead to secondary joint problems and arthritis.

Management can be divided into:

a. Phycological management without clear explanation what is the role of emotional disturbance in the development of such dysfunction

b. Physiological management in the form of muscular exercises, muscle injection of local anesthetic into the trigger area, and appliances to adjust the vertical or horizontal maxillary-mandibular relation

2.2 The TMD dilemma after the development of MRI

The development of MRI is attributed to Lauterbur 1973 [21]. Many studies were made for studying the use of MRI in correlation to TMD [22–25]. Its use for imaging the TMJ leads to directing the explanation of TMD from muscular origin into joint-based problem. For that reason, MRI is used as a diverting point in the dilemma explanation. Instead of studying the relation of the disc to the mandibular condyle in cadaveric anatomical dissection, MRI makes it possible to in vivo study this relation in either normal non-symptomatic subjects or symptomatic TMD patients. One of the changing concepts for TMD as a disease and the way to manage it was proposed by Wilkes [26]. He claimed that the temporomandibular dysfunction symptoms and sign presentations are all due to internal derangement of TMJ, and all his cases share one organic lesion in the form of partial or complete disc anterior displacement, which means that the basic pathological changes for temporomandibular dysfunction are anterior disc displacement, although we know nowadays that there are cases with anterior disc displacement without any significant masticatory dysfunction or symptoms [27, 28]. The hypothesis Wilkes proposed, regard muscular problem is secondary to joint pathology, that the joint internal derangement will lead to secondary muscle spasm called muscle splinting with reduction of the range of motion in term of lateral and vertical opening. Mechanical obstruction due to anterior disc dislocation and with locking in case of anterior disc dislocation without reduction can also be a factor in reduction of mandibular opening. So, the pathogenesis he mentioned is totally based on organic lesion denying totally any psychological role.

Wilkes described the internal derangement of TMJ as a progressive disease with early, intermediate, and late stages [26]. Description of a disease as a progressive one warrants early interference to prevent progression or to manage in the late stage. For that reason, several surgical procedures were proposed as treatment for anterior disc displacement such as disc reposition [29, 30], eminectomy [31], condylotomy [32], arthroplasty with disc reposition [33], arthroplasty without disc reposition [34], and discectomy [35].

Disc displacement and internal derangement confirmed by MRI, plus adopting the hypothetical idea by Wilkes that internal derangement of TMJ is progressive disease which will end with joint degenerative problems and lead to bringing the surgical interference into the surface.

A management conflict between conservative methods which was dominant before MRI, and surgical interference (non-conservative) after MRI images and description of the TMD as prognostic disease.

3. Resolving the debate and dilemma of TMD

The dilemma regarding TMD is caused by confusion in different aspects, from terminology, definition, classification, symptoms pathogenesis, and management.

3.1 Confusion caused by terminology, definition, and classification

The term temporomandibular disorders (TMDs) is defined as an umbrella term involving a group of conditions affecting the masticatory muscles, TMJ/TMJs, and associated structures [36]. This definition means nothing than telling us there are several diseases that can affect the musculoskeletal system of mastication; there can be over 30 kinds of diseases mostly categorized under three main groups:

a. Disorders of the joints including disc disorders

b. Disorders of muscles

c. Headaches associated with TMD

This kind of classification does not clarify the dilemma of TMD, why? It is because there is no clear explanation for the relation between those kind of disorders and the main complaint of TMD patients. The main complaints of TMD patients are pain, limitation of the mouth opening, and clicking. In these complaints, pain is the main cause for the patient to seek treatment [37]. People with clicking without pain are not bothered by it. It is common in our practice to have patients of different ages that during examination we hear the clicking, when we ask those patients about this joint sound, the answer is "this has been for years," and they are not worried about it. They become worried when a doctor tells them that this may progress and destroy their joints. This doctor believes assumptions made by Wilkes who considered clicking as an early phase of a disease that can progress and end with degenerative and destructive changes of the TMJ [26]. The actual problem in such cases is when such a patient is exposed to invasive irreversible treatment such as surgery. Even grinding of the teeth is considered a less invasive procedure to adjust occlusion, but at the same time, it is an irreversible process. For that reason, it is better to classify the management procedure into reversible and irreversible.

Terminology regarding this subject we are dealing with is a reflection of the whole subject confusion. It is used to describe just we propose the name temporomandibular musculoskeletal pain dysfunction syndrome (TMPDS).

3.2 Confusion and dilemma of the etiology

Another dilemma is describing the etiology of TMD. If TMD is an umbrella term for different disorders, so it is logical there is no one cause for several nonspecific disorders, but if we consider the controversy of joint vs. muscle disorders, then occlusion comes into the scene.

The common debate is, does occlusion play a role as an etiological factor for joint and muscle problems?

To answer this question, we should clarify which problem of occlusion we are talking about. If we mean by occlusion, malocclusion like class 2 or class 3 occlusion, then the answer is no. Malocclusion should not be considered as an etiological factor for the development of TMD. The final teeth occluding position is molding process by the orofacial musculature, and it occurs gradually as a result of orchestration between joint, teeth, and muscles. This explains why there are many people with malocclusion who never suffer from TMD and vise verse where there are people with normal occlusion with TMD, so malocclusion is not a main contributing factor in the development of TMD. What we should consider is a change in occlusion. Many factors are playing a role in adaptive capability of the individual including the nervous system and mechanoreceptors in the periodontium, mucosa, and dentition. The degree and location of change are other factors. Changes in lateral guidance (canine or group lateral guidance) have more profound effect than changes in single tooth. High spot restoration will give a warning in the form of hyperemic tooth thermal sensitivity and pain in the periodontium. These symptoms of traumatic occlusion are acute and usually corrected as the etiology is obvious. When the patient tries to avoid a traumatic occluding tooth/teeth or voluntarily puts his teeth in abnormal occlusion (this is seen in patients in class 2 occlusion due to small mandible, and they try to bring the mandible in forward position to camouflage the small chin appearance), the result is strain on muscles and joint ligaments with resultant chronic pain.

The next common debate is bruxism as an etiological factor for TMD. Bruxism is a big issue to be covered here. One of the big mistakes is to discuss bruxism, parafunctional habits, and clenching together as an etiological factor for TMD. Sleep bruxism (SB) can happen at different ages from childhood to adulthood, and the mechanism under it is different accordingly. SB functions as autonomic motor reflex in response to nocturnal arousal [38], this reflex is associated obstruction of the airway [39], and in children, the most common cause for airway obstruction is adenotonsillar hypertrophy [40]. On the other hand, SB in adults could be a protective reflex known as trigeminal cardiac reflex, a reflex that lowers the heart rate and blood pressure during the microarousal stage of sleep that is accompanied by tachycardia and elevation of blood pressure [41]. SB cannot be a main etiological factor for TMD, as it only happens for few seconds during the arousal stage. SB for many years can result in early morning mild restriction of mouth opening, which then becomes normal the rest of the day. The use of the night guard will not stop bruxism, but it will help to protect the teeth attrition from teeth grinding.

On the other hand, awake clenching and parafunctional habits can lead to overuse of the muscles and joints. Parafunctional habits also are considered as an overuse of the masticatory muscles, but it is more a reflection of psychological stress [42, 43], which is considered as an essential part of the pathogenesis of chronic pain as it will be discussed in this chapter. Clenching on the other hand causes an increase in muscle strain and that will leave the muscle open to development of trigger points.

So clenching is considered a main factor in the development of myofascial pain, but does it increase the stress of loading on the TMJ internal structure? To answer this question, we study the mechanical load distribution on the joint. Due to technical limitation for direct measurements of load applied on the TMJ in vivo, experimental model is used instead [44, 45]. The mandible is described during biting as class III lever (**Figures 1** and **2**), where the condyle acts as a fulcrum, the masticatory muscles act as applied force, and the bite pressure acts as the resistance, but this is wrong because this model considered the teeth and the bones of the jaw as one unit, which is not true. There is another joint between the teeth and jawbone. In this case, the biting process will be described as class I lever, where the periodontal ligaments (PL) act as abfulcrum, the masticatory muscles act as applied force, and the bite pressure acts as resistance (**Figures 3** and **4**). Opening the mandible will be class III where the condyle acts as a fulcrum, the muscle tension as the force, and the gravitational weight of the mandible acts as resistance (**Figures 5** and **6**). This is the case also during mandibular resting position. The mechanoreceptors in the PL modulate the muscle forces applied by the teeth. In all the cases, the TMJ is protected from stresses and joint arthritis due to overload as the one that occurs in the knee joint is not expected to occur.

3.3 Confusion and dilemma of TMD symptoms

The three main symptoms of TMD are pain, limitation of mouth opening, and clicking of all of them. Pain is the most driving symptom that forces the patient to seek medical attention [37].

Clicking sound results when the anterior displaced disc overrides the condylar mandibular head during either opening or closing movement. Early clicking during

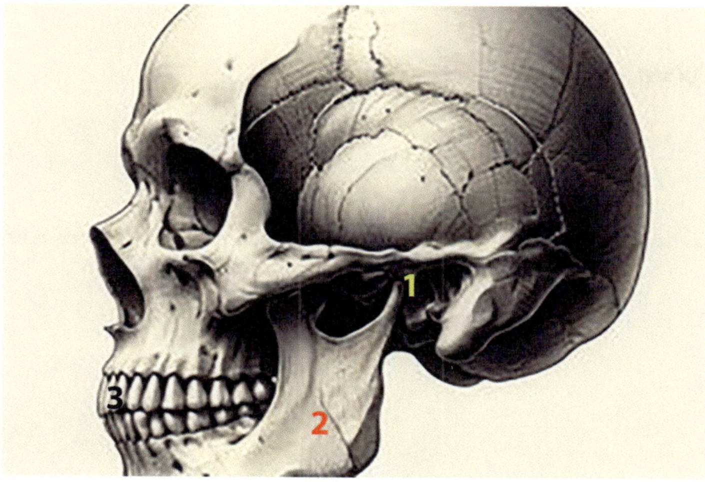

Figure 1.
Mandible as class III lever during biting. 1-Fulcrum (mandibular condyle). 2-Muscle force. 3-Resistance (bite pressure).

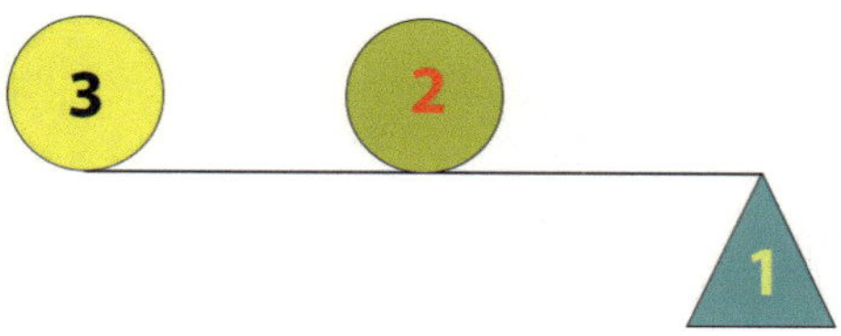

Figure 2.
Mandible as class III lever during biting. 1-Fulcrum (mandibular condyle). 2-Muscle force. 3-Resistance (bite pressure).

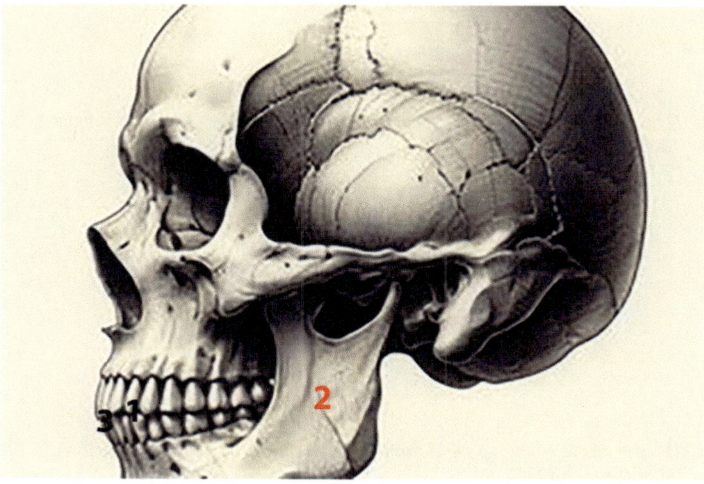

Figure 3.
Mandible as class I lever during biting. 1-Fulcurum (periodontal ligaments). 2-Muscle force. 3- Resistance (bite pressure).

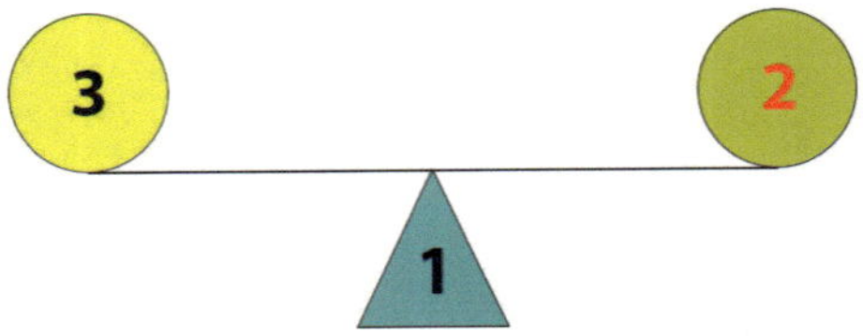

Figure 4.
Mandible as class I lever during biting. 1-Fulcurum (periodontal ligaments). 2-Muscle force. 3- Resistance (bite pressure).

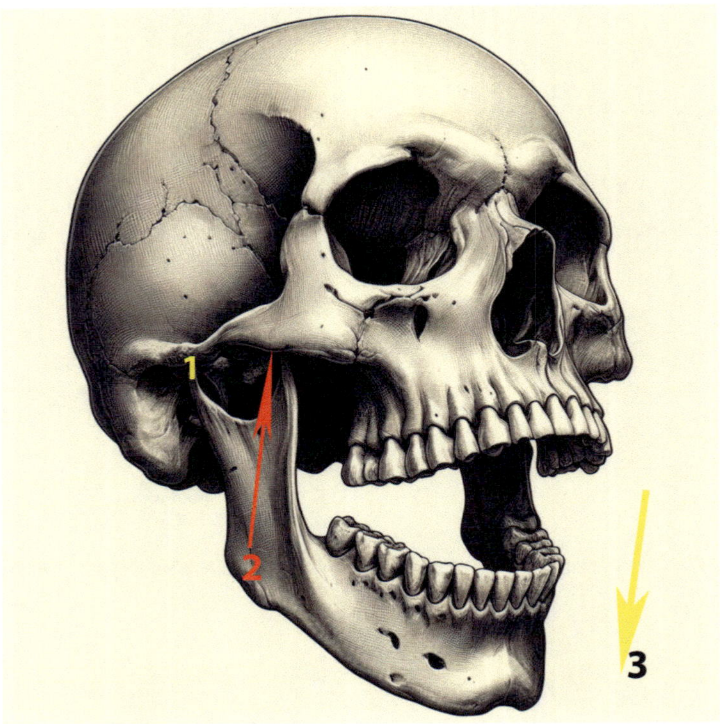

Figure 5.
Mandible as class III lever during opening. 1-Fulcrum (mandibular condyle). 2-Muscle force. 3-Resistance (gravitational weight of the mandible).

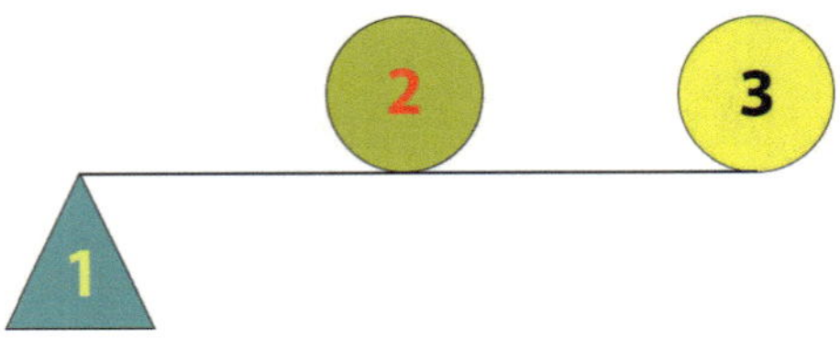

Figure 6.
Mandible as class III lever during opening. 1-Fulcrum (mandibular condyle). 2-Muscle force. 3-Resistance (gravitational weight of the mandible).

opening and late during mouth closing are indications for minimal disc displacement. Clicking sound is an indication of anterior disc displacement. In the case of anterior disc without reduction, the disc keeps its advanced anterior position where it became stuck between the mandibular condyle and the tubercle eminence of zygomatic arch. There are many hypotheses that explain the reason for anterior disc dislocation, for example, hyperactivity of the upper head on lateral pterygoid muscle or stretch of retrodiscal tissue. Talking about the retrodiscal tissue without its components individually is a big mistake or consider the elastic band with vascular and neural tissue representing the retrodiscal tissue. The posterior ligament of the disc that is attaching the disc to the posterior surface of the mandible should be a partpof the ligament that stabilizes the disc over the mandibular condyle. In fact, this is the main ligament when elongated allows the occurrence of anterior disc displacement after mouth being closed, and represents the excess tissue that should be removed during disc reposition surgical procedure. Ligaments in general are tough tissue and non-elastic tissue that cannot be stretched but can be elongated under chronic tensile stress, trauma, or a disease of the collagen tissue.

Pain due to anterior disc displacement was a result of the retrodiscal tissue replacing the disc position and becoming compressed by the condyle producing pain and then due to chronic friction against the tissue. This will become fibrotic and function as a pseudodisc. What against this hypothesis are the followings:

- Not every case of anterior disc displacement is accompanied by pain.
- Pain produced due to nerve friction and compression is a severe neuropathic pain. This is not the kind of pain chronic TMD patients suffer from.
- Ligaments under chronic friction become thickened, so pseudodisc can be explained on the basis of thickening of the posterior disc ligament that takes the place ofbanterior disc displacement.

Can anterior disc displacement result in reduction of the mouth opening?

In fact, patients with anterior disc displacement with reduction continue to open their mouth after clicking. Patients with anterior disc dislocation without reduction have reduced amount of mouth opening when they try to open their mouth to the maximum but not to the degree to stop them from doing functions like chewing, which does not require maximum opening.

Pain is considered a limiting factor for fall range of motion; the patient usually stops opening the mouth further once pain is felt. For that reason, understanding the pathogenesis of pain and the underlying mechanism is essential for better management of TMD. The following section is devoted to pain.

4. Pain, better understanding for better management

Understanding pain has been one of the evolved subjects in the long history of medicine. The last decade witnessed new concepts of pain, especially chronic pain that is considered one of the most disabling factors for patients in general and for TMD cases in specific.

4.1 Pain definition

Defining pain—which is a subjective symptom—was not an easy target in a time that seemed to be impossible, with conflict between psychological and physiological explanation [46]. The obvious relation between a stimulus that causes nerve stimulation with subsequent sensation of pain made it to be classified as a sensation described in terms of receptors and pathways. On the other hand, no one can deny the relation of pain and emotional state.

In 1979, The International Association of Study of Pain (IASP) published the following definition of pain [47].

"An unpleased sensory and emotional experience associated with actual or potential tissue damage, or described in term of such condition".

Wall P.D. raised a question about the nature of pain and considered the description of pain in the definition to be psychologically associated with tissue damage, which is physiological, so what is the relation between psychology and physiology? Describing pain in relation to a stimulus of tissue damage receptors (nociceptive receptors) should then have a threshold and measurable intensity.

The story of the boot nail guy [48]. The story tells us about a worker who presented to the hospital with a long nail penetrating his boot, the worker was in severe pain that the doctor had to sedate him with fentanyl and midazolam in order to be able to take his boot off, and the surprise was that the nail passed between his toes without causing actual tissue damage. This raises the assumption that pain can be based on perception and be exaggerated by the mind.

Melzak attempted to explain the phenomena of phantom pain by formulating a concept called neuromatrix [49]. The neuromatrix is a network of neurons, which is genetically determined and modified by sensory experiences. According to this, pain is considered as an output of the neuromatrix of the brain to the virtual map of the body represented on the body surface known as homunculus (**Figure 4**). The brain will fire this signal whenever it receives a danger message in case of tissue damage or even by emotional stress as in the case of chronic pain [50].

The neuromatrix concept explains many different phenomena regarding pain, such as the absence of correlation between the degree of tissue damage and the degree of pain sensation. It also explains the mechanism of phantom pain and the mechanism by which stress and anxiety play a role in chronic pain (**Figure 7**).

So, we can define pain as unpleasant sensation output from the brain in response to actual or perceptual danger of tissue damage. As such, there are no pain receptors but should always be called nociceptive receptors, not pain receptors, and nociceptive pathway instead of pain pathway.

4.2 Acute vs. chronic pain

In acute pain, the tissue damage and cause are obvious. Stimulation of nociceptive receptors occurs due to release of inflammatory cytokines, and the action of anti-inflammatory drugs is to interfere with production of this cytokines [51]. Dentists and maxillofacial surgeons will train for diagnosing and managing acute pain.

Chronic pain is a totally different story, and it is refractory for treatment if it is managed the same way as acute one. In chronic pain, there is no presence of acute inflammatory cytokines, which explains why the use of such drugs has no/or minimal effect.

The etiology, which triggers the cascade of central sensitization and activation of the neuromatrix, is not easy to find in chronic pain. It is all a suggestion proposed by the doctor or by the patient himself.

Chronic pain and depression have been always linked together with reciprocal effect that chronic pain induces depression and depression causes chronic pain [52].

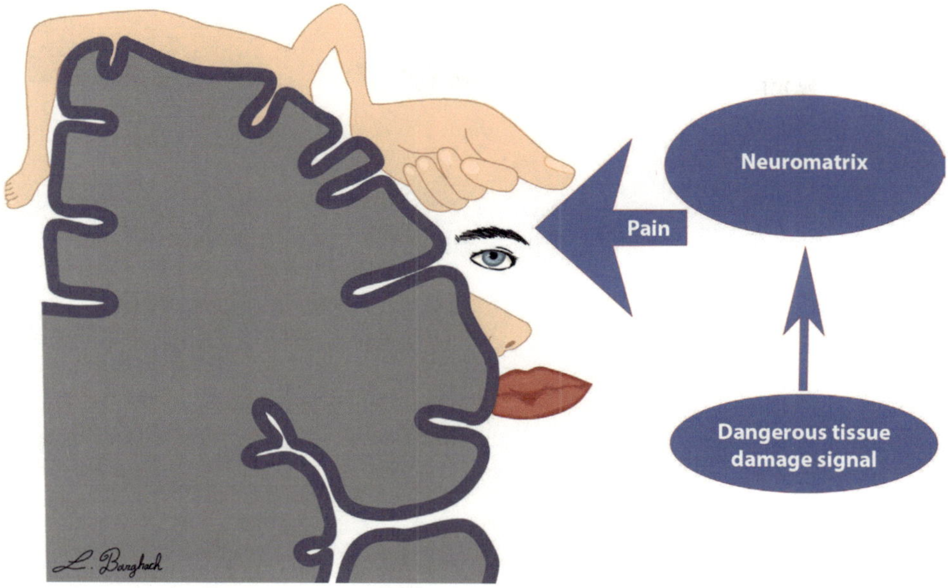

Figure 7.
Neuromatrix concept and mechanism of pain.

So chronic pain is a result of interacting factors that include the following:

- Genetics, which affect the neurons' wiring of the neuromatrix of the brain
- Experience, which will modulate the neurons' connections in the neuromatrix
- Emotional state and sleep quality, a reciprocal relation with chronic pain
- The organic problem as an initiating factor for chronic pain

All these factor together are described as the biopsychosocial model (**Figure 8**).

Genetics, psychological, and social factors are considered as predisposing factors, pathology is considered as the initiator, while psychological and social factors are considered as sustaining factors.

4.3 Reffered pain explained by neuromatrix concept

Referral pain is considered one of the causes of misdiagnosis of pain. Understanding the mechanism of it using the neuromatrix concept could explain the confusion of site vs. source of pain. When we consider pain as an alarming output from the brain, then why does the brain send this alarm to different areas rather than to the area where danger signal is sent?

At this point, we must differentiate between acute and chronic pain. In acute tissue damage, pain must be directed to the area where damage happened, and this is mostly the case, unless there is a missing information about the location of damaged area; example of this is acute pulpitis where nociceptive receptors send signal for tissue damage but the lack of proprioception localization receptors result in pain signal to the teeth sharing the pathway from where danger is coming.

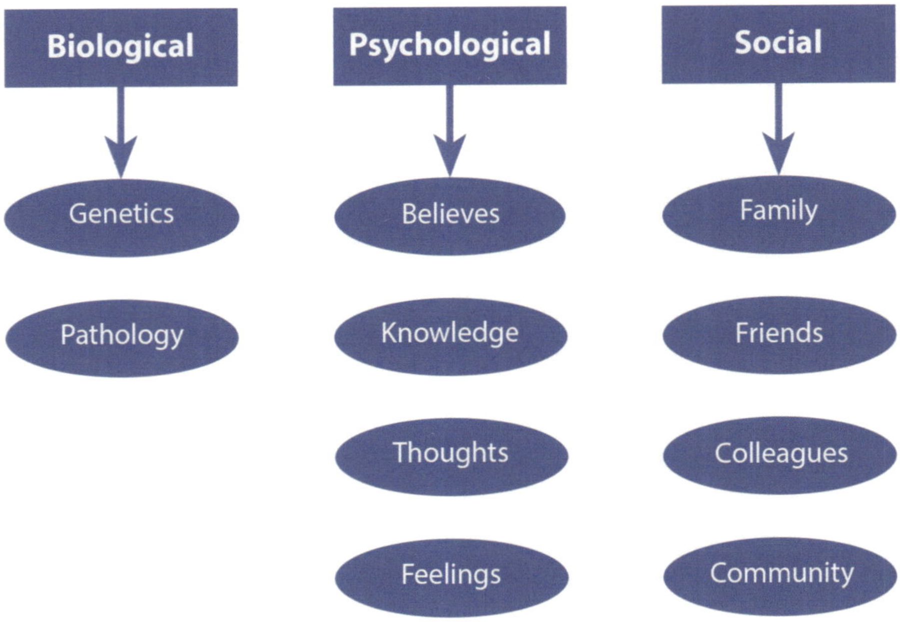

Figure 8.
Biopsychosocial model for TMD chronic pain.

In case of chronic pain, the sustained alarming pain is generated mainly centrally where the brain chose the areas suspected to be the cause of danger according to wired neural network determined by genetics and old experience, which is why there is specific pattern of chronic pain as we noticed in case of pressure on trigger points area or the fluctuating pattern of pain from one area to another. The reflex muscular spasm seen at different muscles can be then a vicious cycle where chronic pain causes impaired unbalanced movement of the jaw and the impaired movement of the jaw causes more strain on muscle with sustained pain, adding to this the emotional effect, making the diagnosis difficult.

5. The confusion and dilemma of TMD management

There are several supposed methods for management of TMD. This includes different surgical procedures, considered as invasive irreversible non-conservative methods. Other methods like occlusal splints, occlusal adjustment, physiotherapy, psychological treatment, and injections (joints or muscles) are considered conservative. Tooth grinding and some types of occlusal splint are also considered non-invasive methods, but they are irreversible. For all these methods, whether conservative or non-conservative, there is no clear indication for when, what, and why it is used. The recommended policy is to try conservative method first for about 6 months; if no improvement, then the last resort is surgical interference. On what basis the 6 months was chosen? What if the surgical interference does not also improve the condition? The lack of rational guidelines for TMD leads to every doctor choosing the method of treatment according to his own beliefs or specialty.

One of the causes of this dilemma is to categorize acute and chronic disorders under one term, TMD. As mentioned before, pain is the most derivative factor for a patient to seek medical treatment [37]. Categorizing acute and chronic pain in the same group is the reason for this confusion and unreliable results. Another cause of the dilemma and confusion is to specify the source of pain, is it joint, muscles, or both.

Acute pain cases, whether it is muscular or joint, are straightforward cases to manage as the cause and effect are clear.

In chronic pain cases, there are no obvious etiological factors, and all explanations of pain are based on assumption. Brain activity is considered the main factor for chronic pain in the absence of tissue damage [53]. In chronic pain, the wired area of the brain becomes sensitized (central sensitization) [54]. Brain reprogramming should be the main step of treatment in any case of chronic pain, including TMD patients. People with chronic pain are trapped in their thoughts worrying about the future; they think how they will go on with this kind of dysfunction, unable to chew, unable to speak, and even unable to do simple tasks like yawing. They use their mouth expecting pain and more tension in the muscles. The subsequent result is a decrease of the mouth opening. The problem of negative thoughts with their reflection on body function is more than a mental process, but about a wired neuron network in the brain generating these thoughts and pain. So, the question is how to stop this neural network from firing?

This process can be done in different ways. Mirror therapy has been used for chronic and phantom pain conditions [55, 56]. Another method is known as pain reprocessing therapy [57]. We applied those principles by using the mirror and engaging active patient brain feedback during mouth opening with gradual stretching of the contracture muscles mainly masseter, medial pterygoids, and temporalis. It is

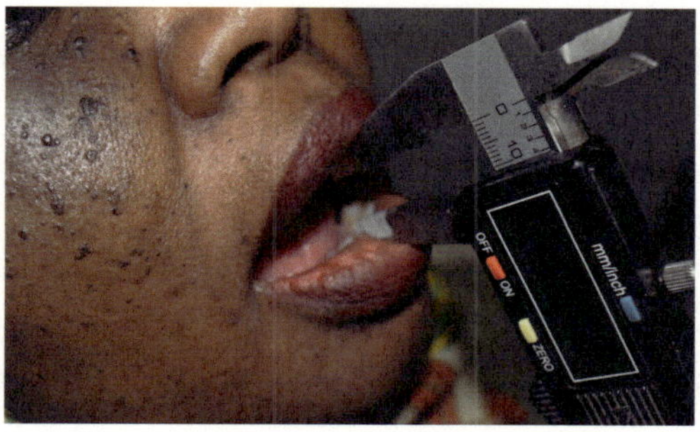

Figure 9.
Before brain reprogramming exercises.

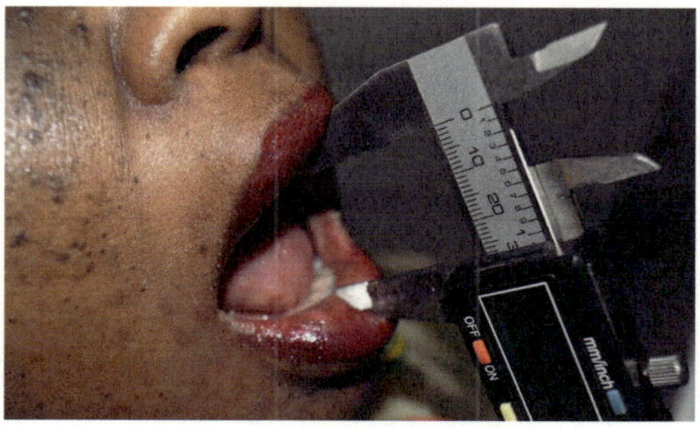

Figure 10.
Two weeks after brain reprogramming exercises.

amazing how this improves patient's pain and the range of mouth that could happen in short period of time, as in this case, a female patient who represented to us suffering from progressive painful mouth limitation since 2 years, with early clicking during mouth opening (**Figure 9**). After 2 weeks of brain reprogramming exercises, the pain and mouth opening improved (**Figure 10**). This method of brain reprogramming exercise is continued by the patient at home after being sure that the patient has understood how to perform it exactly.

6. Protocol for managing TMD patients

After careful history and clinical examination of the patient ensuring no organic pathological conditions or sleep breathing disorders, the following protocol is applied:

a. Patient education, regarding the difference between acute and chronic pain, the role of the brain in chronic pain and brain sensitization, and how abnormal mandibular movements, habits, or body posture play a role in precipitating and aggravating the condition.

b. Training the patient on how to use the mirror for brain reprogramming exercise and follow-up after 2 weeks. Most of the patients, who follow the rules, show improvement.

c. Patient referred to physiotherapy in cases needs assistant exercise or involvement of other body muscles like neck, shoulder, or gross postural adjustment.

d. Patient with advanced degree of depression refers to psychotherapy in addition to brain deprogramming program.

e. Stabilizing appliance therapy is used only in cases of unstable mandibular resting position or occlusion.

- Botox injection is used if there is hypertrophy of masticatory muscles, especially masseter muscle.
- Surgical interference is only applied in the form of TMJ replacement where severe osteoarthritic degenerative changes occur. Most of these cases have undergone disc removal operation in the past.

The duration of treatment for brain deprogramming process depends on many factors like how long the period of suffering was, patient cooperation, and patient psychological condition.

7. Conclusion

Temporomandibular dysfunction is considered a global problem, and chronic pain is a major contributing factor to this disability. For many centuries, etiological factors, pathogenesis, and methods of treatment of TMD have been considered as debatable subjects. Several methods have been applied for treatment, but still no clear indications or rational base for using it. The reason for this dilemma is the missing information and lack of doctors' knowledge, who manage those cases, about the pathogenesis of chronic pain and the role of central mechanism in such conditions. The continuous progress in understanding chronic pain pathogenesis, methods of management, and how it is different from acute pain will improve our management of TMD patients and help to resolve this dilemma.

Acknowledgements

I need to acknowledge the role of my father and my mother in teaching me the value of science. I would like to thank all my colleagues and friends for their support. I would like to extend my thanks to my whole family, especially to my wife Reem Hamadein and my daughter Laila Barghash for helping with drawing and designing this chapter.

Author details

Hossam Barghash
Department of Oral Maxillofacial Surgery, Badran Hospital, Nahda University, Cairo, Egypt

*Address all correspondence to: dr_hossam@gmx.de

References

[1] Benjamin B. Lectures Illustrative of Certain Nervous Local Affections. London: Longman; 1837. pp. 34-37

[2] Annandale T. On displacement of the inter-articular cartilage of the lower jaw, and its treatment by operation. Lancet. 1887;**3313**:411. DOI: 10.1016/S0140-6736(02)28282-3

[3] Lei X, Wang X, Li Y, Liu H, Yan G. Comparison of knee joint and temporomandibular joint development in pig embryos. Animal Biotechnology. 2024;**35**(1):2337760. DOI: 10.1080/10495398.2024.2337760

[4] Wang L et al. Hyaline cartilage cells outperform mandibular condylar cartilage cells in TMJ fibrocartilage tissue engineering application. Osteoarthritis and Cartilage. 2009;**17**(3):346-353. DOI: 10.1016/j.joca.2008.07.004

[5] Singh M et al. Biomechanical properties of the mandibular condylar cartilage and their relevance to the TMJ disc. Journal of Biomechanics. 2009;**42**(4):405-417. DOI: 10.1016/j.jbiomech.2008.12.012

[6] Won KK et al. Biomechanical tissue characterization of the superior joint space of the porcine temporomandibular joint. Annals of Biomedical Engineering. 2003;**31**(8):924-930. DOI: 10.1114/1.1591190

[7] Pringle J. Displacement of the mandibular meniscus and its treatment. British Journal of Surgery. 1918;**23**:385-389. DOI: 10.1002/bjs.1800062307

[8] Monson GS. Impaired function as a result of closed bite. Journal of the American Dental Association. 1921;**October**:833-839. DOI: 10.14219/JADA.ARCHIVE.1921.0186

[9] Goodfriend DJ. Abnormalities of the mandibular articulation. The Journal of the American Dental Association. 1934;**21**(2):204-218. DOI: 10.14219/jada.archive.1934.0035

[10] Costen JB. A syndrome of ear and sinus symptoms dependent upon disturbed function of the temporomandibular joint. The Annals of Otology, Rhinology, and Laryngology. 1934;**106**:805-819. DOI: 10.1177/000348949710601002

[11] Costen JB. Neuralgia and ear symptoms: Associated with disturbed function of the temporomandibular joint. JAMA. 1936;**107**:252-255. DOI: 10.1001/JAMA.1936.02770300006002

[12] Costen JB. Some features of the mandibular articulation as it pertains to medical diagnosis, especially in otolaryngology. The Journal of the American Dental Association. 1937;**24**(9):1507-1511. DOI: 10.14219/jada.archive.1937.0275

[13] Costen JB. Correlation of X-ray findings in the mandibular joint with clinical signs, especially trismus. The Journal of the American Dental Association. 1939;**26**(3):405-407. DOI: 10.14219/jada.archive.1939.0025

[14] Block LS. Diagnosis and treatment of disturbances of the temporomandibular joint especially in relation to vertical dimension. Journal of the American Dental Association (Chicago, IL). 1947;**34**(4):253-260. DOI: 10.14219/jada.archive.1947.0067

[15] Sicher H. Temporomandibular articulation in mandibular overclosure. Journal of the American Dental Association (Chicago, IL).

1948;**36**(2):131-139. DOI: 10.14219/jada.archive.1948.0021

[16] Ireland VE. The problem of "the clicking jaw". Journal of the Royal Society of Medicine. 1951;**44**(5):363-374. DOI: 10.1177/003591575104400507

[17] Travell J, Rinzler SH. The myofascial genesis of pain. Postgraduate Medicine. 1952;**11**(5):425-434. DOI: 10.1080/00325481.1952.11694280

[18] Laszlo Schwartz L. Pain associated with the temporomandibular joint. Journal of the American Dental Association (Chicago, IL). 1955;**51**(4):394-397. DOI: 10.14219/jada.archive.1955.0223

[19] Dolowitz DA et al. The role of muscular incoordination in the pathogenesis of the temporomandibular joint syndrome. The Laryngoscope. 1964;**74**:790-801. DOI: 10.1288/00005537-196406000-00003

[20] Laskin DM. Etiology of the pain-dysfunction syndrome. Journal of the American Dental Association (Chicago, IL). 1969;**79**(1):147-153. DOI: 10.14219/jada.archive.1969.0234

[21] Dreizen P. The nobel prize for MRI: A wonderful discovery and a sad controversy. Lancet. 2004;**363**(9402):78. DOI: 10.1016/S0140-6736(03)15182-3

[22] Emshoff R. Validity of clinical diagnostic criteria for temporomandibular disorders: Clinical versus magnetic resonance imaging diagnosis of temporomandibular joint internal derangement and osteoarthrosis. Oral Surgery oral Medicine, Oral Pathology, Oral Radiology and Endodontics. 2001;**91**(1):50-55. DOI: 10.1067/moe.2001.111129

[23] Emshoff R. Relationship between temporomandibular joint pain and magnetic resonance imaging findings of internal derangement. International Journal of Oral and Maxillofacial Surgery. 2001;**30**(12):118-122. DOI: 10.1054/ijom.2000.0028

[24] Rudish A. Magnetic resonance imaging findings of internal derangement and effusion in patients with unilateral temporomandibular joint pain. Oral Surgery, Oral Medicine, Oral Pathology, Oral Radiology and Endodontics. 2001;**92**(5):566-571. DOI: 10.1067/moe.2001.116817

[25] Barclay P. Comparison of clinical and magnetic resonance imaging diagnosis in patients with disk displacement in the temporomandibular joint. Oral Surgery, Oral Medicine, Oral Pathology, Oral Radiology and Endodontics. 1999;**88**(1):37-42. DOI: 10.1016/s1079-2104(99)70191-5

[26] Wilkes CH. Internal derangements of the temporomandibular joint, pathological variations. Archives of Otolaryngology Head and Neck Surgery. 1989;**115**(4):469-477. DOI: 10.1001/archotol.1989.01860280067019

[27] Katzberg RW et al. Anatomic disorders of the temporomandibular joint disc in asymptomatic subjects. Journal of Oral Maxillofacial Surgery. 1996;**54**(20):147-153. DOI: 10.1016/s0278-2391(96)90435-8

[28] Kircos LT et al. Magnetic resonance imaging of the TMJ disc in asymptomatic volunteers. Journal of Oral and Maxillofacial Surgery. 1987;**45**(10):852-854. DOI: 10.1016/0278-2391(87)90235-7

[29] Mehra P, Wolford LM. Use of the Mitek anchor in temporomandibular joint disc-repositioning surgery. Proceedings (Baylor University,

Medical Center). 2001;**14**:22-26. DOI: 10.1080/08998280.2001.11927726

[30] Goncalves JR, Cassano DS, Wolford LM, et al. Postsurgical stability of counterclockwise maxillomandibular advancement surgery: Affect of articular disc repositioning. Journal of Oral and Maxillofacial Surgery. 2008;**66**:724-738. DOI: 10.1016/j.joms.2007.11.007

[31] Chakraborty SK. Eminectomy for the management of closed lock of temporomandibular joint. Medical Journal, Armed Forces India. 2011;**63**(4):384-385. DOI: 10.1016/S0377-1237(07)80031-1

[32] Hall HD, Nickerson JW Jr, McKenna SJ. Modified condylotomy for treatment of the painful temporomandibular joint with a reducing disc. Journal of Oral and Maxillofacial Surgery. 1993;**51**:133-142. DOI: 10.1016/s0278-2391(10)80009-6

[33] McCarty WL, Farrar WB. Surgery for internal derangements of the temporomandibular joint. The Journal of Prosthetic Dentistry. 1979;**42**:191-196. DOI: 10.1016/0022-3913(79)90174-4

[34] Poswillo D. Experimental investigation of the effects of intra-articular hydrocortisone and high condylectomy on the mandibular condyle. Oral Surgery, Oral Medicine, and Oral Pathology. 1970;**30**:161-173. DOI: 10.1016/0030-4220(70)90355-5

[35] Ângelo DF et al. Unilateral temporomandibular joint discectomy without interposal material in patients with disc perforation or fragmentation: A prospective study. Journal of Oral Maxillofacial Surgery, Medicine and Pathology. 2022;**34**(4):375-380. DOI: 10.1016/j.ajoms.2021.12.005

[36] Schiffman E, Ohrbach R, Truelove E, et al. Diagnostic criteria for temporomandibular disorders (DC/TMD) for clinical and research applications: Recommendations of the international RDC/TMD consortium network* and orofacial pain special interest group, international association for the study of pain. Journal of Oral & Facial Pain and Headache. 2014;**28**(1): 6-27. DOI: 10.11607/jop.1151

[37] Dworkin SF, LeResche L. Research diagnostic criteria for temporomandibular disorders: Review, criteria, examinations and specifications, critique. Journal of Craniomandibular Disorders. 1992;**6**:301-355

[38] Sjoholm TT, Lowe AA, Miyamoto K, Fleetham JA, Ryan CF. Sleep bruxism in patients with sleep-disordered breathing. Archives of Oral Biology. 2002;**45**(10):889-896. DOI: 10.1016/s0003-9969(00)00044-3

[39] Oksenberg A, Arons E. Sleep bruxism related to obstructive sleep apnea: The effect of continuous positive airway pressure. Sleep Medicine. 2002;**3**(6):513-515. DOI: 10.1016/s1389-9457(02)00130-2

[40] Greenfeld M, Tauman R, DeRowe A, Sivan Y. Obstructive sleep apnea syndrome due to adenotonsillar hypertrophy in infants. International Journal of Pediatric Otorhinolaryngology. 2003;**67**(10):1055-1060. DOI: 10.1016/s0165-5876(03)00182-4

[41] Schames SE, Schames J, Schames M, Chagall-Gungur SS. Sleep bruxism, an autonomic self-regulating response by triggering the trigeminal cardiac reflex. Journal of the California Dental Association. 2012;**40**:670-671. DOI: 10.1080/19424396.2012.12220941

[42] Van Selms MK, Lobbezoo F, Visscher CM, et al. Myofascial temporomandibular disorder

pain, parafunctions and psychological stress. Journal of Oral Rehabilitation. 2008;**35**(1):45-52. DOI: 10.1111/j.1365-2842.2007.01795.x

[43] Glaros AG, Williams K, Lausten L. The role of parafunctions, emotions and stress in predicting facial pain. Journal of the American Dental Association (1939). 2005;**136**(4):451-458. DOI: 10.14219/jada.archive.2005.0200

[44] Koolstra JH, van Eijden TM. The jaw open-close movements predicted by biomechanical modelling. Journal of Biomechanics. 1997;**30**:943-950. DOI: 10.1016/S0021-9290(97)00058-4

[45] Langenbach GE, Hannam AG. The role of passive muscle tensions in a three-dimensional dynamic model of the human jaw. Archives of Oral Biology. 1999;**44**:557-573. DOI: 10.1016/s0003-9969(99)00034-5

[46] Merskey H, Spear FG. The concept of pain. Journal of Psychosomatic Research. 1967;**11**(1):59-67. DOI: 10.1016/0022-3999(67)90057-8

[47] Merskey H et al. Pain terms: A list with definitions and notes on usage. Recommended by the IASP Subcommittee on taxonomy. Pain. 1979;**6**(3):247-252. DOI: 10.1016/0304-3959(79)90046-0

[48] Fisher JP, Hassan DT, Connor NO. Minerva. BMJ. 1995;**310**:70. DOI: 10.1136/bmj.310.6971.70

[49] Melzak R. Phantom limbs and the concept of a neuromatrix. Trends Neurosciences. 1990;**13**(3):88-92. DOI: 10.1016/0166-2236(90)90179-e

[50] Moseley GL. A pain neuromatrix approach to patients with chronic pain. Manual Therapy. 2003;**8**(3):130-140. DOI: 10.1016/s1356-689x(03)00051-1

[51] Vane JR, Botting RM. Mechanism of action of antiinflammatory drugs. Scandinavian Journal of Rheumatology. Supplement. 1996;**102**:9-21. DOI: 10.3109/03009749609097226

[52] Kroenke K, Jingwei W, et al. Reciprocal relationship between pain and depression: A 12-month longitudinal analysis in primary care. The Journal of Pain. 2011;**12**(9):964-973. DOI: 10.1016/j.jpain.2011.03.003

[53] Barroso J, Paulo Branco A, Apkarian V. Brain mechanisms of chronic pain: Critical role of translational approach. Translational Research. 2021;**25**(238):76-89. DOI: 10.1016/j.trsl.2021.06.004

[54] Nijs JO, George SZ. Central sensitisation in chronic pain conditions: Latest discoveries and their potential for precision medicine. The Lancet Rheumatology. 2021;**3**(5):E383-E392. DOI: 10.1016/S2665-9913(21)00032-1

[55] Wittkopf PG, Johnson MI. Mirror therapy: A potential intervention for pain management. Revista da Associacao Medica Brasileira (1992). 2017;**63**(11):1000-1005. DOI: 10.1590/1806-9282.63.11.1000

[56] Barbin J, Seetha V, Casillas JM, Paysant J, Pérennou D. The effects of mirror therapy on pain and motor control of phantom limb in amputees: A systematic review. Annals of Physical and Rehabilitation Medicine. 2016;**59**(4):270-275. DOI: 0.1016/j.rehab.2016.04.001

[57] Ashar YK, Gordon A, et al. Effect of pain reprocessing therapy vs placebo and usual care for patients with chronic back pain: A randomized clinical trial. JAMA Psychiatry. 2022;**79**(1):13-23. DOI: 10.1001/jamapsychiatry.2021.2669

Section 3

Artificial Intelligence and Workflow

Chapter 7

Applications of Artificial Intelligence and Machine Learning for Orthodontic Diagnosis

Soukaina Sahim, Moncef Boutissante and Farid El Quars

Abstract

Over the past two decades, artificial intelligence (AI) and machine learning (ML) have undergone significant progress. With advances in the digital technology new possibilities have emerged to improve the orthodontic diagnosis process. AI technology makes it possible to create a virtual patient by assembling all of the patient's clinical data. This technology is applied to identify cephalometric landmarks, to analyze CBCT and to determine the degree of maturation and biological age. Thanks to AI, certain diagnoses are increasingly simple to develop, namely the assessment of the upper airways, the analysis of the temporomandibular joints TMJ and others. This enables more precise analysis, more efficient planning and thus improved treatment results. Artificial intelligence offers many opportunities to improve orthodontic diagnosis. However, it must be used as a decision support tool; clinical expertise and human evaluation remain essential to make informed decisions regarding orthodontic treatment. This chapter highlights different applications of AI for orthodontic diagnosis while assessing the accuracy and the efficiency of this digital technology.

Keywords: artificial intelligence, machine learning, deep learning, orthodontics, diagnosis

1. Introduction

Artificial Intelligence (AI) is a field of computer science that creates systems simulating certain human cognitive functions, such as learning, problem-solving and decision-making. These systems rely on advanced algorithms, often inspired by biological neural networks, which enable them to analyze vast datasets, identify complex correlations and generate accurate predictions or recommendations [1].

Machine Learning (ML) is a subfield of AI that allows computer systems to learn and improve from data without being explicitly programmed for each task. It focuses on developing algorithms capable of analyzing large quantities of data, extracting patterns and structures, and using this knowledge to predict outcomes or make autonomous decisions. In ML, there are four commonly used learning methods, each useful for solving different tasks: supervised, unsupervised, semisupervised and reinforcement learning [2].

Deep Learning (DL), a subset of ML, is inspired by the functioning of the human brain. It employs multiple layers neural networks, to simulate the complex decision-making power of the human brain. Various deep learning algorithms exist, such as convolutional neural networks (CNNs) and artificial neural networks (ANNs). There are also other classification algorithms, including support vector machines (SVMs), regression algorithms (e.g., linear regression, logistic regression), random forests, and others [3].

Artificial intelligence has revolutionized many fields, including orthodontics. AI facilitates the processing and analysis of extensive patient datasets, including radiographs, dental impressions, and cephalometric tracings. It plays a crucial role in the early detection and prediction of dental and facial anomalies. AI also assists orthodontists in determining residual growth potential and biological age by analyzing cephalometric data and growth patterns and enables accurate diagnosis of Upper airways, TMJ pathologies and others [4, 5].

Despite notable advancements, integrating AI into orthodontics faces several challenges. Overcoming these challenges is essential to fully harness the potential of AI in orthodontics, providing more personalized and efficient care to patients. The main purpose of this chapter is to provide an overview of existing data on the use of artificial intelligence and machine learning in orthodontic diagnosis, and to assess the accuracy and the efficiency of this digital technology.

2. Methods

2.1 Research strategy

The research strategy adopted was the PICO method (Patient, Intervention, Comparison, Outcome), which allowed for the formulation of precise research questions and the development of an effective bibliographic search strategy.

- *P (Patient/Population)*: Patients who were candidates for or undergoing orthodontic treatment.

- *I (Intervention)*: Application of artificial intelligence for orthodontic diagnosis.

- *C (Comparison)*: Comparison between different algorithms or between conventional methods and AI-based methods.

- *(Outcome)*: Accuracy and efficiency of AI algorithms.

2.1.1 Identification of databases

Our research was conducted using various databases to select relevant articles related to the application of artificial intelligence in orthodontic diagnosis.

The databases chosen for our bibliographic research were the following: Medline, Science Direct, Web of Science and EBSCO for the period between 2018 and 2024.

2.1.2 Keywords and search equations

The keywords (MeSH) used were as follows:

- Orthodontics
- Artificial intelligence
- Machine Learning
- Deep Learning
- Orthodontic diagnosis
- Cephalometrics
- Bone age
- Dental age

The keywords combined with the Boolean words generated the search equations on the different databases (**Table 1**).

2.1.3 Selection criteria

2.1.3.1 Inclusion criteria

- Articles published between 2018 and 2024.
- Articles published in English.
- Clinical studies on the application of artificial intelligence in orthodonticdiagnosis.
- Any clinical study comparing an AI-based method with a conventional orthodontic method or approach.
- Retrospective and prospective clinical studies.

Database	Search equation
PubMed	• *(Orthodontic diagnosis) AND ((Artificial Intelligence) OR (Machine Learning) OR (Deep Learning))* • *(Cephalometrics)AND ((Artificial Intelligence) OR (Machine Learning) OR (Deep Learning))* • *((Bone age) OR (Dental age)) AND (Orthodontics) AND ((Artificial Intelligence) OR (Machine Learning) OR (Deep Learning))*
ScienceDirect/EBSCOhost/Web of Science	• *Orthodontic diagnosis AND Artificial Intelligence* • *Cephalometrics AND Artificial Intelligence* • *Bone age AND Orthodontics AND Artificial intelligence* • *Dental age AND Orthodontics AND Artificial intelligence* • *Filters:2018–2024*

Table 1.
Search equations on the different databases.

2.1.3.2 Exclusion criteria

- Articles published in languages other than English.
- Meta-analyses and systematic reviews.
- Case-control studies, case reports, or case series.

2.2 Study selection

After identifying the articles in the different databases, duplicates were removed, and the titles and abstracts of potentially relevant studies were reviewed to exclude articles that did not meet the inclusion criteria. In case of doubt, studies were included, and their full texts were assessed for eligibility in the next stage. Studies were included if they met all the inclusion criteria and were excluded for reasons of irrelevance or unavailability of full text. The extracted data included:

- Author name and publication date.
- Study objective.
- Method used in the study.
- AI algorithm utilized.
- Analysis method.
- Study results.

3. Results

3.1 Study selection process

The sequence of literature search in various databases using the aforementioned keywords and Boolean equations followed the Preferred Reporting Items for Systematic Reviews and Meta-Analyses (PRISMA) flowchart (**Figure 1**).

3.2 Description of results

3.2.1 AI and cephalometric analysis

AI revolutionized the identification of cephalometric landmarks. Many studies evaluated the effectiveness of AI in cephalometric analysis, by comparing different algorithms or by comparing AI-based methods to conventional methods (**Table 2**).

The integration of AI into cephalometric analysis opened the door to applications other than cephalometric identification. AI made it possible to generate lateral radiographs from CBCT, to develop automated diagnostic systems and to classify maxillofacial morphology (**Table 3**).

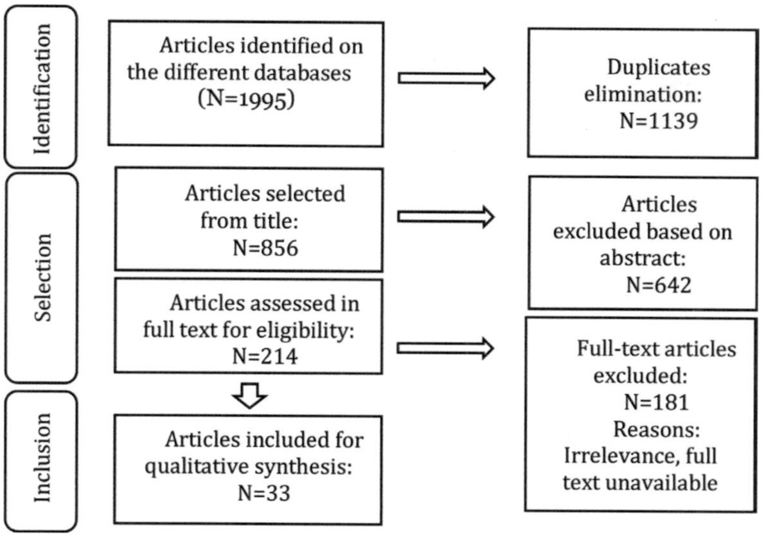

Figure 1.
PRISMA flowchart.

3.2.2 AI applications for CBCT and CT interpretation and segmentation

The integration of artificial intelligence (AI) into 3D segmentation of images obtained through CBCT et CT scans represents a significant advancement reducing the time required for analysis and enhancing the accuracy. Numerous studies have evaluated the effectiveness of AI-based methods in CBCT and CT interpretation and segmentation (**Table 4**).

3.2.3 AI and upper airway assessment

Artificial intelligence (AI) plays an increasingly important role in diagnosing upper airway (UA) pathologies. Numerous studies have evaluated the effectiveness of AI-based methods in the segmentation of the upper airways (**Table 5**).

3.2.4 AI and determination of biological age

AI has advanced the determination of biological age, including bone age and dental age, in the field of orthodontics. Bone age, essential for evaluating residual growth and prescribing orthopedic treatments, can be measured using various methods, including the Greulich and Pyle method and vertebral maturation. For dental age estimation, the Cameriere and Demirjian methods are the most commonly used. Numerous studies have evaluated the effectiveness of AI-based methods in identifying biological age (**Table 6**).

4. Discussion

The integration of artificial intelligence (AI) in orthodontics represents a major advance in daily clinical practice. Thanks to sophisticated algorithms and the analysis of large data sets, AI systems can provide accurate diagnosis and thus effectively guide orthodontic therapies [39].

Study	Objective	Imaging modality	Method	Algorithm	Analysis method	Results
Hwang et al. [6]	Comparison of the accuracy of YOLOv3 and the manual method in cephalometric landmark identification	Lateral cephalogram (LC)	• 1028 LC • 80 landmarks • Manual annotation by an examiner	You-Only-Look-Once version 3 (YOLOv3)	• Learning data: 1028 LC • Test data: 283 LC	• AI method had a mean detection error better than human examiner in 14 points out of 46.
Park et al. [7]	Comparison of the accuracy of 2 AI algorithms for cephalometric landmark identification	Lateral cephalogram (LC)	• 1028 LC • 80 landmarks	• You-Only-Look-Once version 3 (YOLOv3) • Single Shot Multibox Detector (SSD)	• Learning data: 1028 LC • Test data: 283 LC	• YOLOv3 outper-formedSSD in accuracy for 38 out of 80 landmarks. • YOLOv3 was faster (0.05 seconds vs. 2.89 sec-onds for SSD).
Kang et al. [8]	Evaluation of the performance of a deep reinforcement learning model for cephalometric landmark identification	Computerized tomography (CT)	• 28 adults with Class I • 16 landmarks • 5 bilateral points and the rest unilateral	Deep reinforcement learning (DRL): • Multi-stage • Single-stage	• Training dataset: 20 patients. • Test dataset: 8 patients	The system studied showed a low level of detection error and low interindividual variation (1.96 ± 0.78 mm).
Kim et al. [9]	Evaluation of the accuracy of a CNN in anatomical landmark identification compared to the manual method.	Lateral cephalogram (LC)	• 950 LC • 13 landmarks • Manual annotation using Ortho Vision software.	CNN: ROI + PNS + ELU	Mean radial error (MRE) to evaluate accuracy	• The A-point, LIB, UIB, and ANS showed lower MRE values with the AI model than experts.
Jeon et al. [10]	Comparison of cephalometric analysis using CephX™ and the conventional method	Lateral cephalogram (LC)	• LC of 35 patients analyzed by: o *CephXTM o *V-Ceph • 26 cephalometric measurements	CephXTM.	• Paired t test • Bland–Altman plots to compare measurements	• Any significant differ-ence between the two methods for soft tissue measurements. • Additional manual adjust-ment is needed for dental measurements.

Study	Objective	Imaging modality	Method	Algorithm	Analysis method	Results
Kim et al. [11]	Evaluation of the validity of an automatic landmark prediction system on posteroanterior (PA) cephalograms	PA cephalograms from CBCT.	• 430 PA cephalograms derived from CBCT. • 23 landmarks.	Multi-stage CNN model	Mean radial error (MRE) to evaluate accuracy	• The model did not adequately achieve the clinically acceptable error range < 2 mm.
Tanikawa et al. [12]	Evaluation of the accuracy of CNN models for cephalometric landmark identification	Digital lateral cephalogram (LC)	• 1785 patients • 8 groups based on: o *Dental age. o *Cleft lip and/or palate. o *Orthodontic appliance o *Overjet	• Landmark patch classification (CNN-PC) • Landmark point estimation by regression (CNN-PE)	• Learning data: • 1755 LC • Test data: 30 LC	• Skeletal landmarks showed success rates >90%. • Dental landmarks (U6, L6) showed success rates of 73% and 76%.
Çoban et al. [13]	Comparison of cephalometric analysis using WebCeph with the digital manual (DM) method	Lateral cephalogram (LC)	• 105 LC manually traced using Dolphin software. • 10 linear measurements • 12 angular measurements.	WebCeph.	Intraclass correlation coefficient (ICC) for accuracy measurement	Significant differences between the AI method and the DM method in most measurements but no "clinically significant."
El -Dawlatly et al. [14]	Evaluation and comparison of the accuracy and efficiency of AI in performing cephalometric measurements	Lateral cephalogram (LC)	• 200 LC • Three methods: o AI method o AI method with manual modifications o Use of OnyxCeph software.	WebCeph	• The results of the measurements by the three methods were compared • The time required	• The use of AI alone was not accurate enough. • The modified AI was successful. • The AI method was the fastest, followed by the modified AI method and OnyxCeph.

Study	Objective	Imaging modality	Method	Algorithm	Analysis method	Results
Gupta et al. [15]	Evaluation of the accuracy of a Web-Based AI method and a smartphone application for cephalometric analysis compared to manual analysis	Lateral cephalogram (LC)	• 40 LC o Group A: Manual tracing. o Group B: Tracing assisted by smartphone application o Groups C and D: Automated tracing.	WebCeph.	Intraclass correlation coefficient (ICC) for accuracy measurement	• Very good to excellent agreement in accuracy between Web-based AI systems and smartphone application compared to manual tracing (ICC between 0.707 and 0.9).

Table 2.
AI for identification of cephalometric landmarks.

Study	Objective	Method	Algorithm	Analysis method	Results
Chung et al. [16]	Comparison of the consistency of 2D lateral cephalograms (LC) and AI-generated cephalograms using CBCTs	Thirty patients divided into two groups: • Group 1: Conventional LC • Group 2: LC generated by CBCT.	WebCeph.	• The one-way analysis of variance (ANOVA) • Tukey's post hoc test	• No significant difference between 2D cephalometric measurements and those generated from CBCT images, demonstrating the effectiveness of the algorithm.
Ali et al. [17]	Prediction of cephalometric variables *via* a lateral photograph in skeletal classes I, II, and III patterns.	• 94 patients (15–20 years) • Skeletal classes divided into three groups. • Correlation between lateral photographs and cephalograms.	ANN	Predictive Power R to evaluate the accuracy	The algorithm demonstrated excellent predictive power R = 0.99 and a limited estimation error for each malocclusion class (classes I, II, and III).
Kim et al. [18]	Comparison of DenseNet's performance for classifying sagittal skeletal relationships with an existing AI model	• 1574 lateral cephalograms classified based on ANB angle (Class I).	• DenseNet (dense CNN) • V-Ceph	• 1334 images for training • 120 for validation • 120 for testing	The AI model based on DCNN classified with an accuracy of 0.96, which was higher than the automated tracing AI software (V-Ceph).
Ueda et al. [19]	Classification of maxillofacial morphology using cephalometric analysis	• 220 patients (18 years or older) • Three orthodontists classified the morphologies using 8 cephalometric measurements.	• Random Forest Classifier (RF). • Logistic Regression (LR). • Support Vector Classification (SVC).	• Training and testing performed 5 separate times • Outcome measured and averaged for overall performance	Accuracy of facial classification: • Anteroposterior classification: 0.986 ± 0.011 • Vertical classification: 0.850 ± 0.037

Table 3.
Other applications of AI in cephalometric analysis.

Study	Objective	Method	Algorithm	Analysis method	Results
Xu et al. [20]	Evaluation of automated segmentation of 3D dental models acquired by CT scanning	• Segmentation achieved by labeling each mesh. • Two levels of segmentation: o Interdental labeling o teeth and gum labeling	Two-level hierarchical CNNs	• Training set: 1000. • Validation set: 50 • Test set: 150	• The algorithm enabled segmentation of dental models with an excellent accuracy of 99.06% (applicable in computer-aided design systems).
Kim et al. [21]	Comparison of skeletal malocclusion identification accuracy between multichannel models and single-channel DL models.	• 218 CBCT-Division into three classes: Class I, Class II, Class III. • Each 3D CBCT image was projected into three views creating 2D images.	• 2 Multi-channel models: "Ensemble" and "Synchronized multi-channel" • Single channel DL models	• 173 CBCTs for training set • 45 CBCTs for test set.	Multi-channel models perform significantly better overall (accuracy greater than 93%), compared to single-channel DL models.
Lo Guidice et al. [22]	Evaluation of the accuracy of a DL method for fully automatic segmentation of the mandible in comparison with manual segmentation	• 40 CBCT • Manual mandible segmentation was carried out by using Mimics software	CNN model	• Training set: 20 CBCT • Test Set: 20 CBCT. • ICC • Dahlberg's formula (method error) • Model superimposition	• High correlation of measurements between automatic and manual segmentation of the mandible (ICC of 0.937). • Acceptable accuracy of AI method (error of 0.24 mm 3).
Wang et al. [23]	Validation of MS-D network to simultaneously segment the jaw and the teeth in CBCT scans.	• 30 CBCT (9507 slices) • To acquire gold standard labels, all 30 CBCT scans were segmented into three classes: jaw, teeth, and background	MS-D (mixed scale dense): used for segmentation	• Dice similarity coefficient (DSC) • Surface deviations between the MS-D network and the gold standards	• MS-D exhibited minor surface deviations from the Gold Standard 3D models • To segment 1 CBCT: • 25 seconds for MS-D / 5 hours for manual segmentation.

Study	Objective	Method	Algorithm	Analysis method	Results
Ahn et al. [24]	Evaluation of the accuracy and efficiency of an AI system combining facial profile analysis algorithm and DL models.	• 200 CBCT • 13 geometric parameters • detection and segmentation of regions of interest by extracting facial profile and applying Mask-RCNN	• VGG-net CNN for landmark detection • Mask-RCNN for tooth segmentation • decentralized CNN for evaluation of incisor inclination	• 170 cases for training set • 30 cases for validation set.	• High consistency of measurements by AI and manual method • Measuring time reduced: 30 minutes for manual approach / 30 seconds for AI method.
Duman et al. [25]	Morphological classification of sella turcica in CBCT images using AI	• 188 CBCT • 1977 sagittal slices: o *199 sella turcica-flattened images o *629 sella turcica-oval images o * 1149 sella turcica-round images	• Pytorch -library supported UNet: for segmentation • The TensorFlow 1-supported Google Net Inception V 3: to classify the sella turcica.	• Training set: 537 images. • Test set: 60 images.	• The model segmented and classified the sella turcica with high accuracy: o Flattened sella turcica: 98% o Oval sella turcica: 92% o Round sella turcica: 90%.
Zhu et al. [26]	Comparison between the performance of ML models in assessing midpalatal suture (MPS) maturation stage.	• 785 CBCT • 2371 images containing the complete MPS o 263 slices: stage A o 256 slices: stage B o 1007 slices: stage C o 392 slices: stage D o 453 slices: stage E	• ResNet50 • ResNet18, • RessNet101, • Inception-v3, • Efficientnetv2-	• Validation set: 70 participants • Test set: 70 participants.	• CNN models accurately distinguished between stages C and D (the turning points for whether the MPS was calcified or not).

Table 4.
AI for CBCT and CT interpretation and segmentation.

Study	Objective	Method	Algorithm	Analysis method	Results
Sin et al. [27]	Evaluation of automatic segmentation of upper airways (UA) in comparison with manual method	• 306 CBCTs • Semi-automatic software (ITK-SNAP) used to manually generate the UA	U-Net: Deep Learning model.	• 214 images for training set. • 46 images for validation • 46 images for testing.	• The AI model performed UA segmentation with an accuracy of 96.01%. • Average UA volume 18.08 cm^3 by human examiner/17.32 cm3 by AI.
Yoon et al. [28]	Evaluation of the accuracy of automatic detection of UA soft tissue landmarks compared with the skeletal landmarks.	• 600 LC • 16 landmarks (7 skeletal-9 UA) • UA landmarks: o posterior pharyngeal wall (AD1, AD2, and Ss) o soft palate (Sb, St) o tongue (Tb, Td), o * epiglottis (Eb, Et)	Cascaded two-stage CNN model	• 428 training datasets • 72 validation datasets • 100 test datasets	• Compared with mean interexaminer difference, AI showed better accuracies for nasopharynx landmarks AD2 and Ss and lower accuracies for Td, Sb and St. • Less accurate performance for three skeletal landmarks.
Chu et al. [29]	Comparison of automatic UA segmentation by four AI-based models.	• 201 2D UA images acquired using CBCT. • The regions of interest (ROI) were segmented into three regions: o nasopharynx, o retropalatal pharynx o retroglossal pharynx	• UNet18, • UNet36, • DeepLab5 • DeepLab101	• Training set: 161 images. • Validation set: 40 images.	• All four models demonstrated excellent accuracy in automatic UA segmentation (accuracy greater than 90%). • AI processing was more efficient than manual processing.
Jeong et al. [30]	Evaluation of a DL model for the diagnosis of UA obstruction in comparison with other AI models.	• 1219 LC o Number of cases with UA obstruction: 610 o Number of cases without UA obstruction: 609.	• DCNN model based on ResNet backbone structure • VGG16.	• 1099 images for training • 120 images for testing.	• Compared to VGG16, DCNN showed better performance with a sensitivity of 0.86. • The DCNN model provided rapid and accurate diagnoses of UA obstruction.

Table 5.
AI and upper airway assessment.

Study	Objective	Method	Algorithm	Analysis method	Results
Reddy et al. [31]	Evaluation of AI automatic prediction of bone age (BA) from radiographs using only the index finger rather than the whole hand.	• 12,811 hand X-rays. • The index was cut to create a second dataset. • Three radiologists determined the BA from the whole-hand and index-finger radiographs	CNN model.	• Training set: 12611 hand radiographs • Test set: 200 radiographs	• The mean absolute difference between ground truth and CNN-BA for the whole hand and index finger was similar (4.7 months vs. 5.1 months). • Both values were significantly lower than radiologists.
Booz et al. [32]	Evaluation of the accuracy and efficiency of an AI model for BA assessment compared to Greulich Pyle (GP) method.	• X-rays of 514 patients • BA was assessed by three radiologists using the GP method and AI software.	BoneXpert version 2.1 (Multi-layer neural network)	• Root mean square deviation (RMSD) for model accuracy	• The algorithm enabled a highly accurate BA assessment (RMSD of 0.38 years for AI/RMSD of 0.89 years for the GP method). • Mean reading times reduced by 87% using AI system.
Shen et al. [33]	Prediction of dental age using AI and comparison with age determined by Cameriere method.	• Panoramic radiographs of 748 children (5–15 years) • Dental age estimated using the Cameriere method (7 left mandibular permanent teeth excluding third molars)	• Random Forest (RF) • Support Vector Machine (SVM) • Linear regression (LR)	• 598 images: training set • 150 images: test set	• ML models were more accurate than the traditional Cameriere formula. • SVM model and the RF model had the highest accuracy.
Galibourg et al. [34]	Comparison of the ability of ML algorithms to predict dental age against reference methods.	• A total of 3605 panoramic radiographs of patients (2–24 years) • Seven left permanent mandibular teeth and four third molars evaluated using Demirjian and Willems stages.	10 ML algorithms	• Training set: 80% of the sample. • Test set: • 20% of the sample • Mean absolute error (MAE) for model accuracy	• All ML methods based on the maturation stages defined by Demirjian were accurate in estimating dental age (MAE < 0.811 years).

Study	Objective	Method	Algorithm	Analysis method	Results
Li et al. [35]	Comparison of the performance of four CNN models in the classification of cervical vertebral maturation (CVM)	• LC of patients (5–18 years) • 2 orthodontists manually grouped images into six stages: (CS1), (CS2), (CS3), (CS4), (CS5), and (CS6).	• VGG16, • Google Net • DenseNet161 • ResNet152.	• Training set: 70% of the sample • Validation set: 15% of the sample • Test set: 15% of the sample.	• ResNet 152 outperformed other algorithms in terms of accuracy in classifying CVM ResNet 152 > DenseNet161> Google Net > VGG16.
Kim et al. [36]	Evaluation of DL-based BA prediction model by comparing it with a GP-based DL model.	• A total of 21,036 hand radiographs of Korean children and adolescents • All labels were manually annotated by an experienced radiologist	• ResNet 50. • VUNO Med-BoneAge (GP-based model)	• Mean absolute error (MAE) • Root mean square error (RMSE)	Compared with the GP-based model: the Korean model showed a lower RMSE and MAE (8.2 vs. 10.5 months).
Kök et al. [37]	Evaluation of the performance of an artificial neural network in determining growth periods.	• 419 patients • LC were divided into six cervical vertebrae stages. • 27 cervical reference points and 32 linear measurements	ANN: artificial neural network	• Training set: 70% of the sample • Test set: 15% of the sample • Validation set: 15% of the sample	• The ANN-7 model (32 linear measurements and age) had the highest model accuracy with 0.9427.
Wang et al. [38]	Comparison of the performance of two ML models in dental age estimation	• A total of 9586 panoramic radiographs of patients (6–20 years) • Demirjian method was used for the manual method.	• VGG 16 • ResNet 101	• Training set: 70% of the sample • Validation set: 20% of the sample • Test set: 10% of the sample.	• The VGG16 network performed better than the ResNet101 network in terms of prediction.

Table 6.
AI and determination of biological age.

The fields of application of AI for orthodontic diagnosis have been increasingly developed. AI can be used for various diagnostic purposes, namely cephalometric landmark identification, individualized radiological interpretation, CBCT and CT segmentation, upper airway assessment and biological age determination. Other applications can also be achieved using AI algorithms, including precise analysis of TMJs, determination of facial symmetry, morphological classification of exobuccal photographs, etc. [4, 40].

AI is increasingly being used to facilitate cephalometric analysis. Many studies have focused on evaluating the effectiveness of AI-based models compared to traditional manual tracing methods in cephalometry. Kim et al. [9] compared the detection performed by two orthodontists against a neural network model. They found that the AI model can perform fully automatic identification of cephalometric landmarks and achieve better results than examiners for some landmarks such as the A-point, the incisal tip of the maxillary and mandibular incisors, and ANS.

Jeon et al. [10] used CephXTM, a CNN model, and compare it with the conventional method using V-Ceph. The saddle angle, linear measurements of maxillary incisor to NA line and mandibular incisor to NB line showed statistically significant differences. They suggested an additional manual adjustment for dental measurements regarding tooth structures for higher accuracy.

Among the innovative software for cephalometric analysis, WebCeph stands out by offering a comprehensive analysis of cephalometric data. Various studies have evaluated its performance. El-Dawlatly et al. [14] compared AI method using WebCeph software, the modified AI method using WebCeph software after manual modification of the landmarks' position, and the use of OnyxCeph software. They found that the AI method followed by fine tuning of the location of landmarks was successful and can be used as an alternative to ordinary digital landmark identification for lateral cephalometric analysis. They also found that measurements were generated fastest using the AI method, followed by the modified AI method, and finally the conventional digital method. Gupta et al. [15] enriched this comparison by assessing a mobile application, finding a satisfactory agreement between the accuracies of the AI model and the mobile application (ICC between 0.707 and 0.9) compared to the manual method.

YOLO (You Only Look Once) v3, an improved version of a real-time object detection algorithm, is particularly appreciated for its ability to detect and localize multiple objects accurately and quickly. Hwang et al. [6] found that YOLOv3 outperformed the human examiner in terms of detection, with a better average error in 14 of the 46 landmarks evaluated. Park et al. [7] also found that Single YOLOv3 outperformed Shot Multibox Detector SSD in accuracy for 38 out of 80 landmarks and was found to be faster (0.05 seconds vs. 2.89 seconds for SSD).

The application of AI in cephalometric analysis was not limited to lateral cephalograms only; it was also extended to CBCT and CT images for automated annotation. Tanikawa et al. [12] evaluated the accuracy of CNN models for cephalometric landmark identification in digital lateral cephalograms. They found that skeletal landmarks showed success rates >90% and dental landmarks (U6, L6) showed success rates of 73% and 76%. Kang et al. [8] also evaluated the performance of a deep reinforcement learning model for cephalometric landmark identification on CT images, and they found that the AI system showed a low level of detection error and low interindividual variation (1.96 ± 0.78 mm).

The integration of AI in the analysis of lateral cephalograms goes far beyond the identification of cephalometric landmarks. Indeed, various applications are emerging, such as the automatic classification of maxillofacial morphology. Kim et al. [18] evaluated the accuracy of DenseNet, a neural network designed for the classification of sagittal skeletal relationships. The software achieved an accuracy of 96% outperforming other automatic tracing softwares. Ueda et al. [19] assessed the accuracy of Random Forest, Logistic Forest, as well as a Support Vector Classifier. They found that the DL models successfully classified the morphologies of 220 patients with accuracies of 82% for combined facial classification, 98.6% for anteroposterior classification and 85% for vertical classification. Ali et al. [17] employed the ANN for the prediction of skeletal parameters for full orthodontic diagnosis using lateral photographs. The algorithm demonstrated excellent predictive power R = 0.99 and a limited estimation error for each malocclusion class (classes I, II, and III). Therefore, ANNs could be an alternative approach for the cephalometric radiographs for measuring angular and linear variables.

AI software can also be used for the generation of lateral cephalograms from CBCT, as demonstrated by Chung et al. [16] using WebCeph.

The use of AI for orthodontic diagnosis can also be applied for the interpretation of 3D radiological images as well as CT and CBCT segmentation. This not only allows the segmentation of dental models with high accuracy but also enables various applications such as the classification of the sella turcica, the assessment of skeletal development, the creation of virtual models and the determination of malocclusions.

Xu et al. [20] evaluated the accuracy of automated segmentation of 3D dental models and showed that the algorithm achieved segmentation with an excellent accuracy of 99.06%, making it applicable in computer-aided design (CAD) systems. Lo Giudice et al. [22] evaluated of the accuracy of a DL method for fully automatic segmentation of the mandible in comparison with manual segmentation. They found a high correlation between the two methods with acceptable accuracy of the AI method used (error of 0.24 mm^3). Wang et al. [23] also highlighted the impact of AI on reducing procedure time through their M-SD network, which was able to simultaneously segment the jaw and the teeth in CBCT scans in just 25 seconds, while manual methods required approximately 5 hours.

Furthermore, integrating AI into CBCT analysis enables other promising applications. Duman et al. [25] used TensorFlow to classify the sella turcica into three distinct categories: flattened, oval, and round, with accuracies of 0.98, 0.92, and 0.90, respectively. This accurate classification contributes to a better understanding of the anatomical variations of the sella turcica, which is essential for various diagnoses. Zhu et al. [26] used CNN models to determine the maturation stage of the midpalatal suture (MPS). They found that the models accurately distinguished between stages C and D, the turning points for whether the MPS was calcified or not. Therefore, they can help orthodontists avoid the side effects of using RME in calcified MPS and avoid unnecessary SARME for patients whose MPS is uncalcified.

AI also helps in determining malocclusions on CBCT. The study by Kim et al. [21] revealed that a multichannel model achieved 93% accuracy in detecting malocclusions, compared to a single-channel model. Ahn et al. [24] introduced a hybrid system that combines a facial profile analysis with deep-learning methods (Mask-RCNN and decentralized CNN). The system could calculate cephalometric measurements representing sagittal, coronal analyses, occlusal cant, facial asymmetry, and anterior teeth inclination for orthodontic diagnosis on 3D CBCT images. The system also enabled time savings by reducing the measuring time from about 30 min to about 30 s.

Other applications of AI in orthodontics include the use of algorithms for upper airway (UA) assessment and diagnosis of respiratory pathologies. Sin et al. [27]

evaluated the accuracy of AI in UA segmentation using a Deep Learning U-Net model, which achieved an accuracy of 96.01%. In fact, the human examiner estimated the average UA volume to be 18.08 cm^3 while the artificial intelligence estimated 17.32 cm^3. Chu et al. [29] evaluated the ability of AI models to localize the minimum cross-sectional area (CSAmin), which denotes the region with the greatest constriction. They found that the AI models accurately segmented UA and were able to predict 3D CSAmin information for screening out potential airway problems. Jeong et al. [30] also evaluated a DL model for the diagnosis of UA obstruction. Compared to VGG16, DCNN showed better performance with a sensitivity of 0.86. The model provided rapid and accurate diagnoses of UA obstruction. Therefore, AI could play a crucial role in early detection of some respiratory pathologies such as obstructive sleep apnea. AI would not only allow better identification of patients at risk, but also personalization of therapeutic strategies.

The integration of artificial intelligence (AI) in growth potential assessment offers fascinating prospects by automating processes and increasing the accuracy of results. Growth potential assessment in orthodontics can be performed by determining bone age. The latter could be estimated using various methods, the most commonly used being the Greulich-Pyle method and cervical maturation estimation. With advances in ML and DL algorithms, AI has helped automate and improve laborious processes of bone age estimation, reducing human errors. Booz et al. [32] evaluated the accuracy and efficiency of BoneXpert software for automated BA assessment compared to the Greulich-Pyle (GP) method. They found that the AI model enabled highly accurate and objective BA assessment, regardless of gender with a root mean square deviation (RMSD) of 0.38 years for AI versus 0.89 years for the GP method. The AI method was also efficient with mean reading times being reduced by 87%. A study by Kim et al. [36] compared two AI models, the ResNet 50 and a Greulich-Pyle (GP) based model. The results showed that the ResNet 50 model performed better, with a mean absolute error of 8.2 months, compared to 10.5 months for the GP-based model.

Li et al. [35] compared the performance of four CNN models in the classification of cervical vertebral maturation (CVM). They found that CNN models were a convenient, fast, and reliable method for CVM analysis and ResNet152 proved to be the best model among the four models. Kök et al. [37] evaluated the performance of an ANN in determining growth periods from the cervical vertebrae. The ANN-7 model (32 linear measurements and age) had the highest model accuracy highlighting the effectiveness of neural networks in identifying bone maturation stages.

The use of artificial intelligence is also promising in estimating dental age traditionally determined by manual methods such as Dermijian and Cameriere methods. Shen et al. [33] evaluated the effectiveness of ML models in estimating dental age by comparing their performance with the Cameriere method. The results showed that the ML models were more accurate than the traditional Cameriere formula with the Support Vector Machine (SVM) model and the Random Forest (RF) model having the highest accuracy. Galibourj et al. [34] assessed the accuracy of 10 ML algorithms in predicting dental age compared to Demirjian and Willems methods. They found that all ML methods based on the maturation stages defined by Demirjian were accurate in estimating dental age with a mean absolute error (MAE) under 0.811 years. These results support the use of ML algorithms instead of using standard population tables.

The future of AI in orthodontic diagnosis holds immense potential for innovation and advancement. With the continued development of machine learning algorithms and imaging technologies, it will become possible to achieve more precise and early diagnoses, even in complex or atypical cases. Moreover, the digital technology is expected to redefine the standards of orthodontic diagnosis, making it faster, more reliable, and increasingly personalized.

5. Conclusion

The integration of artificial intelligence (AI) in orthodontics represents a major technological advance, revolutionizing clinical practices by opening up new diagnostic perspectives.

The results of this study showed that AI has significantly improved the accuracy and efficiency of orthodontic diagnosis. Indeed, deep learning models often outperform traditional methods in localizing cephalometric landmarks, segmenting complex anatomical structures, segmenting the upper airways, and also in estimating growth potential and biological age.

However, despite these advances, limitations remain. Ethical and practical challenges related to the integration of these technologies into clinical routine must be addressed, particularly in terms of cost, practitioner training and patient data management.

Acknowledgements

Special thanks to the department of orthodontics of the faculty of dentistry of the University Hassan II of Casablanca. We would also like to acknowledge the support of Professor Farid Bourzgui for the realization of this work and for sharing and discussing the ideas of the project.

Conflict of interest

The authors declare they have no conflict of interest.

Author details

Soukaina Sahim[1*], Moncef Boutissante[2] and Farid El Quars[1]

1 Department of Orthodontics, Faculty of Dentistry, University Hassan II of Casablanca, Morocco

2 Dental Private Practice, Casablanca, Morocco

*Address all correspondence to: souki-2s@hotmail.fr

References

[1] Khalifa M, Albadawy M. Artificial intelligence for clinical prediction: Exploring key domains and essential functions. Computer Methods and Programs in Biomedicine-Update. 2024;**5**(100148):1-11. DOI: 10.1016/j.cmpbup.2024.100148

[2] Choi RY, Coyner AS, Kalpathy-Cramer J, Chiang MF, Campbell JP. Introduction to machine learning, neural networks, and deep learning. Translational Vision Science & Technology. 2020;**9**(2):14. DOI: 10.1167/tvst.9.2.14

[3] Taye MM. Understanding of machine learning with deep learning: Architectures, workflow, applications and future directions. Computers. 2023;**12**(5):91. DOI: 10.3390/computers12050091

[4] Bichu YM, Hansa I, Bichu AY, Premjani P, Flores-Mir C, Vaid NR. Applications of artificial intelligence and machine learning in orthodontics: A scoping review. Progress in Orthodontics. 2021;**22**(1):18. DOI: 10.1186/s40510-021-00361-9

[5] Liu J, Zhang C, Shan Z. Application of artificial intelligence in orthodontics: Current state and future perspectives. Healthcare (Basel). 2023;**11**(20):2760. DOI: 10.3390/healthcare11202760

[6] Hwang HW, Park JH, Moon JH, Yu Y, Kim H, Her SB, et al. Automated identification of cephalometric landmarks: Part 2-might it be better than human? The Angle Orthodontist. 2020;**90**(1):69-76. DOI: 10.2319/022019-129.1

[7] Park JH, Hwang HW, Moon JH, Yu Y, Kim H, Her SB, et al. Automated identification of cephalometric landmarks: Part 1—Comparisons between the latest deep-learning methods YOLOV3 and SSD. The Angle Orthodontist. 2019;**89**(6):903, 9. DOI: 10.2319/022019-127.1

[8] Kang SH, Jeon K, Kang SH, Lee SH. 3D cephalometric landmark detection by multiple stage deep reinforcement learning. Scientific Reports. 2021;**11**(1):17509. DOI: 10.1038/s41598-021-97116-7

[9] Kim YH, Lee C, Ha EG, Choi YJ, Han SS. A fully deep learning model for the automatic identification of cephalometric landmarks. Imaging Science in Dentistry. 2021;**51**(3):299-306. DOI: 10.5624/isd.20210077

[10] Jeon S, Lee KC. Comparison of cephalometric measurements between conventional and automatic cephalometric analysis using convolutional neural network. Progress in Orthodontics. 2021;**22**(1):14. DOI: 10.1186/s40510-021-00358-4

[11] Kim MJ, Liu Y, Oh SH, Ahn HW, Kim SH, Nelson G. Evaluation of a multi-stage convolutional neural network-based fully automated landmark identification system using cone-beam computed tomography synthesized posteroanterior cephalometric images. The Korean Journal of Orthodontics. 2021;**51**(2):77-85. DOI: 10.4041/kjod.2021.51.2.77

[12] Tanikawa C, Lee C, Lim J, Oka A, Yamashiro T. Clinical applicability of automated cephalometric landmark identification: Part I-patient-related identification errors. Orthodontics & Craniofacial Research. 2021;**24**(Suppl. 2):43-52. DOI: 10.1111/ocr.12501

[13] Çoban G, Öztürk T, Hashimli N, Yağci A. Comparison between cephalometric measurements using digital manual and web-based artificial intelligence cephalometric tracing software. Dental Press Journal of Orthodontics. 2022;**27**(4):e222112. DOI: 10.1590/2177-6709.27.4.e222112.oar

[14] El-Dawlatly M, Attia KH, Abdelghaffar AY, Mostafa YA, Abd E-GM. Preciseness of artificial intelligence for lateral cephalometric measurements. Journal of Orofacial Orthopopedics. May 2024;**85**(Suppl. 1):27-33. DOI: 10.1007/s00056-023-00459-1

[15] Gupta S, Shetty S, Natarajan S, Nambiar S, Mv A, Agarwal S. A comparative evaluation of concordance and speed between smartphone app-based and artificial intelligence web-based cephalometric tracing software with the manual tracing method: A cross-sectional study. Journal of Clinical and Experimental Dentistry. 2024;**16**(1):e11-e17. DOI: 10.4317/jced.60899

[16] Chung EJ, Yang BE, Park IY, Yi S, On SW, Kim YH, et al. Effectiveness of cone-beam computed tomography-generated cephalograms using artificial intelligence cephalometric analysis. Scientific Reports. 2022;**12**(1):20585. DOI: 10.1038/s41598-022-25215-0

[17] Ali SM, Saloom HF, Tawfeeq MA. Cephalometric variables prediction from lateral photographs between different skeletal patterns using regression artificial neural networks. Turkish Journal of Orthodontics. 2022;**35**(2):101-111. DOI: 10.5152/TurkJOrthod.2022.21087

[18] Kim HJ, Kim KDK, Kim DH. Deep convolutional neural network-based skeletal classification of cephalometric image compared with automated-tracing software. Scientific Reports. 2022;**12**(1):11659. DOI: 10.1038/s41598-022-15856-6

[19] Ueda A, Tussie C, Kim S, Kuwajima Y, Matsumoto S, Kim G, et al. Classification of maxillofacial morphology by artificial intelligence using cephalometric analysis measurements. Diagnostics. 2023;**13**(13):2134. DOI: 10.3390/diagnostics13132134

[20] Xu X, Liu C, Zheng Y. 3D tooth segmentation and labeling using deep convolutional neural networks. IEEE Transactions on Visualization and Computer Graphics. 2019;**25**(7):2336-2348. DOI: 10.1109/TVCG.2018.2839685

[21] Kim I, Misra D, Rodriguez L, Gill M, Liberton DK, Almpani K, et al. Malocclusion classification on 3D cone-beam CT craniofacial images using multi-channel deep learning models. In: Annual International Conference of the IEEE Engineering in Medicine and Biology Society. Annual International Conference. Vol. 2020. IEEE Engineering in Medicine and Biology Society; Jul 2020. pp. 1294-1298. DOI: 10.1109/EMBC44109.2020.9176672

[22] Lo Giudice A, Ronsivalle V, Spampinato C, Leonardi R. Fully automatic segmentation of the mandible based on convolutional neural networks (CNNs). Orthodontics & Craniofacial Research. 2021;**24**((S2) Suppl. 2):100-107. DOI: 10.1111/ocr.12536

[23] Wang H, Minnema J, Batenburg KJ, Forouzanfar T, Hu FJ, Wu G. Multiclass CBCT image segmentation for orthodontics with deep learning. Journal of Dental Research. 2021;**100**(9):943-949. DOI: 10.1177/00220345211005338

[24] Ahn J, Nguyen TP, Kim YJ, Kim T, Yoon J. Automated analysis of three-dimensional CBCT images taken in

natural head position that combines facial profile processing and multiple deep-learning models. Computer Methods and Programs in Biomedicine. 2022;**226**:107123. DOI: 10.1016/j.cmpb.2022.107123

[25] Duman ŞB, Syed AZ, Celik Ozen DC, Bayrakdar İŞ, Salehi HS, Abdelkarim A, et al. Convolutional neural network performance for Sella turcica segmentation and classification using CBCT images. Diagnostics. 2022;**12**(9):2244. DOI: 10.3390/diagnostics12092244

[26] Zhu M, Yang P, Bian C, Zuo F, Guo Z, Wang Y, et al. Convolutional neural network-assisted diagnosis of midpalatal suture maturation stage in cone-beam computed tomography. Journal of Dentistry. 2024;**141**:104808. DOI: 10.1016/j.jdent.2023.104808

[27] Sin Ç, Akkaya N, Aksoy S, Orhan K, Öz U. A deep learning algorithm proposal to automatic pharyngeal airway detection and segmentation on CBCT images. Orthodontics and Craniofacial Research. 2021;**24**(S2):117-123. DOI: 10.1111/ocr.12480

[28] Yoon HJ, Kim DR, Gwon E, Kim N, Baek SH, Ahn HW, et al. Fully automated identification of cephalometric landmarks for upper airway assessment using cascaded convolutional neural networks. European Journal of Orthodontics. 2022;**44**(1):66-77. DOI: 10.1093/ejo/cjab054

[29] Chu G, Zhang R, He Y, Ng CH, Gu M, Leung YY, et al. Deep learning models for automatic upper airway segmentation and minimum cross-sectional area localisation in two-dimensional images. Bioengineering (Basel, Switzerland). 2023;**10**(8):915. DOI: 10.3390/bioengineering10080915

[30] Jeong Y, Nang Y, Zhao Z. Automated evaluation of upper airway obstruction based on deep learning. BioMed Research International. 2023;**2023**:8231425. DOI: 10.1155/2023/8231425

[31] Reddy NE, Rayan JC, Annapragada AV, Mahmood NF, Scheslinger AE, Zhang W, et al. Bone age determination using only the index finger: A novel approach using a convolutional neural network compared with human radiologists. Pediatric Radiology. 2020;**50**(4):516-523. DOI: 10.1007/s00247-019-04587-y

[32] Booz C, Yel I, Wichmann JL, Boettger S, Al Kamali A, Albrecht MH, et al. Artificial intelligence in bone age assessment: Accuracy and efficiency of a novel fully automated algorithm compared to the Greulich-Pyle method. European Radiology Experimental. 2020;**4**(1):6. DOI: 10.1186/s41747-019-0139-9

[33] Shen S, Liu Z, Wang J, Fan L, Ji F, Tao J. Machine learning assisted Cameriere method for dental age estimation. BMC Oral Health. 2021;**21**(1):641. DOI: 10.1186/s12903-021-01996-0

[34] Galibourg A, Cussat-Blanc S, Dumoncel J, Telmon N, Monsarrat P, Maret D. Comparison of different machine learning approaches to predict dental age using Demirjian's staging approach. International Journal of Legal Medicine. 2021;**135**(2):665-675. DOI: 10.1007/s00414-020-02489-5

[35] Li H, Chen Y, Wang Q, Gong X, Lei Y, Tian J, et al. Convolutional neural network-based automatic cervical vertebral maturation classification method. Dento-Maxillo Facial Radiology. 2022;**51**(6):20220070. DOI: 10.1259/dmfr.20220070

[36] Kim PH, Yoon HM, Kim JR, Hwang JY, Choi JH, Hwang J, et al. Bone age assessment using artificial intelligence in Korean pediatric population: A comparison of deep-learning models trained with healthy chronological and Greulich-Pyle ages as labels. Korean Journal of Radiology. 2023;**24**(11):1151-1163. DOI: 10.3348/kjr.2023.0092

[37] Kök H, Izgi MS, Acilar AM. Determination of growth and development periods in orthodontics with artificial neural network. Orthodontics & Craniofacial Research. 2021;**24**((S2) Suppl. 2):76-83. DOI: 10.1111/ocr.12443

[38] Wang J, Dou J, Han J, Li G, Tao J. A population-based study to assess two convolutional neural networks for dental age estimation. BMC Oral Health. 2023;**23**(1):109. DOI: 10.1186/s12903-023-02817-2

[39] Kazimierczak N, Kazimierczak W, Serafin Z, Nowicki P, Nożewski J, Janiszewska-Olszowska J. AI in orthodontics: Revolutionizing diagnostics and treatment planning—A comprehensive review. Journal of Clinical Medicine. 2024;**13**(2):344. DOI: 10.3390/jcm13020344

[40] Gracea RS, Winderickx N, Vanheers M, Hendrickx J, Preda F, Shujaat S, et al. Artificial intelligence for orthodontic diagnosis and treatment planning: A scoping review. Journal of Dentistry. 2025;**152**:105442. DOI: 10.1016/j.jdent.2024.105442

Chapter 8

Computerized Workflow in Cranio-Maxillofacial Surgery for Skeletal Class III

Orazio Bennici and Gloria Francesca Pia Bennici

Abstract

The implementation of a digital workflow in cranio-maxillofacial surgery has revolutionized the management of skeletal Class III malocclusion. This chapter outlines a comprehensive approach that integrates orthodontic and orthognathic interventions with advanced digital planning tools. Post-treatment records demonstrate significant skeletal and dentoalveolar improvements, including normalization of hyperdivergent skeletal patterns and enhanced facial esthetics adhering to the golden facial proportions. Detailed cephalometric analysis confirms the achievement of optimal sagittal and vertical relationships, alongside a well-balanced soft tissue profile. The combination of traditional and digital approaches, including three-dimensional (3D) imaging, virtual surgical planning, and customized surgical guides, ensures predictable outcomes tailored to patient-specific anatomical and functional needs. This protocol facilitates not only precise execution of complex interventions but also minimizes procedural errors, reduces operative time, and enhances patient satisfaction. Post-operative follow-up protocols are essential to monitor skeletal stability, soft tissue adaptation, and long-term occlusal harmony. The integration of cone beam computed tomography (CBCT), digital models, and advanced imaging aids in evaluating the alignment between surgical outcomes and preoperative plans. Studies underscore the role of personalized surgical guides and digital tools in reducing relapse rates and improving stability in Class III cases. Advances in artificial intelligence (AI), augmented reality, robotics, and imaging technologies further extend the capabilities of cranio-maxillofacial surgery, paving the way for more personalized, minimally invasive, and precise interventions. This paradigm shift underscores the ongoing evolution in surgical practice, fostering outcomes that are functional, esthetic, and sustainable over time.

Keywords: skeletal class III, digital workflow, cranio-maxillofacial surgery, virtual surgical planning, customized surgical guides, 3D imaging, cephalometric analysis

1. Introduction

Conventional orthognathic surgery planning integrates clinical examinations with diagnostic tools, such as lateral cephalometric radiographs, dental casts, facebow transfers, articulators, and photographs. However, traditional planning approaches based on plaster models often overlook anatomical details of the entire craniofacial structure. In patients with severe craniofacial deformities, this limitation can lead to discrepancies with undesirable outcomes and potentially significant complications.

Skeletal Class III malocclusions continue to pose challenges for both orthodontists and maxillofacial surgeons. These challenges arise from the combined presence of a maxillary component, often characterized by transverse constriction, and a hypertrophic mandibular component, frequently exhibiting asymmetry.

1.1 Epidemiological and clinical background, incidence, prevalence, and distribution of narrow palate

A narrow palate, defined as a reduced transverse width of the maxillary arch, significantly impacts patient's quality of life, contributing to respiratory issues, masticatory inefficiencies, and increased susceptibility to malocclusion and occlusal dysfunctions. This anatomical condition is particularly relevant in orthodontics and maxillofacial surgery due to its association with complex clinical scenarios. Prevalence estimates for narrow palate range between 7 and 20% in the general population, with significant variations across age, gender, and ethnic groups. In children and adolescents, narrow palate incidence is strongly linked to oral breathing, often secondary to tonsillar hypertrophy, adenoidal enlargement, or chronic allergic conditions. Studies suggest that oral breathing adversely affects the growth and development of the maxilla, compromising palatal width and predisposing individuals to future malocclusions. Geographical distribution highlights a higher prevalence in urban and industrialized areas, where environmental pollutants exacerbate chronic respiratory disorders, a well-recognized predisposing factor for narrow palate [1].

1.2 Incidence, prevalence, and distribution of skeletal class III malocclusion

Skeletal Class III malocclusion represents one of the most challenging conditions in orthodontics and maxillofacial surgery, characterized by mandibular prominence relative to the maxilla, resulting in a prognathic profile and significant masticatory dysfunction. Its prevalence varies significantly across populations: approximately 10–15% in Asian ethnic groups compared to 1–5% in Western and Caucasian populations [2]. This dysmorphia exhibits a strong genetic predisposition, often inherited in an autosomal dominant pattern, as documented in numerous studies. In addition to genetic factors, Class III malocclusions are often associated with growth disturbances, where excessive mandibular growth relative to the maxilla leads to anteroposterior (AP) misalignment. Early diagnosis in pediatric cases can mitigate the progression of deformity through interceptive orthodontic interventions. Conversely, in adolescents and adults with a mature skeletal structure, combined surgical and orthodontic approaches are essential for correcting Class III discrepancies [3].

1.3 Association between narrow palate and skeletal class III malocclusion

The coexistence of a narrow palate and skeletal Class III malocclusion represents one of the most intricate challenges for maxillofacial surgeons. These conditions often exacerbate each other, complicating treatment. While the prevalence of this combination remains poorly documented, it is frequently observed in patients with chronic respiratory anomalies and swallowing dysfunctions, which predispose them to develop both conditions [4]. In adult patients, the combination of a narrow palate and prognathic mandible often leads to compromised respiratory function, affecting sleep quality and overall life satisfaction. Recent studies emphasize that addressing only one of these conditions often fails to achieve optimal esthetic and functional outcomes. Consequently, combined treatment protocols, including palatal expansion and mandibular prognathism correction, have become a cornerstone of advanced orthodontic and surgical management strategies [5].

1.4 Therapeutic alternatives for correcting narrow palate and skeletal class III

The management of narrow palate and skeletal Class III malocclusion requires a personalized approach, tailored to the patient's age and skeletal maturity.

1.4.1 Traditional orthodontic approaches

In growing patients, non-surgical palatal expansion is a first-line option to correct the transverse maxillary deficiency. Rapid palatal expanders (RPEs) are utilized in orthodontics to achieve gradual midpalatal suture separation. However, in adults with mature palatal bones and ossified midpalatal sutures, this approach is ineffective due to the lack of suture flexibility [6].

1.4.2 Traditional orthognathic procedures without SARPE (surgically assisted rapid palatal expansion)

In skeletal Class III cases, bimaxillary osteotomy is a well-established surgical solution to correct anteroposterior discrepancies. However, this procedure does not address the transverse dimension of the maxilla. When applied to patients with both narrow palate and Class III malocclusion, it may improve dental arch alignment but fails to resolve the transverse deficiency, leaving palatal expansion unaddressed [7].

1.4.3 Advanced technologies and computerized workflows

The combination of miniscrew-assisted rapid palatal expansion (MARPE) and digitally planned orthognathic surgery offers a comprehensive solution for narrow palate associated with skeletal Class III malocclusion. Computerized workflows represent the most advanced approach, ensuring precise planning and predictable outcomes [8]. The integration of cone beam computed tomography (CBCT) and 3D models allows for accurate design of both palatal expansion and corrective surgery, reducing intraoperative risks and enhancing post-operative stability. The use of 3D printing and patient-specific surgical guides further improves surgical accuracy, resulting in superior esthetic and functional outcomes [9].

2. Traditional vs. computerized workflows in surgical planning

Orthognathic surgery demands meticulous and precise planning to achieve optimal functional and esthetic results. Traditionally, surgical planning has relied on a comprehensive patient assessment involving clinical examinations and key diagnostic tools, including lateral cephalometric radiographs, plaster models, facebow transfers, articulators, and extra- and intraoral photographs. For decades, these tools have formed the foundation of orthognathic planning, enabling a two-dimensional (2D) evaluation of skeletal structure and dental relationships [10].

2.1 Lateral cephalometric radiographs and photographs

Lateral cephalometric radiographs are essential in traditional planning, providing a lateral view of the skull to analyze anteroposterior and vertical skeletal proportions. However, their 2D nature limits the visualization of the complete craniofacial anatomy. Extra- and intraoral photographs serve as complementary visual aids, facilitating the evaluation of facial esthetics and smile harmony. However, these images fail to deliver detailed insights into deeper skeletal structures [11].

2.2 Plaster models and articulators

Plaster models, created from traditional dental impressions, have long been the primary method for occlusal analysis and planning dental and skeletal movements. Mounted on mechanical articulators, these models enable the simulation of masticatory movements and the analysis of interocclusal relationships. While effective for assessing occlusion, these models have significant limitations in cases involving severe craniofacial deformities. Manual manipulation of plaster models does not provide precise insights into cranial structures or the skeletal interactions between the mandible and maxilla, often neglecting critical details necessary for comprehensive planning [12]. By addressing these limitations, computerized workflows and advanced technologies represent a transformative evolution in orthognathic surgical planning (**Figure 1**).

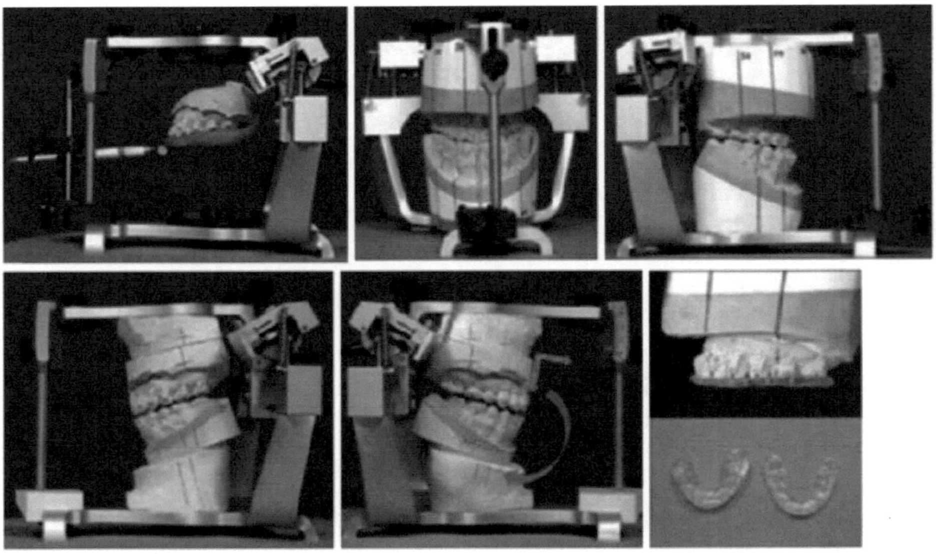

Figure 1.
Plaster models and articulators.

2.2.1 Facebow and articulator mounting

The facebow is employed to transfer the spatial position of the maxilla relative to the cranial base. This tool facilitates the mounting of plaster models in an articulator, replicating the patient's occlusal orientation. However, this procedure is prone to errors, as the facebow does not account for complex three-dimensional asymmetries that may be present in patients with severe craniofacial deformities [13].

2.2.2 Limitations of traditional planning in severe deformities

Conventional planning based on plaster models and two-dimensional tools has significant limitations when applied to patients with severe craniofacial deformities. In complex cases where skeletal structures are severely compromised or asymmetrical, two-dimensional planning and simulation using plaster models often fail to incorporate the complete anatomical information of the entire craniofacial skeleton. The lack of a global, three-dimensional perspective can result in errors in assessing the position and movement of skeletal structures, leading to undesirable variations in surgical outcomes. These errors, arising from the limited ability of plaster models to accurately replicate the patient's anatomical complexity, may cause unfavorable consequences, such as discrepancies in intermaxillary relationships, occlusal plane alignment, post-operative asymmetries, and patient dissatisfaction with the esthetic results [14]. Furthermore, the intricate correction process necessitates the fabrication of one or more surgical splints to guide the repositioning of the maxilla and mandible after their detachment from the cranial base. These splints often exhibit inaccuracies and low reproducibility due to the challenges in managing repositioning lines on plaster models, especially when adjusted based on two-dimensional planning from surgical or orthodontic treatment objectives (virtual treatment objectives (VTO)/surgical treatment objectives (STO)) [15].

2.2.3 The need for advanced solutions

The limitations of traditional planning highlight the necessity for more advanced techniques that incorporate three-dimensional representations of the patient's anatomy.

2.2.4 Digital innovations for comprehensive planning

- Imaging advances: Cone beam computed tomography (CBCT) provides a highly detailed three-dimensional visualization of skeletal structures, enabling an in-depth evaluation of anatomical relationships.

- 3D modeling: Digital models allow for precise simulation of surgical interventions, encompassing assessments of soft tissues, jaw positioning, and dental structures.

- Preoperative digital planning: Advanced digital techniques improve planning accuracy, minimize errors, and enhance the predictability of surgical outcomes.

- Custom surgical splints: Splints fabricated using 3D printing based on virtual models demonstrate superior precision and reliability compared to those created through traditional methods.

2.2.5 Integration of soft tissue analysis

A comprehensive planning approach must extend beyond skeletal evaluation to include facial soft tissues, jaw positioning, and the underlying skeletal structures. This integrated analysis ensures optimal functional and esthetic outcomes, ultimately enhancing patient satisfaction and surgical precision [16].

The adoption of computer-aided workflows represents the future of orthognathic surgery, providing a more comprehensive, precise, and predictable alternative to traditional techniques [17].

2.2.6 Advantages of digitalization

The introduction of digitalization in the field of orthognathic surgery has opened new horizons, making the planning and surgical process more efficient and secure. Beyond the primary benefits already mentioned, several additional clinical and operational advantages can be highlighted.

2.2.7 Enhanced precision and error reduction

Digital planning eliminates many human variables associated with the manual manipulation of models and two-dimensional tools. Advanced algorithms integrated into software platforms enable precise calculations of skeletal movements and allow for accurate predictions of both functional and esthetic outcomes. For instance, in cases involving complex asymmetries or three-dimensional rotations of skeletal bases, digital software provides highly accurate simulations that significantly reduce the risk of post-operative occlusal discrepancies [18].

2.2.8 Customized treatment plans

The digital workflow allows for treatments tailored to the specific needs of each patient. Every surgical intervention is planned according to the patient's unique morphology, incorporating considerations, such as mandibular biomechanics, joint function, and airway dimensions [19]. For example, in patients with obstructive sleep apnea (OSA), digital simulations can evaluate the impact of mandibular advancement on airway patency. This predictive capability ensures that the planned surgical intervention addresses both skeletal discrepancies and functional impairments, resulting in a comprehensive treatment strategy. Digitalization enhances the ability to foresee potential outcomes, providing a level of customization and precision unattainable through traditional methods. This paradigm shift not only improves surgical outcomes but also enhances patient satisfaction and confidence in the treatment process (**Figure 2**).

2.2.9 Speed and time optimization

The automation of multiple stages of treatment planning through digital workflows significantly reduces the time required for preoperative preparation. This translates into the ability to treat a greater number of patients and achieve better organization of surgical schedules. Additionally, rapid simulations enable real-time discussions with patients, improving communication and facilitating shared decision-making [19].

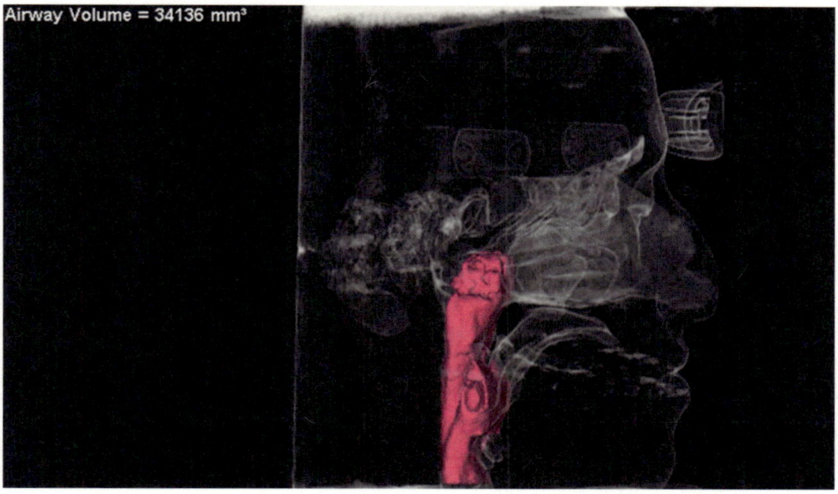

Figure 2.
Customized treatment plans.

2.2.10 Predictability and effective communication

The ability to present patients with a three-dimensional simulation of the planned procedure enhances their understanding of the expected results. This improves patient confidence and actively involves them in the treatment process. Furthermore, the increased predictability of outcomes reduces the likelihood of post-operative revisions, leading to greater overall satisfaction.

2.2.11 Summary of benefits

- Enhanced precision and error reduction
- Customized treatment plans
- Speed and time optimization
- Predictability and effective communication

2.3 Advanced imaging and diagnostic techniques

The use of advanced imaging techniques is a cornerstone of digital treatment planning. These tools provide detailed representations of anatomical structures, enabling precise diagnosis and meticulous surgical planning [20].

2.3.1 CBCT (cone beam computed tomography)

CBCT is considered the gold standard for craniofacial imaging due to its ability to capture high-resolution, three-dimensional images with a lower radiation dose compared to traditional computed tomography. This imaging modality allows for the evaluation of:

- The three-dimensional skeletal morphology.
- The relationships between the maxilla, mandible, and cranial base.
- The airway passages and dental structures with exceptional clarity.

2.3.2 3D intraoral and facial scans

Intraoral scans, obtained using digital scanners, provide virtual models of the dental arches, eliminating the need for traditional physical impressions. These datasets can be integrated with 3D facial scans, which realistically capture the patient's facial features, creating a comprehensive model that combines both skeletal and esthetic morphology [21].

2.3.3 Multimodal integration

The integration of data from CBCT, intraoral scanners, and facial scans results in a unified digital model. This comprehensive model serves as the foundation for surgical analysis and planning, offering a global, three-dimensional view of anatomical structures and occlusal relationships [22]. This advanced approach ensures an accurate and personalized treatment strategy, significantly enhancing the predictability and success of orthognathic surgery (**Figure 3**).

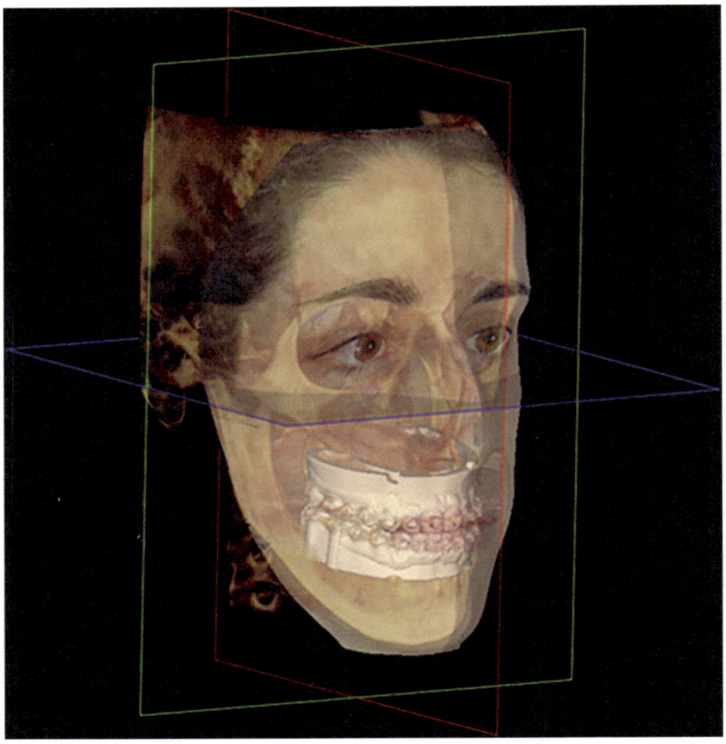

Figure 3.
Multimodal integration.

3. Digital workflow for simulation

3.1 Orthognathic surgery planning for skeletal class III malocclusion

The surgical correction of skeletal Class III malocclusion represents a significant challenge in cranio-maxillofacial surgery. Digital planning has revolutionized the approach to these cases, providing advanced tools to enhance precision, efficiency, and predictability of both esthetic and functional outcomes. This chapter explores the planning techniques, surgical procedures, and key clinical considerations in managing such patients [23–25].

3.2 3D model design for bimaxillary osteotomy

The creation of a three-dimensional (3D) virtual facial model is the foundational step in modern surgical planning. This model integrates data from advanced imaging techniques, allowing for a detailed visualization of craniofacial morphology and precise simulation of the necessary skeletal movements.

3.2.1 Required data inputs

- CBCT of the full craniofacial region
- STL files of the dental arches (3D model)
- 2D frontal facial photographs or facial scans

3.2.2 3D model creation process

1. CBCT (cone beam computed tomography): Provides high-resolution images of skeletal and dental structures while reducing radiation exposure compared to traditional CT scans.
2. STL of the arches: Intraoral scans deliver highly accurate models of dental arches, eliminating the need for physical impressions and improving overall precision.
3. Facial scans: Facial scanners complete the digital dataset by providing surface morphology that integrates seamlessly with CBCT imaging.

Specialized software, such as Dolphin Imaging with its surgical module, combines CBCT data with dental and facial scans to generate a virtual facial model. This model accurately represents the anatomical relationships between hard and soft tissues [26].

3.2.3 Anatomical model segmentation and surgical simulation

In the subsequent step, anatomical 3D models (virtual replicas of the patient's skeletal and dental structures) are segmented, mobilized, and repositioned according to the surgical plan. This involves:

- Precisely identifying osteotomy sites.
- Simulating skeletal movements.
- Evaluating both functional and esthetic impacts of the planned corrections.

The enhanced anatomical detail offered by this workflow minimizes intraoperative errors. The repositioning of anatomical structures is guided by esthetic and functional references (see the section on esthetic analysis), ensuring the restoration of proper functional, esthetic, and dental balance [27].

3.2.4 Real-time simulation and optimization

Digital planning software allows for real-time visualization of three-dimensional surgical simulations, including soft tissue predictions. This capability enables surgeons to simulate and optimize surgical outcomes while improving communication with patients. One of the key advantages of digital planning is its ability to predict esthetic and functional changes, aligning surgical objectives with the patient's specific needs and expectations.

3.2.5 Surgical splint fabrication

The final stage involves the production of a surgical splint (wafer), which is initially generated virtually and then fabricated using 3D printing technologies. These splints, made from biocompatible materials such as photopolymeric resins, serve as precise guides for maxillary and mandibular repositioning. This ensures the safety and efficacy of the surgical procedure [28–30]. The digital workflow not only enhances surgical precision but also streamlines the preoperative process, ultimately improving patient outcomes and satisfaction.

3.2.6 Advantages of the digital workflow

This method offers several advantages:

- Millimetric precision in osteotomies.
- Extreme personalization for patients with complex morphologies.
- Reduced operating times due to detailed preoperative planning.

3.3 Esthetic analysis

The correction of skeletal Class III malocclusion requires complex surgical interventions involving both the maxilla and the mandible. The primary goal is to restore esthetic and functional balance through precise and personalized techniques [31–33].

3.3.1 Role of 3D simulation

3D simulation enables:

- Visualization of facial proportions before and after surgery.

- Identification of disharmonies not evident in 2D examinations.
- Customization of surgical plans to optimize overall facial esthetics.

The visual representation of expected outcomes enhances doctor-patient communication, improving treatment understanding and overall satisfaction. Most importantly, it ensures that the correction of facial proportions, profile balance, and soft tissue harmony aligns with the achievable corrections and patient expectations. Furthermore, it emphasizes the adjustment and stabilization of occlusion, which, according to the author, represents the key element of stability. Achieving a final mandibular position that respects the primary components of the masticatory system, teeth, muscles, and temporomandibular joints (TMJs) is essential.

3.4 Facial proportions

Three-dimensional (3D) simulation is an indispensable tool for analyzing and harmonizing facial proportions. It ensures that surgical outcomes extend beyond skeletal corrections to achieve a balanced and esthetically pleasing appearance [34].

3.5 Facial proportions analysis

3.5.1 Vertical lines

According to Arnett and Gunson, the face is divided into vertical thirds:

- Upper third: From the trichion (hairline) to the glabella.
- Middle third: From the glabella to the base of the nose.
- Lower third: From the base of the nose to the menton.

A disproportionate lower third is a common characteristic in patients with skeletal Class III malocclusion and can be addressed through mandibular and/or maxillary repositioning.

3.5.2 Transverse relationships

The symmetry of the dental arches and the position of the zygomatic bones are assessed to ensure equilibrium between the two sides of the face.

3.5.3 Frontal balance

- The dental midline is compared with the facial midline.
- The width of the nasal base, zygomatic bones, and upper dental arch should be proportional to the lower third of the face.

This comprehensive analysis guarantees that the surgical approach not only corrects skeletal discrepancies but also achieves optimal esthetic and functional outcomes.

3.6 Facial profile

The facial profile is a critical parameter in esthetic evaluation. Orthognathic surgery, particularly in patients with skeletal Class III malocclusion, aims to enhance the projection of the nasolabial profile, chin, and lips [35, 36].

3.6.1 Reference lines

1. Ricketts' esthetic line

   - A line drawn from the nasal tip to the chin tip. Ideally, the upper lip should lie 4 mm behind this line, and the lower lip 2 mm behind [24].

2. Arnett-Gunson analysis

   - Upper lip position: The position of the upper lip relative to the nasal base and the projection of the upper incisors.
   - Chin-neck line: The line connecting the menton to the neck, crucial for assessing the cervico-mental angle, which should range between 105° and 120°.
   - Maxillary position: The position of the maxilla relative to the central face, essential for nasolabial harmony.
   - Soft tissue thickness: The thickness of soft tissues in the perioral and chin regions must be evaluated to predict esthetic outcomes.
   - Dynamic smile analysis: A dynamic assessment of the smile is essential to ensure that movement does not compromise esthetic results.
   - Symmetry and balance: Soft tissues should appear symmetric and harmonized with the underlying skeletal structures.

3. Facial mask

   - Marquardt beauty analysis: Based on biological and mathematical principles, this approach evaluates human visual esthetics.

3.7 Surgical objectives

Virtual skeletal movements were performed according to the following parameters:

- Correction of excessive mandibular projection or maxillary retrusion.
- Achieving balance between the upper and lower lips relative to the esthetic line.
- Improving chin projection, harmonizing the cervico-mental angle.
- Correction of midline discrepancies.

- Correction of the occlusal plane: a downward inclination of the maxilla.
- Adjustment of the anteroposterior position of the maxilla. Specific cephalometric parameters, such as the sella-nasion-A (SNA) angle, were monitored during movement simulations using the software.
- Adjustment of the anteroposterior and vertical position of the mandible.
- Correction of anterior facial proportions.
- Attainment of soft tissue balance.

This systematic approach ensures that both skeletal corrections and soft tissue harmony are achieved, optimizing esthetic and functional outcomes.

3.8 Impact on soft tissues

Skeletal changes induced by orthognathic surgery inevitably influence soft tissues, particularly in the perioral, nasal, and chin regions. A thorough analysis of soft tissue response is essential to ensure an esthetically satisfactory outcome [33, 34].

3.9 Preoperative simulation and evaluation

3.9.1 Perioral tissues

- The projection of the upper and lower lips is simulated based on the repositioning of the maxillary and mandibular incisors.
- The nasolabial angle is optimized during maxillary repositioning to enhance facial harmony.

3.9.2 Nasal tissues

- Maxillary advancement may alter the width of the nasal base. Surgical techniques should account for these changes, potentially integrating rhinoplasty to refine the nasal structure.

3.9.3 Chin region

- Mandibular repositioning affects the position and projection of the chin. Soft tissue analysis is critical to prevent undesirable outcomes, such as an overly prominent or recessed chin [34, 37].

3.9.4 Airway management and soft tissue considerations

- Mandibular setback can reduce airway volume. During planning, airway patency must be evaluated using volumetric analysis software to minimize the risk of post-operative complications.

4. Case report

4.1 Diagnosis and etiology

A 23-year-old female patient presented for orthodontic consultation to address craniofacial dysmorphosis and improve facial appearance and smile esthetics.

Extraoral examination revealed:

- A moderate skeletal Class III malocclusion.
- Pronounced elongation of the lower third of the face, contributing to an aged appearance.
- Thin lips with minimal vermilion show an underdevelopment of the midface region.
- Facial asymmetry in frontal view, characterized by:
  - o Higher labial commissure on the right side.
  - o Chin displacement toward the right.
  - o Hemimandibular elongation on the left side (**Figure 4**).

4.2 Intraoral examination

The intraoral examination revealed a Class III malocclusion with a complete crossbite involving the entire arch, transverse maxillary deficiency, and dental crowding in both arches. The upper midline was centered, while the lower midline was shifted to the right (**Figure 5**: intraoral photographs taken post-expansion achieved with miniscrews). No clinically evident signs or symptoms of temporomandibular dysfunction were reported. A 3D model analysis (TRIOS, 3Shape A/S, Copenhagen, Denmark) was conducted to evaluate occlusal characteristics and identify potential abnormal contacts (**Figure 6**: intraoral scans, post-expansion achieved with miniscrews).

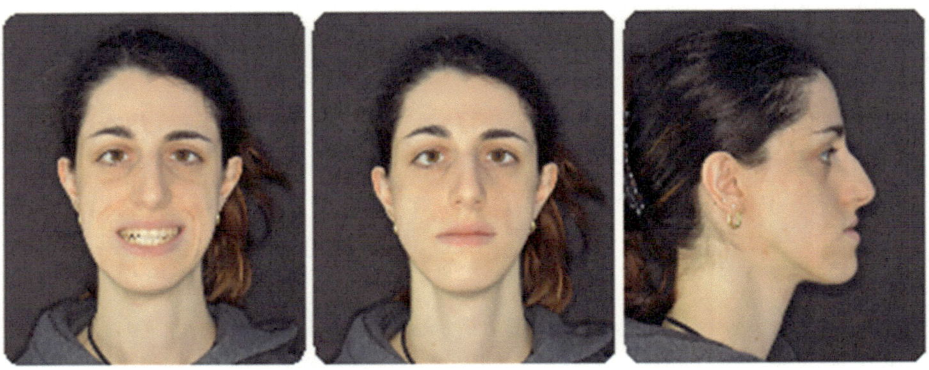

Figure 4.
Intraoral examination.

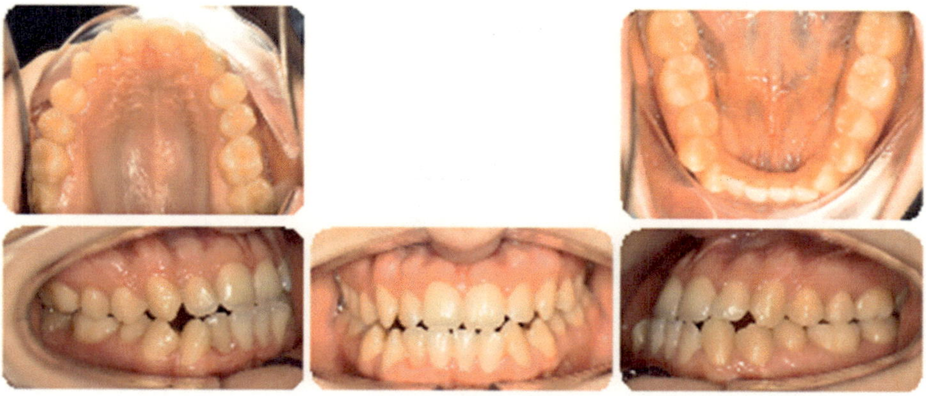

Figure 5.
Intraoral photographs taken post-expansion achieved with miniscrews.

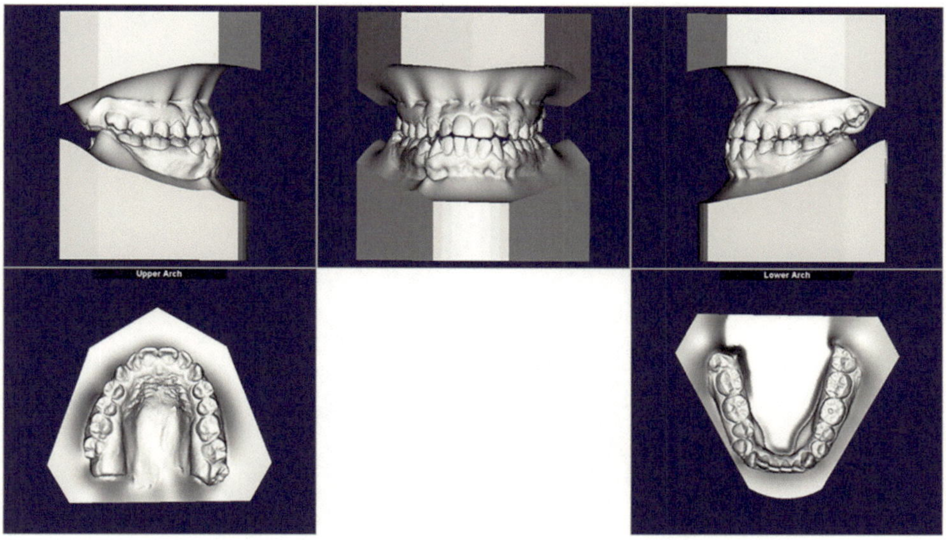

Figure 6.
Intraoral scans, post-expansion achieved with miniscrews.

The panoramic radiograph revealed impaction of both maxillary and mandibular third molars (**Figure 7**). Cephalometric analysis confirmed a severe skeletal Class III malocclusion in a hyperdivergent patient, with the following measurements:

SNA 82°,
SNB 85.2°,
ANB −3.2°,
WITS −9.9,
FMA (MP-FH) 28.1°,
IMPA 77.2°,
MP-SN 39.9°.

A soft tissue cephalometric analysis was also performed to assess the vertical and anteroposterior projection of the lips and other soft tissue components (**Figures 8** and **9**: cephalometric radiograph).

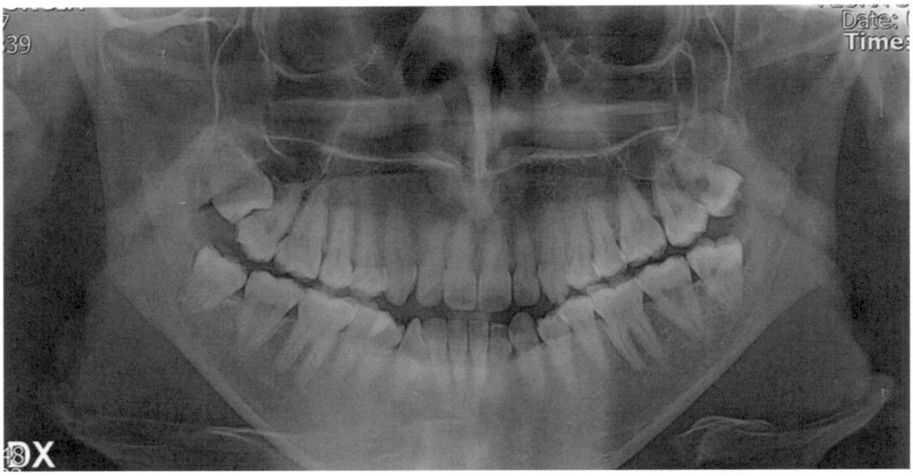

Figure 7.
High-definition intraoral scan with TRIOS (3Shape A/S, Copenhagen, Denmark).

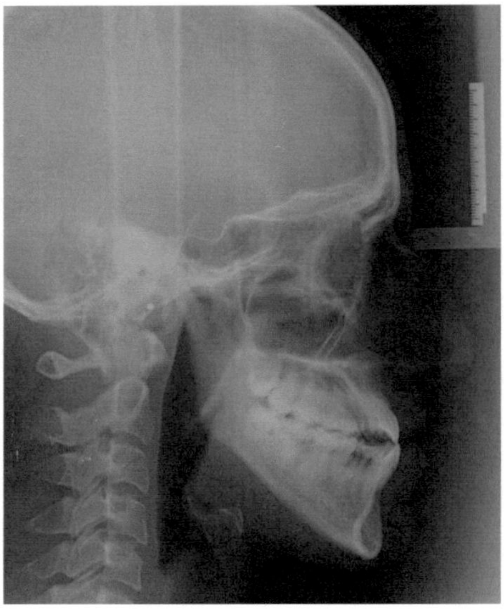

Figure 8.
High-definition intraoral scan with TRIOS (3Shape A/S, Copenhagen, Denmark).

4.3 Treatment objectives

The treatment objectives included:

- Correction of maxillary and mandibular dental crowding.
- Correction of sagittal and transverse skeletal discrepancies to achieve a Class I relationship.
- Enhancement of smile esthetics and facial profile.

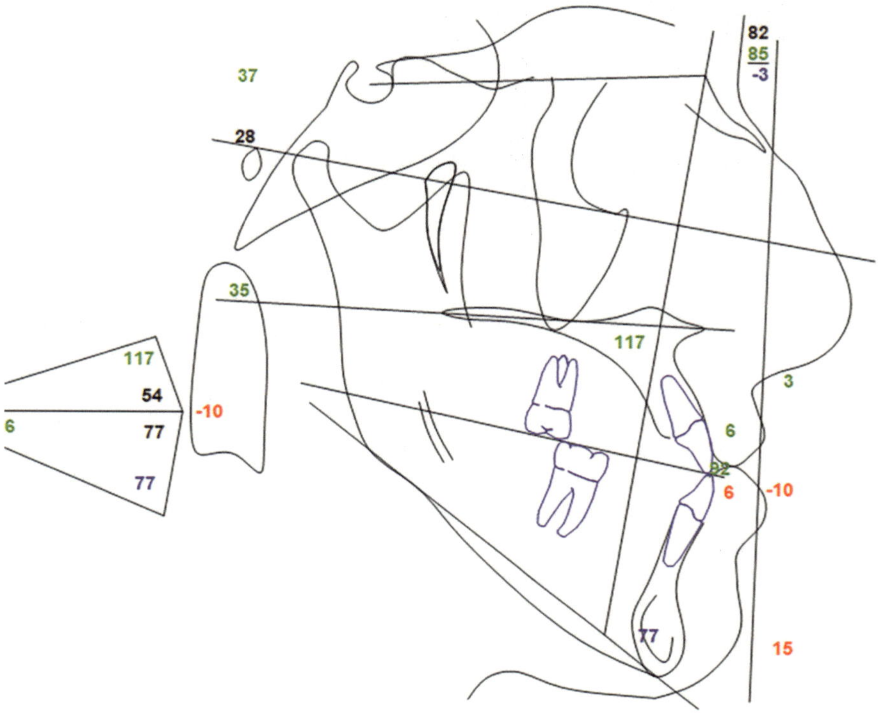

Group/Measurement	Value	Norm	Std Dev	Dev Norm
* HORIZONTAL SKELETAL *				
SNA (°)	82.0	82.0	3.5	-0.0
SNB (°)	85.2	80.0	3.0	1.7 *
ANB (°)	-3.2	2.0	2.4	-2.2 **
Maxillary Skeletal (A-Na Perp) (mm)	3.5	1.0	3.1	0.8
Mand. Skeletal (Pg-Na Perp) (mm)	15.2	-2.0	5.3	3.2 ***
Wits Appraisal (mm)	-9.9	-1.0	1.0	-8.9 ********
* VERTICAL SKELETAL *				
FMA (MP-FH) (°)	28.1	26.0	5.0	0.4
MP - SN (°)	39.9	33.0	6.0	1.2 *
Palatal-Mand Angle (°)	35.0	28.0	6.0	1.2 *
Palatal-Occ Plane (PP-OP) (°)	9.2	10.0	4.0	-0.2
Mand Plane to Occ Plane (°)	25.8	17.4	5.0	1.7 *
Mx occlusal plane (MxOP-Na Perp) (°)	92.3	95.6	1.8	-1.8 *
* ANTERIOR DENTAL *				
U-Incisor Protrusion (U1-APo) (mm)	5.6	6.0	2.2	-0.2
L1 Protrusion (L1-APo) (mm)	6.1	1.0	2.3	2.2 **
U1 - Palatal Plane (°)	116.7	110.0	5.0	1.3 *
U1 - Occ Plane (°)	54.1	57.5	7.0	-0.5
L1 - Occ Plane (°)	77.0	72.0	5.0	1.0 *
IMPA (°)	77.2	95.0	7.0	-2.5 **
Subnasale - ST Menton	63.6	N/A	N/A	N/A
Soft tissue A pt to SnV (mm)	4.3	-2.0	N/A	N/A
Soft tissue B pt to SnV (mm)	-5.0	-5.0	N/A	N/A
Upper lip anterior (ULA - Sn Vertical) (mm)	0.2	3.0	1.0	-2.8 **
Lower lip anterior (LLA - Sn Vertical) (mm)	0.0	1.0	1.0	-1.0 *
Soft tissue Lower lip - Sn-7 (mm)	74.9	N/A	N/A	N/A
Soft tissue Pogonion - Sn-7 (mm)	96.1	N/A	N/A	N/A

Figure 9.
Comprehensive assessment of the patient's craniofacial structures.

4.4 Therapeutic options

Option 1: Orthodontic treatment with multibracket appliances, involving extraction of teeth 3.4 and 4.4, followed by space closure and resolution of maxillary dental crowding. However, this option would not improve the midface profile or address the skeletal Class III discrepancy as required by the patient.

Option 2: Miniscrew-assisted rapid maxillary expansion (MARPE) to correct the transverse maxillary deficiency, combined with the application of miniplates in the lower arch to manage the Class III correction using intermaxillary elastics. However, given the extent of sagittal discrepancy and the patient's age, this approach would not meet the patient's esthetic expectations.

Option 3: Combined orthodontic-surgical treatment, beginning with multibracket therapy to decompensate the skeletal discrepancy, followed by maxillofacial surgery including Le Fort I and bilateral sagittal split osteotomy (BSSO) for skeletal correction. However, this option would not provide adequate transverse expansion of the midface, limiting treatment to sagittal and vertical skeletal imbalances.

Option 4: Surgically assisted rapid palatal expansion (SARPE) to address transverse maxillary dimensions, followed by combined orthodontic-surgical treatment with maxillofacial surgery (Le Fort I and BSSO).

Patient's decision. The patient, supported by her parents, opted for the fourth treatment option to address dentoskeletal discrepancies, asymmetry, esthetic concerns, and dental crowding. Informed consent was obtained for the chosen treatment plan and the use of sensitive data. As part of the preparatory phase, the maxillary and mandibular third molars were extracted to facilitate surgical osteotomies, as well as repositioning and fixation maneuvers.

5. Orthodontic sequence

5.1 Phase 1: Maxillary expansion with MARPE

The initial phase of treatment involved miniscrew-assisted rapid palatal expansion (MARPE), which utilizes skeletal anchorage for expansion without surgical release of resistance sites, combined with the application of orthopedic forces [38, 39]. Virtual insertion of the miniscrews was planned using Dolphin software. Subsequently, Appliance Designer (TRIOS, 3Shape A/S, Copenhagen, Denmark) was used to design a surgical guide for precise miniscrew placement. Concurrently, intraoral scans (TRIOS, 3Shape A/S, Copenhagen, Denmark) were sent to a digital orthodontic laboratory for the fabrication of a HYRAX maxillary expander. The device featured bands on teeth 1.6 and 2.6, with extended arms reaching the second molars, positioned 1 mm above the gingival margin. The procedure was conducted in the surgical unit of a private dental clinic in Catania. Conscious intravenous sedation, administered by an experienced anesthesiologist, was utilized to minimize intraoperative stress. Local infiltration anesthesia with articaine was applied in the retroincisal area. Following this, the surgical guide was used for pilot drilling at 200 rpm (revolutions per minute) with irrigation and a torque of 60 N/m. Two miniscrews, measuring 2 mm in diameter and 13 mm in length (HDC, Thiene, Italy), were inserted using a surgical micromotor at 50 rpm and a torque of 20 N/m. No osteotomies were performed. The device was cemented with glass ionomer cement (KETAC, 3 M, Saint Paul, MN, USA) immediately after the miniscrew insertion. Post-operatively, the expander screw was activated four times, followed by one daily activation until the screw was fully opened (10 mm). Upon completion of activation, the screw was secured with 0.010-inch passive stainless-steel ligatures. After a six-month retention period, the appliance and miniscrews were removed. A comprehensive orthodontic follow-up was performed, including intraoral and extraoral photographs, intraoral scanning, and radiographic evaluations (panoramic and lateral cephalometric radiographs) [40, 41]. A self-ligating 0.022-inch fixed appliance with Damon prescription (Ormco, Orange, CA, USA) was placed on the labial surface of all erupted teeth. Both maxillary and mandibular arches were treated using the same archwire sequence: 0.014 Cu 155 NiTi, 0.018 Cu NiTi, 0.014 × 0.025 Cu NiTi, 0.018 × 0.025 NiTi, 0.017 × 0.025 TMA, and 0.019 × 0.025 SS with stops (**Figure 10**). This wire sequence facilitated alignment, leveling, and coordination of the arches, preparing them for the presurgical phase with rigid stainless steel (SS) archwires. The combination of self-ligating brackets and thermally activated NiTi wires created a biomechanical system that delivered low-force levels, enabling dentoalveolar discrepancy correction without causing iatrogenic damage to the periodontal tissues. Once the orthodontic archwire sequence was completed—ensuring full transfer of the bracket prescription and correcting all dentoalveolar compensations in both transverse and sagittal planes—a thorough presurgical diagnostic workup was initiated. This critical step included high-definition intraoral scans with TRIOS (3Shape A/S, Copenhagen, Denmark) (**Figures 7** and **8**) and a CBCT scan with a large field of view (FOV) to obtain a comprehensive assessment of the patient's craniofacial structures (**Figure 9**).

5.2 Acquisition and integration of patient data

The acquired data were imported into the Dolphin 3D Surgery module, where high-resolution intraoral scans and CBCT images were meticulously aligned to create a detailed virtual model of the patient's craniofacial anatomy, integrated with high-resolution dental arches. This integration combines all anatomical and dental

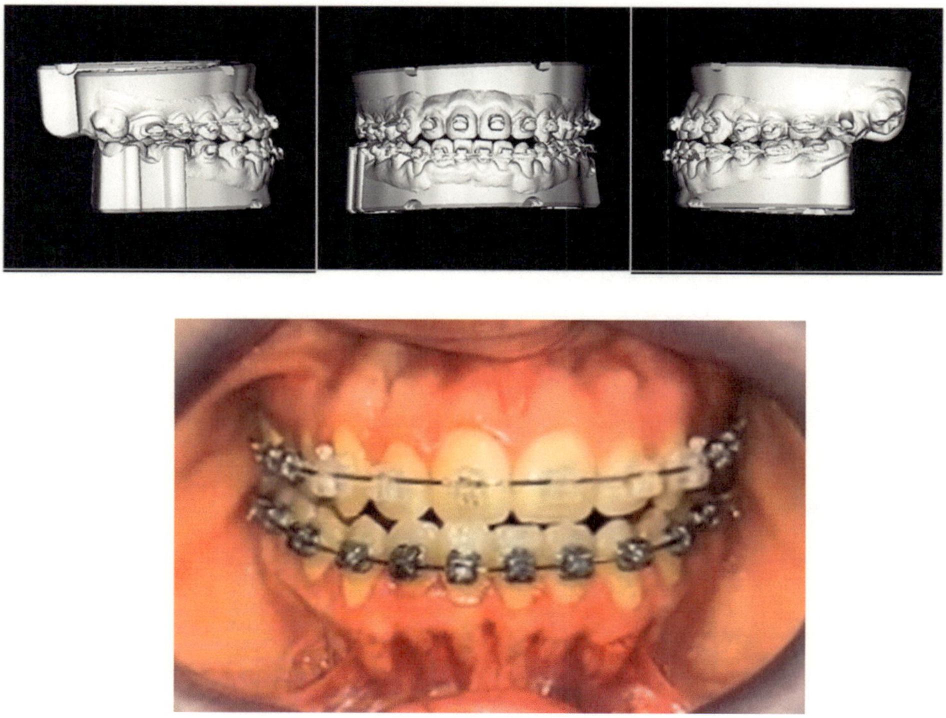

Figure 10.
Splints.

information into a single representation, providing the surgical team with a comprehensive foundation for treatment planning.

5.3 Integration of photographs and patient feature assessment

An additional level of detail was achieved by integrating the patient's extraoral frontal photographs with the 3D reconstructed cranial model. This approach facilitates a holistic assessment of skeletal and soft tissue characteristics (Supplementary Figures 2–4). This functionality allowed the team to accurately simulate jaw movements and predict the esthetic and functional impact of the surgical procedure, thus enhancing the precision of the planning process.

5.4 Virtual treatment objectives (VTO)

The virtual planning was executed using the Dolphin 3D Surgery module, guided by the objectives outlined by the orthodontist and surgeon. A complete iconographic workflow of the digital orthognathic surgery planning process using Dolphin 3D Surgery software has been documented comprehensively [42, 43].

6. Design and prototyping of surgical splints

Once the optimal final positions of the maxilla and mandible were determined, the "Splint Tool" in Dolphin 3D software was used to design intermediate and final digital splints. These splints included specific fixation holes for intermaxillary fixation (**Figure 10(a)**) and were customized according to the treatment plan

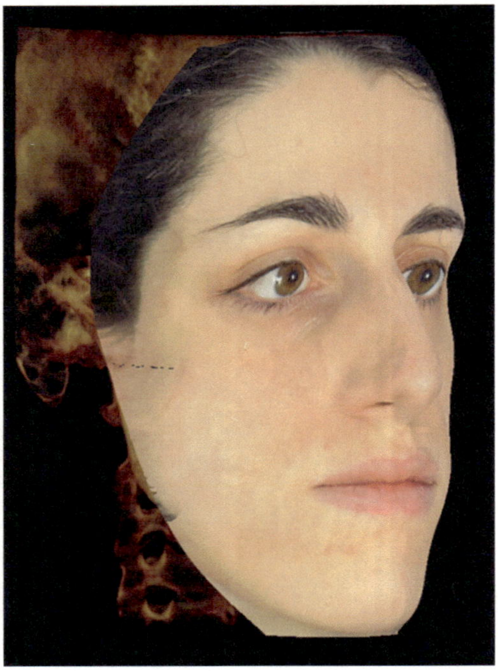

Figure 11.
The STL files exported for final prototyping.

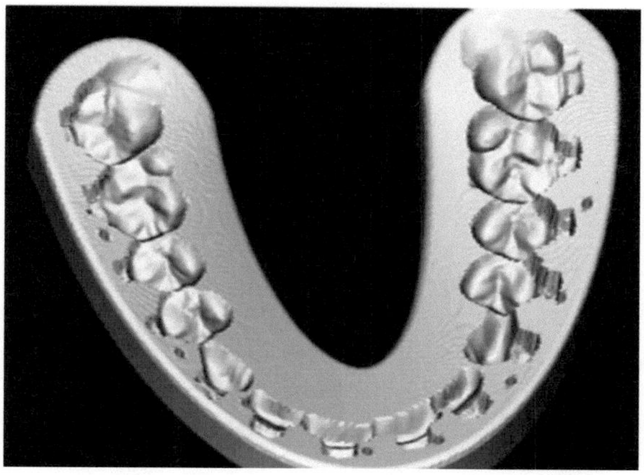

Figure 12.
Digital splints were prototyped using a FORMLAB 3D printer (SLA technology, FORMLAB, Somerville, MA, USA) with a biocompatible transparent resin (Surgical Guide Resin) at a layer thickness of 50 μm.

parameters, such as width, thickness, and other functional characteristics. The STL files generated were exported for final prototyping (**Figure 11**). Custom surgical guides, essential for transferring the virtual plan to the operating table, were designed using advanced software and fabricated with 3D printing technology. These tools significantly enhance surgical precision and efficacy. Digital splints were prototyped using a FORMLAB 3D printer (SLA technology, FORMLAB, Somerville, MA, USA) with a biocompatible transparent resin (Surgical Guide Resin) at a layer thickness of 50 μm (**Figure 12**). The post-curing process followed the manufacturer's guidelines to ensure the stability and safety of the surgical instruments.

7. Surgical procedure and post-operative rehabilitation

The surgical intervention followed the detailed digital plan, employing Le Fort I and BSSO (bilateral sagittal split osteotomy) approaches to correct skeletal dysmorphisms. Final stabilization was achieved using rigid plates and screws to ensure long-term stability [44, 45].

7.1 Pre-surgical preparation

The digitization process streamlines and optimizes intraoperative workflows, ensuring accurate alignment between the virtual plan and the surgical procedure. Surgical guides were sterilized, adapted to the patient before surgery, and cross-verified against the virtual model and surgical plan (**Figures 13** and **14**). The guides were temporarily fixed to dental structures using fixation wires, guiding the precise angle and depth of osteotomy cuts.

8. Bimaxillary osteotomy techniques

8.1 Le fort I osteotomy procedure

An intraoral incision provided access to the maxilla. The osteotomy was performed above the dental apices to separate the maxilla from the cranial base, improving soft

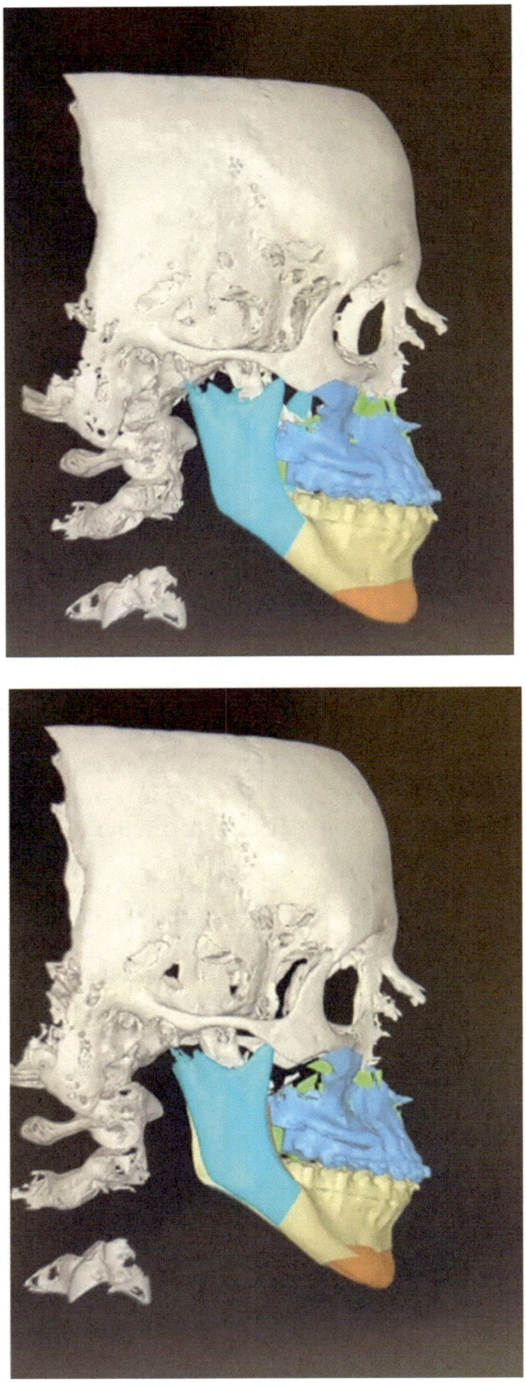

Figure 13.
Pre-surgical preparation.

tissue support, correcting the occlusal relationship, and optimizing facial esthetics. Additionally, lateral cuts extending through the zygomatic process of the maxilla were made to achieve three-dimensional enhancement of the zygomatic region, resulting in volumetric improvement (**Figure 15**).

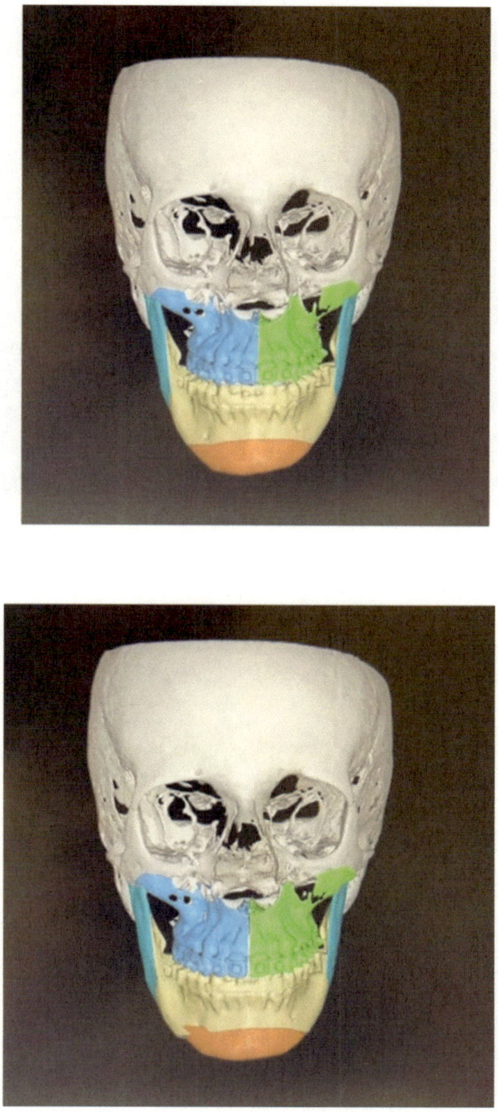

Figure 14.
Pre-surgical preparation.

8.2 Bilateral sagittal split osteotomy (BSSO). Procedure

The osteotomy was performed along the mandibular ramus, enabling anteroposterior repositioning of the mandible. Stability of the osteotomized segments was ensured with rigid plates and miniscrews, achieving ideal occlusion, maintaining facial symmetry, and ensuring long-term stability. Simultaneous genioplasty involved repositioning the symphysis, secured with plates and screws. The esthetic impact on soft tissues, particularly in the chin and lower lip region, was evaluated during 3D simulations to ensure harmonious outcomes. Following soft tissue healing, the patient underwent a personalized 8-week home physiotherapy program aimed at improving phonation, mastication, and joint mobility. This regimen was complemented by progressive exercises to restore joint function and enhance neuromuscular adaptation (**Figure 16**).

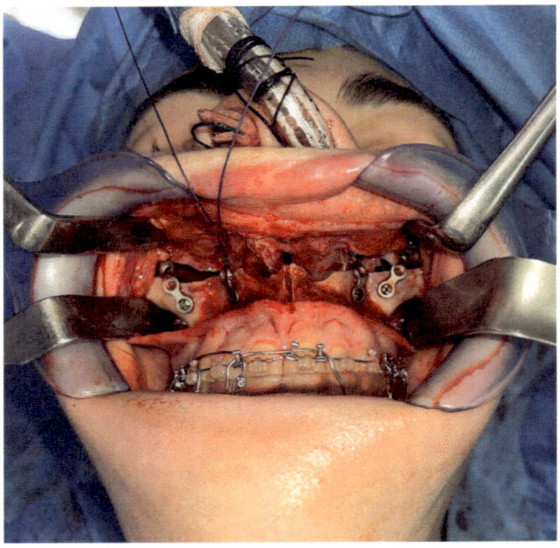

Figure 15.
Lateral cuts extending through the zygomatic process of the maxilla were made to achieve three-dimensional enhancement of the zygomatic region, resulting in volumetric improvement.

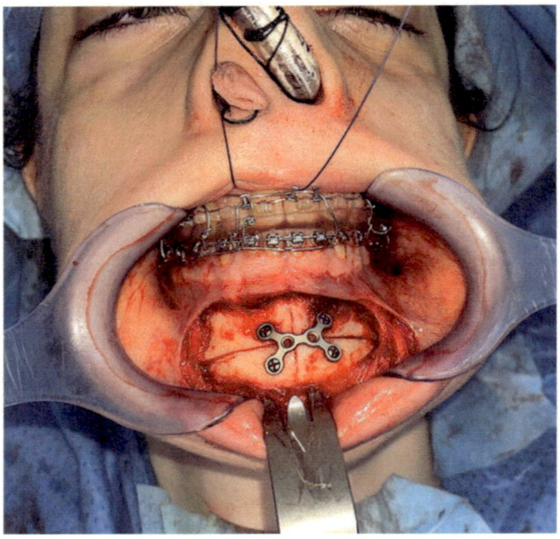

Figure 16.
Bilateral sagittal split osteotomy (BSSO).

9. Post-operative management

- Skin quality and soft tissue retraction were monitored to ensure optimal recovery.
- Complementary esthetic treatments, such as fillers or non-invasive lifting, were considered to optimize outcomes (**Figure 17**).

10. Final phase and retention

Post-treatment records highlighted significant improvements in both skeletal and dentoalveolar parameters. Specifically, facial photographs demonstrated a notable

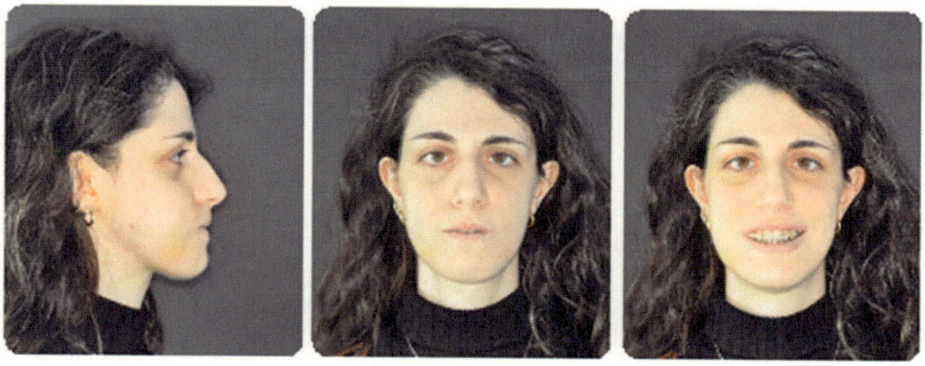

Figure 17.
Post-operative management.

enhancement in the patient's smile and overall facial esthetics (**Figures 11–15**). A comparison between pre- and post-treatment lateral cephalometric radiographs revealed that the hyperdivergent skeletal pattern (long face) was corrected to a normodivergent sagittal plane, with a significant improvement in the ratio of anterior to posterior facial heights. On the frontal plane, facial proportions now adhere to the facial golden ratio (**Figure 16**). Final cephalometric analysis illustrated the treatment's impact through both orthodontic and surgical interventions. Corrections and normalization of previously aberrant cephalometric values were achieved:

- SNA: 83° (82°)
- SNB: 83.7° (85.2°)
- ANB: 0.2° (−3.2°)
- WITS: −7.2 (−9.9)
- FMA (MP-FH): 28.1° (28.1°)
- IMPA: 83.7° (77.2°)
- MP-SN: 31.9° (39.9°)

These improvements extended beyond skeletal components, encompassing esthetic and soft tissue enhancements. Soft tissues are now well proportioned and aligned with current standards. The superimposition of pre- and post-treatment radiographs demonstrates the effectiveness of combining orthognathic surgery and orthodontic treatment in this case (**Figure 17**). Final panoramic radiographs reveal adequate root parallelism and the absence of significant root resorption (**Figure 15**). Final models and intraoral photographs confirm Class I canine relationships with normalized overjet and overbite, achieving proper incisal and canine guidance. The resolution of crowding was accomplished without proclination of incisors or periodontal compromise (**Figure 18A,B**). The new maxillary position improved the frontal exposure of the incisal group and restored muscle tone to the upper lip, which now appears well balanced in both frontal and lateral views, with preserved and enhanced lip competence. Ten months post-surgery, the treatment was concluded with intermaxillary elastics to optimize intercuspation and occlusal harmony, complemented

(a)

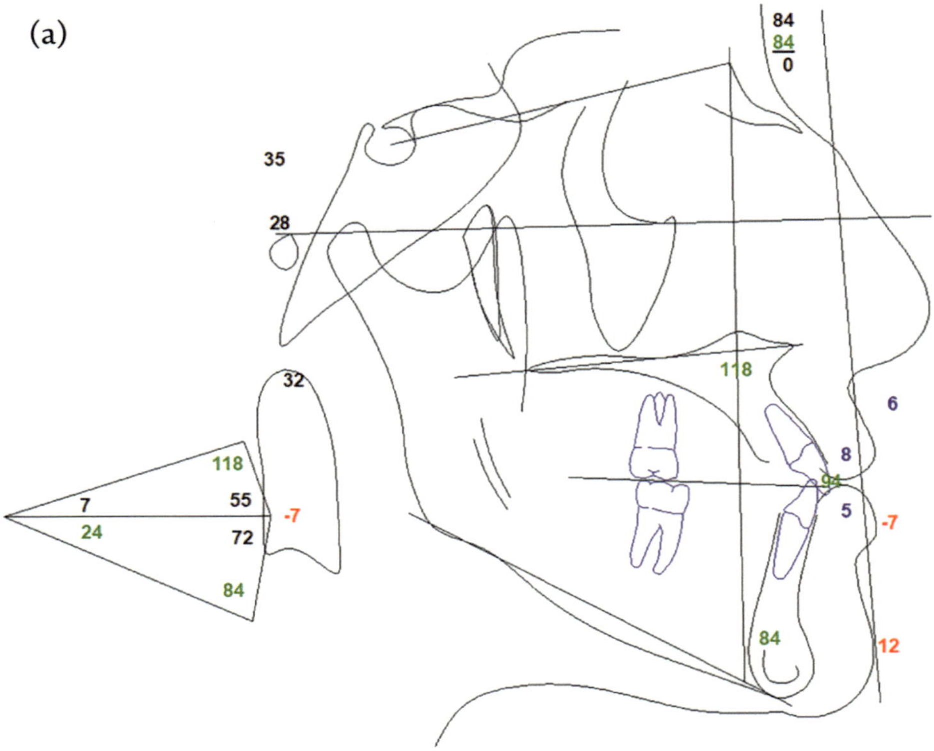

(b)

Group/Measurement	Value	Norm	Std Dev	Dev Norm
* HORIZONTAL SKELETAL *				
SNA (°)	83.8	82.0	3.5	0.5
SNB (°)	83.7	80.0	3.0	1.2 *
ANB (°)	0.2	2.0	2.4	-0.8
Maxillary Skeletal (A-Na Perp) (mm)	6.0	1.0	3.1	1.6 *
Mand. Skeletal (Pg-Na Perp) (mm)	12.2	-2.0	5.3	2.7 **
Wits Appraisal (mm)	-7.2	-1.0	1.0	-6.2 ******
* VERTICAL SKELETAL *				
FMA (MP-FH) (°)	28.1	26.0	5.0	0.4
MP - SN (°)	40.1	33.0	6.0	1.2 *
Palatal-Mand Angle (°)	31.9	28.0	6.0	0.7
Palatal-Occ Plane (PP-OP) (°)	7.5	10.0	4.0	-0.6
Mand Plane to Occ Plane (°)	24.4	17.4	5.0	1.4 *
Mx occlusal plane (MxOP-Na Perp) (°)	93.7	95.6	1.8	-1.1 *
* ANTERIOR DENTAL *				
U-Incisor Protrusion (U1-APo) (mm)	7.5	6.0	2.2	0.7
L1 Protrusion (L1-APo) (mm)	5.4	1.0	2.3	1.9 *
U1 - Palatal Plane (°)	118.0	110.0	5.0	1.6 *
U1 - Occ Plane (°)	54.5	57.5	7.0	-0.4
L1 - Occ Plane (°)	71.9	72.0	5.0	-0.0
IMPA (°)	83.7	95.0	7.0	-1.6 *
Subnasale - ST Menton	64.3	N/A	N/A	N/A
Soft tissue A pt to SnV (mm)	5.6	-2.0	N/A	N/A
Soft tissue B pt to SnV (mm)	0.3	-5.0	N/A	N/A
Upper lip anterior (ULA - Sn Vertical) (mm)	3.5	3.0	1.0	0.5
Lower lip anterior (LLA - Sn Vertical) (mm)	3.8	1.0	1.0	2.8 **
Soft tissue Lower lip - Sn-7 (mm)	83.2	N/A	N/A	N/A
Soft tissue Pogonion - Sn-7 (mm)	106.0	N/A	N/A	N/A

Figure 18.
The resolution of crowding was accomplished without proclination of incisors or periodontal compromise.

by finishing arches to refine occlusal details. For retention, permanent splints were placed in both the upper and lower arches, and an Essix® retainer was prescribed for nighttime use to ensure maintenance of the achieved results (**Figure 19**). This combination of traditional and digital approaches enabled predictable, personalized outcomes, significantly enhancing the patient's experience and optimizing clinical results. The comprehensive treatment plan successfully met all objectives, leaving the patient satisfied with the esthetic, functional, and masticatory outcomes. The total treatment duration was 30 months (**Figure 20**). Post-operative monitoring and follow-up are critical phases for the long-term success of orthognathic surgery. Digital technologies not only facilitate outcome evaluation but also provide predictive and corrective tools to further enhance treatment efficacy. Post-surgery, it is essential to monitor healing and evaluate the correspondence between planned and achieved results (**Figure 21**). Outcome verification and any discrepancies between planning workflows and surgical execution are analyzed using post-operative CBCT scans or traditional orthodontic radiographic kits (panoramic radiographs, lateral cephalograms, and posteroanterior (PA) cephalograms), facial scans or photographs, and dental scans [46, 47].

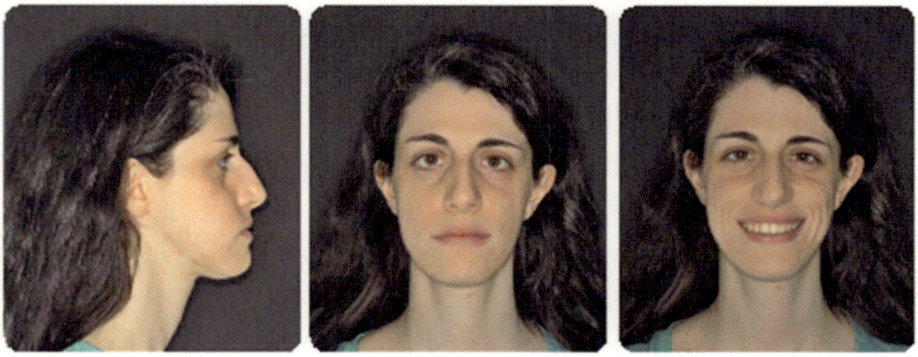

Figure 19.
Retention.

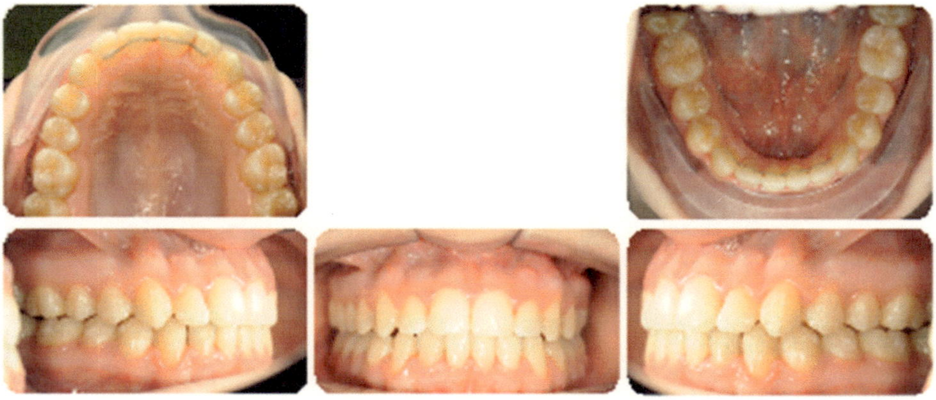

Figure 20.
Treatment duration.

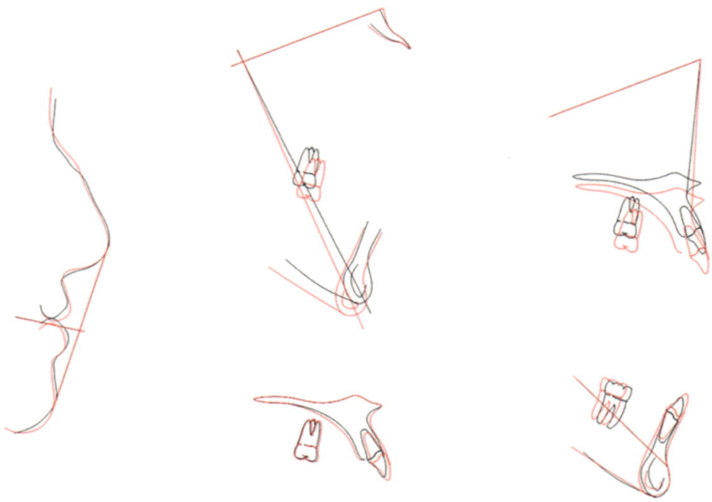

Figure 21.
Monitoring healing.

Our surgical protocols include the following follow-up procedures:

1. Initial follow-up (1–2 weeks post-operatively): Verification of incision healing and initial skeletal stability.

2. Intermediate follow-up (3–6 months): Evaluation of bone consolidation and adaptation of soft tissues.

3. Long-term assessment (1 year or more): Monitoring of skeletal stability and final esthetic results.

Surgical outcome stability is influenced by biomechanical, biological, and behavioral factors. Digital planning provides significant advantages in predicting and managing long-term stability.

11. Stability analysis

- Skeletal movements: Monitoring potential relapses through comparative analysis of pre- and post-operative 3D models.

- Soft tissue adaptation: Evaluation of soft tissue response relative to the new skeletal morphology.

- Dental occlusion: Occlusal control plays a vital role in overall stability.

11.1 Clinical studies

Numerous studies demonstrate that digital planning reduces relapse risk in patients with skeletal Class III malocclusion. Authors have highlighted that the use of customized surgical guides improves mandibular positioning accuracy, enhancing long-term stability [48, 49].

12. Conclusions

The application of a digitized workflow represents a true revolution in cranio-maxillofacial surgery, enabling precise planning and safe execution of complex procedures. Through the use of customized guides and advanced digital tools, predictable and optimized outcomes tailored to individual patient needs are ensured.

12.1 Enhancing treatment quality

- Operational precision: Planning and simulating each procedural phase minimizes errors and improves surgical outcomes.
- Reduced timelines: Digital processes, such as the production of customized surgical guides via 3D printing, shorten preparation and operative times.
- Minimized invasiveness: Detailed planning allows for more conservative approaches, limiting the impact on both soft and skeletal tissues.
- Lower complication rates: Advanced technologies enable more effective management of intra- and post-operative risks.
- Personalized treatment: Patients benefit from a highly tailored approach that accounts for their specific anatomical characteristics and esthetic expectations, increasing satisfaction and trust in the surgeon.

The landscape of cranio-maxillofacial surgery is undergoing dynamic evolution, driven by the integration of digital technologies. Innovations in diagnostics, planning, and clinical application provide new opportunities to enhance accuracy, efficiency, and safety in surgical interventions, paving the way for increasingly predictable and individualized outcomes.

12.2 Future perspectives

- Artificial intelligence (AI): AI applications promise to optimize surgical planning, providing more accurate simulations through machine learning algorithms.
- Augmented reality (AR) and virtual reality (VR): Emerging tools enable surgeons to visualize and interact with 3D models in real time during procedures.
- Robotic assistance: Robotic surgery, already used in some fields, could be further implemented to enhance precision and reduce invasiveness.
- Advanced imaging technologies: High-resolution imaging systems and dynamic scanning technologies may offer even more detailed visualization of craniofacial structures and soft tissues.

The future of cranio-maxillofacial surgery lies in the continued integration of digital technologies, with the potential to redefine standards of care. Advances toward more interactive, personalized, and precise approaches will not only improve clinical efficacy but also strengthen the surgeon's role as a guide in an increasingly patient-centered process.

Acknowledgements

True success is never achieved in isolation; it is the result of unwavering determination, the pursuit of excellence, and the support of a strong foundation. To my family, whose steadfast encouragement and belief in my journey have been my anchor, I owe my deepest gratitude. Your presence has been the silent force behind every milestone. As Aristotle wisely said, *"We are what we repeatedly do. Excellence, then, is not an act but a habit."* This work is a testament to the relentless dedication to that principle, guided by a vision of continuous improvement and an unyielding commitment to progress. To my mentors, colleagues, and collaborators, who have inspired and challenged me to refine my skills and expand my horizons, thank you for sharing in this journey of growth and discovery. Together, we create not just success, but a legacy of excellence.

Conflict of interest

The authors declare no conflict of interest.

Abbreviations

SARPE	surgically assisted rapid palatal expansion
VTO	virtual treatment objectives
CBCT	cone beam computed tomography
BSSO	bilateral sagittal split osteotomy
3D	three-dimensional
CAD-CAM	computer-aided drafting-computer-aided manufacturing
FOV	field of view
AP	anteroposterior
SS	stainless steel
MARPE	microimplant-assisted rapid palatal expansion.

Author details

Orazio Bennici[1*] and Gloria Francesca Pia Bennici[2]

1 Orthodontics, Private Practice, Catania, Italy

2 Independent Researcher, Catania University, Italy

*Address all correspondence to: odontomax@tiscali.it

References

[1] Plooij JM, Maal TJ, Haers P, Borstlap WA, Kuijpers-Jagtman AM, Berge SJ. Digital three-dimensional image fusion processes for planning and evaluating orthodontics and orthognathic surgery. A systematic review. International Journal of Oral and Maxillofacial Surgery. 2011;**40**(4):341-352

[2] Tonin RH, Iwaki Filho L, Yamashita AL, et al. Accuracy of 3D virtual surgical planning for maxillary positioning and orientation in orthognathic surgery. Orthodontics and Craniofacial Research. 2020;**23**(2):229-236

[3] Chen Z, Mo S, Fan X, You Y, Ye G, Zhou N. A meta-analysis and systematic review comparing the effectiveness of traditional and virtual surgical planning for orthognathic surgery: Based on randomized clinical trials. Journal of Oral and Maxillofacial Surgery. 2021;**79**:471 e471-471 e419

[4] Baan F, van Meggelen EM, Verhulst AC, Bruggink R, Xi T, Maal TJJ. Virtual occlusion in orthognathic surgery. International Journal of Oral and Maxillofacial Surgery. 2021;**50**(9):1219-1225

[5] Arnett GW, Jelic JS, Kim J, et al. Soft tissue cephalometric analysis: Diagnosis and treatment planning of dentofacial deformity. American Journal of Orthodontics and Dentofacial Orthopedics. 1999;**116**(3):239-253

[6] Elnagar MH, Aronovich S, Kusnoto B. Digital workflow for combined orthodontics and orthognathic surgery. Oral and Maxillofacial Surgery Clinics of North America. 2020;**32**(1):1-14

[7] Alkhayer A, Piffko J, Lippold C, Segatto E. Accuracy of virtual planning in orthognathic surgery: A systematic review. Head and Face Medicine. 2020;**16**(1):34

[8] Schneider D, Kammerer PW, Hennig M, Schon G, Thiem DGE, Bschorer R. Customized virtual surgical planning in bimaxillary orthognathic surgery: A prospective randomized trial. Clinical Oral Investigations. 2019;**23**(7):3115-3122

[9] Steinbacher DM, Kontaxis KL. Does simultaneous third molar extraction increase intraoperative and perioperative complications in orthognathic surgery? The Journal of Craniofacial Surgery. 2016;**27**(4):923-926

[10] Hernandez-Alfaro F, Mareque Bueno J, Diaz A, Pagés CM. Minimally invasive surgically assisted rapid palatal expansion with limited approach under sedation: A report of 283 consecutive cases. Journal of Oral and Maxillofacial Surgery. 2010;**68**(9):2154-2158

[11] Tecco S, Di Iorio D, Cordasco G, Verrocchi I, Festa F. An in vitro investigation of the influence of self-ligating brackets, low friction ligatures, and archwire on frictional resistance. European Journal of Orthodontics. 2007;**29**(4):390-397

[12] Cozzani M, Sadri D, Nucci L, Jamilian P, Pirhadirad AP, Jamilian A. The effect of Alexander, Gianelly, Roth, and MBT bracket systems on anterior retraction: A 3-dimensional finite element study. Clinical Oral Investigations. 2020;**24**(3):1351-1357

[13] Carlson C, Sung J, Mccomb RW, Machado AW, Moon W. Microimplant-assisted rapid palatal expansion appliance to orthopedically correct

transverse maxillary deficiency in an adult. American Journal of Orthodontics and Dentofacial Orthopedics. 2016;**149**(5):716-728

[14] Baik H-S, Kang Y-G, Choi YJ. Miniscrew-assisted rapid palatal expansion: A review of recent reports. Journal Case Reports in Dentistry of the World Federation of Orthodontists. 2020;**9**(3S):S54-S58

[15] Carvalho PHA, Moura LB, Trento GS, et al. Surgically assisted rapid maxillary expansion: A systematic review of complications. International Journal of Oral and Maxillofacial Surgery. 2020;**49**(3):325-332

[16] Ludlow JB, Timothy R, Walker C, et al. Effective dose of dental CBCT-a meta-analysis of published data and additional data for nine CBCT units. Dentomaxillofacial Radiology. 2015;**44**(1):20140197

[17] Leonardi R, Aboulazm K, Lo Giudice A, et al. Evaluation of mandibular changes after rapid maxillary expansion: A CBCT study in youngsters with unilateral posterior crossbite using a surface-to-surface matching technique. Clinical Oral Investigations. 2021;**25**(4):1775-1785

[18] Lo Giudice A, Ronsivalle V, Spampinato C, Leonardi R. Fully automatic segmentation of the mandible based on convolutional neural networks (CNNs). Orthodontics and Cranio-Facial Research. 2021;**24**(S2):100-107

[19] Lin H-H, Lonic D, Lo L-J. 3D printing in orthognathic surgery—A literature review. Journal of the Formosan Medical Association. 2018;**117**(7):547-558

[20] Leonardi R, Muraglie S, Lo Giudice A, Aboulazm KS, Nucera R. Evaluation of mandibular symmetry and morphology in adult patients with unilateral posterior crossbite: A CBCT study using a surface-to-surface matching technique. European Journal of Orthodontics. 2020;**pii**:cjz106

[21] Leonardi R, Muraglie S, Bennici O, Cavallini C, Spampinato C. Three-dimensional analysis of mandibular functional units in adult patients with unilateral posterior crossbite: A cone beam study with the use of mirroring and surface-to-surface matching techniques. The Angle Orthodontist. 2019;**89**(4):590-596. DOI: 10.2319/081718-607.1. Epub 2019 Apr 23

[22] Chin SJ, Wilde F, Neuhaus M, Schramm A, Gellrich NC, Rana M. Accuracy of virtual surgical planning of orthognathic surgery with aid of CAD/CAM fabricated surgical splint-a novel 3D analyzing algorithm. Journal of Cranio-Maxillo-Facial Surgery. 2017;**45**(12):1962-1970

[23] Bennici O, Malgioglio A, Moschitto S, Spagnuolo G, Greco Lucchina A, Ronsivalle V, et al. Case report, a full computerized workflow for planning surgically assisted rapid palatal expansion and orthognathic surgery in a skeletal class III patient. Case Reports in Dentistry (Hindawi). 2022;**2022**:6413898, 18

[24] Ricketts RM. The wisdom of the bioprogressive philosophy. Seminars in Orthodontics. 1998;**4**(4):201-209. DOI: 10.1016/s1073-8746(98)80025-x

[25] Ronsivalle V, Venezia P, Bennici OM, D'Antò V, Leonardi R, Giudice AL. Accuracy of digital workflow for placing orthodontic miniscrews using generic and licensed open systems. A 3d imaging analysis of non-native. Stl files for guided protocols. BMC Oral Health. 2023;**23**:494

[26] Lerario F, Roncati M, Gariffo A, et al. Non-surgical periodontal treatment of peri-implant diseases with the adjunctive use of diode laser: Preliminary clinical study. Laser in Medical Science. 2016;**31**(1):1-6

[27] d'Apuzzo F, Minervini G, Grassia V, Rotolo RP, Perillo L, Nucci L. Mandibular coronoid process hypertrophy: Diagnosis and 20-year follow-up with CBCT, MRI and EMG evaluations. Applied Sciences. 2021;**11**(10):4504

[28] Lo Giudice A, Quinzi V, Ronsivalle V, Martina S, Bennici O, Isola G. Description of a digital workflow for CBCT-guided construction of micro-implant supported maxillary skeletal expander. Materials (Basel). 2020;**13**(8):1815. DOI: 10.3390/ma13081815

[29] De Felice ME, Nucci L, Fiori A, Flores-Mir C, Perillo L, Grassia V. Accuracy of interproximal enamel reduction during clear aligner treatment. Progress in Orthodontics. 2020;**28**(21):28

[30] Arnett GW, Gunson MJ, McLaughlin RP. The future of Orthognathic surgery: Computer-assisted 3D planning. International Journal of Oral and Maxillofacial Surgery. 2008;**37**(4):323-334

[31] Raffaini M, Magri A. Stability of class III orthognathic surgery: Digital planning versus traditional approaches. Journal of Cranio-Maxillofacial Surgery. 2021;**49**(7):905-912

[32] Swennen GRJ et al. Three-dimensional cephalometric analysis: A novel method for orthognathic surgery planning. Journal of Oral and Maxillofacial Surgery. 2009;**67**(11):2192-2208

[33] Heufelder M, Kessler P. Advancements in digital workflow for orthognathic surgery. Oral and Maxillofacial Surgery Clinics of North America. 2015;**27**(4):527-543

[34] Hatcher DC. CBCT imaging in orthognathic surgery. Seminars in Orthodontics. 2010;**16**(2):79-90

[35] Marzola C, Raffaini M. 3D planning in orthognathic surgery: The path to predictability. Craniofacial Surgery Updates. 2020;**15**(2):125-134

[36] Chng C, Gandedkar N, Liou E. Surgery-First Orthodontic Management: A Clinical Guide to a New Treatment Approach. 2019. DOI: 10.1007/978-3-030-18696-8

[37] Raffaini M, Magri A. Advanced technologies in orthognathic surgery. Journal of Oral and Maxillofacial Surgery. 2021;**79**(4):678-689

[38] Gateno J, Xia JJ, Teichgraeber JF, et al. A new protocol for three-dimensional cephalometry: The anatomical interactive approach. American Journal of Orthodontics and Dentofacial Orthopedics. 2007;**132**(4):468-479

[39] Heufelder M et al. Accuracy of computer-assisted surgery in orthognathic treatment: A systematic review. International Journal of Oral and Maxillofacial Surgery. 2014;**43**(4):610-619

[40] Jacobs R, Quirynen M, et al. Digital planning and 3D printing for guided surgery. Clinical Oral Implants Research. 2018;**29**(3):23-38

[41] Arnett GW, Gunson MJ. Facial planning for orthognathic surgery. American Journal of Orthodontics and Dentofacial Orthopedics. 2004;**126**(3):290-295

[42] Proffit WR, White RP, Sarver DM. Contemporary Treatment of Dentofacial Deformity. Mosby; 2007

[43] Schendel SA, Carlotti AE. Changes in the soft tissue facial profile following mandibular advancement surgery. American Journal of Orthodontics and Dentofacial Orthopedics. 1991;**100**(3):213-222

[44] Stokbro K, Aagaard E, Torkov P, et al. Virtual planning in orthognathic surgery. International Journal of Oral and Maxillofacial Surgery. 2018;**47**(6):748-754

[45] Arnett GW, Gunson MJ. Facial and Dental Planning for Orthodontists and Oral Surgeons. Elsevier; 2010

[46] Raffaini M, Magri A. Advances in digital planning for orthognathic surgery. International Journal of Oral and Maxillofacial Surgery. 2021;**50**(6):789-800

[47] Xia JJ, Gateno J, Teichgraeber JF. Three-dimensional computer-assisted surgical simulation for maxillofacial surgery. Atlas of the Oral and Maxillofacial Surgery Clinics of North America. 2009;**17**(2):59-70

[48] Heufelder M et al. Accuracy of computer-assisted surgery in orthognathic treatment. International Journal of Oral and Maxillofacial Surgery. 2014;**43**(4):610-619

[49] Verweij JP et al. Clinical applications of 3D printing in orthognathic surgery. Oral Surgery, Oral Medicine, Oral Pathology and Oral Radiology. 2018;**126**(3):217-225

Chapter 9

Role of 3D Image Processing and Printing in the Diagnosis and Treatment Planning for Maxillofacial Surgery

Ruchi Pathak Kaul and Sushma Sagar

Abstract

Visualization plays an important role in diagnosis and treatment planning for patient care. To provide state-of-the-art care for individuals, especially for secondary reconstruction in cases of trauma, tumor or congenital defects, 3D image processing, and 3D printing play a significant role. For the past 45 years, 3D printing has been used by engineers to build innovative products. With the Industrial Revolution 4.0, technology has penetrated almost every sector and has enabled the possibility of solving complex problems. In the healthcare sector, especially for maxillofacial surgery, 3D printing and 3D image processing plays a vital role in the visualization of complex patient scenarios to planning difficult surgical procedures using different tools. This chapter discusses the successful application of 3D printing in maxillofacial surgery for the creation of patient specific models, guides/splints, and implants to enable better visualization, leading to better surgical planning. These procedures can be replicated by other surgeons to build more long-term scientific literature on this subject.

Keywords: 3D printing, image processing, maxillofacial surgery, surgical planning, visualization

1. Introduction

This chapter explores the transformative impact of 3D image processing and 3D printing on maxillofacial surgery. It delves into how these technologies enhance diagnosis, improves treatment planning, and optimizes surgical outcomes. This entire chapter is divided into five key sections including:

- An overview of 3D image processing and 3D printing
- The application of 3D image processing and 3D printing in maxillofacial surgery

 IntechOpen

- The benefits of 3D image processing and 3D printing in maxillofacial surgery
- Few case studies
- Future prospects with emerging technologies.

2. Overview of 3D image processing and 3D printing

2.1 Overview of 3D image processing

3D image processing refers to the techniques and methodologies used to analyze, manipulate, and visualize three-dimensional data obtained from various imaging modalities. These modalities can include computed tomography (CT), magnetic resonance imaging (MRI), and 3D ultrasound. The primary objective of 3D image processing is to transform raw data into meaningful and interpretable information that can be utilized for medical diagnosis, treatment planning, and research. Various software tools used in this process include Materialize MIMICS, Synopsys Simpleware, Slicer3D, Embodi3D, etc. [1, 2].

The principals involved in 3D image processing include:

- Image acquisition—This uses devices like CT scanners, 3D cameras, and MRI machines
- Image processing
- Image analysis
- Image visualization
- 3D model reconstruction and analysis.

3. History of 3D image processing

3.1 The beginning

The history of 3D image processing can be traced back to the early 1960s with the advent of computer graphics and the development of algorithms for rendering 3D objects. Early pioneers like Ivan Sutherland, who created the first interactive computer graphics program called Sketchpad in 1963, laid the groundwork for future advancements in 3D visualization [1–4].

3.2 1970s: Progress in imaging technologies

The introduction of CT scans and MRI in the 70s provided the first glimpses into the human body in three dimensions, revolutionizing medical diagnostics. This resulted in significant progress. Researchers began developing algorithms to process and visualize these 3D images, leading to the emergence of digital image processing.

3.3 1980s: Integration with computers

The 1980s marked a turning point with the widespread adoption of personal computers and the development of more sophisticated software for image processing. This era saw the introduction of techniques such as volume rendering and surface rendering, which allowed for more detailed and accurate 3D visualizations. The field of medical imaging benefited greatly from these advancements, enabling better diagnosis and treatment planning.

3.4 1990s: Growth of 3D modeling and printing

The 1990s witnessed the growth of 3D modeling and printing technologies. The invention of stereolithography (SLA) by Chuck Hull in 1984 and the subsequent development of other 3D printing technologies like fused deposition modeling (FDM) and selective laser sintering (SLS) opened new possibilities for creating physical models from digital data. These technologies were quickly adopted in various fields, including medicine, for creating anatomical models and surgical guides.

3.5 2000s: Enhanced processing power and algorithms

The 2000s brought significant improvements in processing power and the development of advanced algorithms for 3D image processing. With the rise of parallel computing and GPUs, it became possible to process large datasets more efficiently, leading to faster and more accurate 3D reconstructions. This era also saw the integration of artificial intelligence and machine learning techniques, further enhancing the capabilities of 3D image processing.

3.6 2010s: Democratization of 3D technologies

The 2010s marked the democratization of 3D image processing and printing technologies. The expiration of key patents and the emergence of low-cost, open-source 3D printers made these technologies more accessible to researchers, clinicians, and even hobbyists. This period also saw the development of bioprinting and the use of 3D printing for creating patient-specific implants and prosthetics.

3.7 Techniques used in 3D image processing

i. *Segmentation*: Segmentation involves dividing a 3D image into different regions or objects for focused analysis. Each segment corresponds to a distinct anatomical structure, tissue type, or organ. Various segmentation techniques include thresholding, region growing, clustering, and machine learning algorithms.

ii. *Registration*: Image registration aligns multiple 3D images obtained at different times, from different devices, or under different conditions, into a single coherent framework. Various techniques include rigid, affine, and non-rigid transformations. Advanced methods leverage feature-based and intensity-based approaches.

iii. *Visualization*: Visualization converts processed 3D data into comprehensible visual formats, enabling easier interpretation and analysis. Techniques include volume rendering, surface rendering, and maximum intensity projection (MIP).

iv. *Reconstruction*: 3D reconstruction involves creating a 3D model from 2D images or slice data. Techniques include tomographic reconstruction, such as filtered back projection (FBP) and iterative reconstruction.

v. *Quantification*: Quantification involves measuring anatomical or pathological features within a 3D image. The process includes calculating volume, surface area, shape analysis, and texture analysis.

vi. *Denoising*: Denoising reduces noise and artifacts in 3D images to improve image quality. Techniques include Gaussian filtering, median filtering, and more advanced methods like wavelet transform and deep learning-based approaches.

4. Overview of 3D printing

4.1 Definition of 3D printing

3D printing, also known as additive manufacturing, is a process of creating three-dimensional objects from a digital model by sequentially adding material layer by layer. Unlike traditional subtractive manufacturing methods, which remove material from a solid block, 3D printing builds objects from the ground up, allowing for complex geometries and intricate designs [1, 3, 5, 7, 10].

4.2 Principles of 3D printing

1. Digital design creation

    - Computer-aided design (CAD): The process begins with creating a digital 3D model using CAD software. Designers can create intricate models from scratch or use existing digital scans of real-world objects.

    - STL file format: The CAD model is then converted into an stereolithography (STL) file, which contains the geometric information of the object.

2. Slicing the model

    - Slicing software: The STL file is processed using slicing software, which divides the 3D model into thin horizontal layers. The slicing software also generates the instructions (G-code) that guide the 3D printer on how to build each layer.

    - Layer thickness: The thickness of each layer can vary depending on the desired resolution and the capabilities of the 3D printer.

3. Material selection

    - Variety of materials: 3D printing can utilize a wide range of materials, including plastics, metals, ceramics, and even biological tissues. The choice of material depends on the application and the specific 3D printing technology being used.

    - Filament, resin, powder: Materials can come in different forms, such as filament (for FDM printing), liquid resin (for SLA printing), or powder (for SLS printing).

4. Printing process

    - Layer-by-layer construction: The 3D printer constructs the object layer by layer, following the instructions provided by the slicing software. Each layer is added sequentially, with precise control over the material deposition.

    - Bonding layers: The printer ensures that each new layer bonds adequately with the previous one, forming a cohesive and solid structure.

5. Postprocessing

    - Removing supports: Some 3D printing techniques require support structures to stabilize the object during printing. After printing, these supports are removed.

    - Finishing touches: Additional postprocessing steps, such as sanding, painting, or curing (for resin-based prints), may be needed to achieve the desired surface finish and mechanical properties.

5. Historical background of 3D printing

5.1 Early beginnings

The concept of 3D printing dates to the early 1980s. In 1981, Dr. Hideo Kodama from the Nagoya Municipal Industrial Research Institute published a paper detailing a rapid prototyping technique using a photopolymer that could be polymerized by UV light. Although Kodama did not secure a patent, his work laid the foundation for future developments [1, 6, 7, 9].

5.2 The birth of stereolithography (SLA)

In 1984, Chuck Hull invented stereolithography (SLA), the first 3D printing technology. Hull founded 3D systems and released the SLA-1, the first commercial 3D printer, in 19,871. SLA uses a UV laser to cure a photosensitive resin layer by layer, creating highly detailed objects.

5.3 Expansion of technologies

The late 1980s and early 1990s saw the emergence of other 3D printing technologies, such as fused deposition modeling (FDM) by Scott Crump in 1989 and selective laser sintering (SLS) by Carl Deckard in 1988. These technologies expanded the range of materials and applications for 3D printing.

5.4 Democratization and open-source movement

The 2000s brought significant changes with the expiration of key patents and the rise of open-source initiatives like the RepRap Project in 2005. This project aimed to create a self-replicating 3D printer, making 3D printing more accessible and affordable. Companies like MakerBot further popularized 3D printing by introducing low-cost, user-friendly printers.

6. Advancements in 3D printing technology

6.1 Multi-material and multi-color printing

Recent advancements have enabled 3D printers to use multiple materials and colors simultaneously. This innovation allows for the creation of more complex and functional parts, such as wearable devices with integrated electronics.

6.2 Increased print speeds

Technologies like continuous liquid interface production (CLIP) and two-photon lithography have significantly reduced print times by enabling layer-less printing. These methods improve the quality and strength of the finished products.

6.3 Large-scale 3D printing

Advances in large-scale 3D printing are paving the way for constructing entire buildings and large infrastructure components. This technology has the potential to revolutionize the construction industry by reducing labor costs, construction time, and material waste.

6.4 Integration of AI and machine learning

Artificial intelligence and machine learning are being integrated into 3D printing software to optimize designs, reduce material usage, and ensure successful printing. Cloud-based platforms enable collaborative design, allowing teams to work together in real time from different locations.

6.5 Bioprinting and tissue engineering

3D printing is making significant strides in bioprinting and tissue engineering, with the development of bio-inks composed of living cells and biomaterials. This technology holds promise for creating tissue-like structures for medical and research applications.

3D printing has come a long way from its early days, transforming various industries and opening up new possibilities for innovation and customization.

6.6 Common 3D printing technologies

6.6.1 Fused deposition modeling (FDM)

- Principle: FDM works by extruding thermoplastic filament through a heated nozzle. The nozzle moves layer by layer, depositing the material to build up the object (**Figure 1**) [2–4, 7, 8, 10–13].
- Materials: Common materials include PLA, ABS, PETG, and other thermoplastics (**Figure 2**).
- Advantages: Cost-effective, user-friendly, suitable for a wide range of applications.

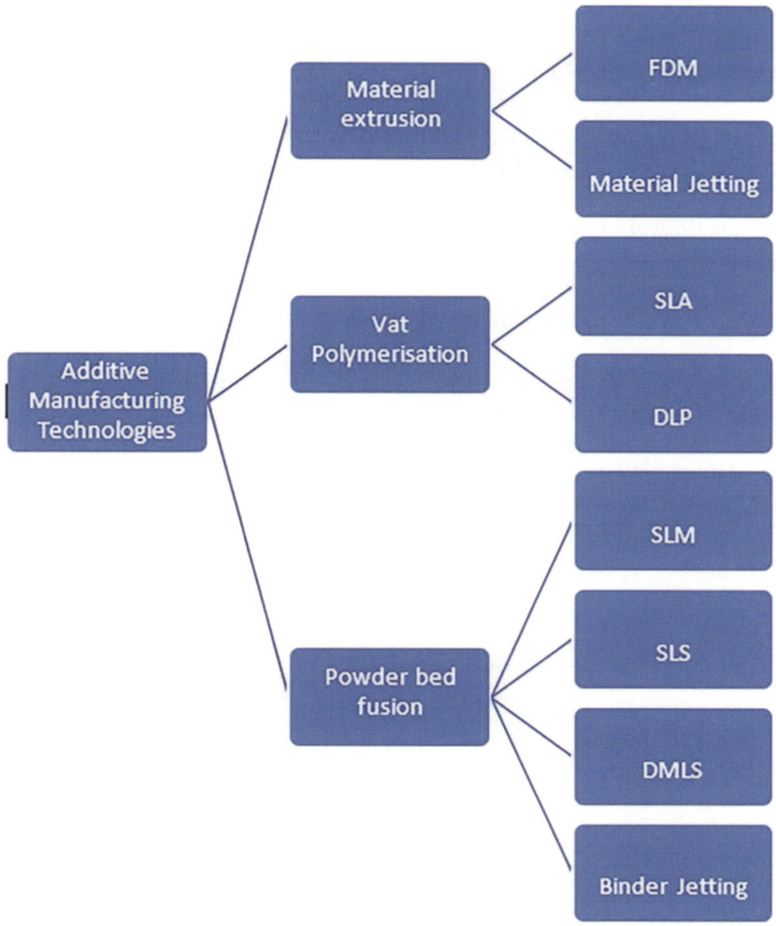

Figure 1.
Common 3D printing technologies.

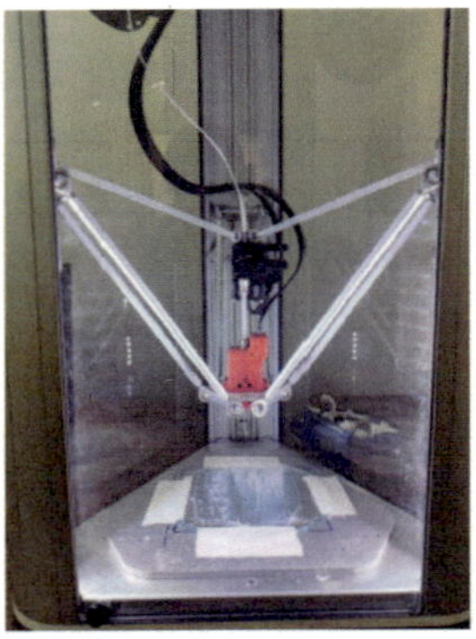

Figure 2.
FDM printer.

- Disadvantages: Lower resolution compared to other methods, visible layer lines, and limited material strength.
- Applications: Most medical models except soft tissues are made using this technology.

6.6.2 Stereolithography (SLA)

- Principle: SLA uses a UV laser to cure a photosensitive resin layer by layer. The laser selectively solidifies the resin to form the object (**Figure 3**).
- Materials: Photopolymer resins with various properties (e.g., flexible, rigid, and transparent).
- Advantages: High resolution, smooth surface finish, capable of fine details.
- Disadvantages: Expensive resins, postprocessing required to remove excess resin and cure the final object.
- Applications: Medical guides and splints along with implant template and molds can be made in biocompatible material using this technology.

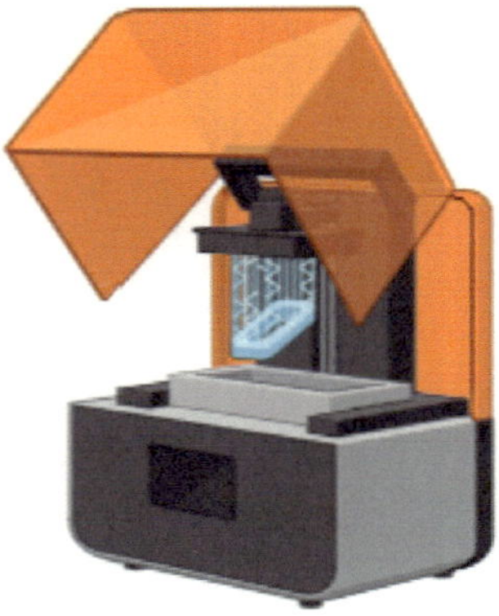

Figure 3.
SLA printer.

6.6.3 Selective laser sintering (SLS)

- Principle: SLS uses a high-powered laser to sinter powdered material, fusing the particles together layer by layer to create a solid object.
- Materials: Nylon, polyamide, and other powdered materials.
- Advantages: High strength, no need for support structures, suitable for complex geometries.
- Disadvantages: Expensive equipment and materials, rough surface finish, and powder handling considerations.

6.6.4 Digital light processing (DLP)

- Principle: DLP is similar to SLA but uses a digital light projector to cure the resin. The projector displays a complete layer at once, curing it in a single step.
- Materials: Photopolymer resins.
- Advantages: Faster than SLA, high resolution, smooth surface finish.
- Disadvantages: Limited build volume, expensive resins, postprocessing required.

6.6.5 Binder jetting

- Principle: Binder jetting involves depositing a liquid binding agent onto a bed of powdered material. The binder fuses the powder together to form each layer.
- Materials: Metal, sand, ceramics, and other powders.
- Advantages: Can produce large parts, variety of materials, no need for support structures.
- Disadvantages: Brittle parts, lower strength compared to other methods, and additional postprocessing needed for metal parts.

6.6.6 Direct metal laser sintering (DMLS)/selective laser melting (SLM)

- Principle: DMLS and SLM use a laser to fully melt metal powder, creating dense and robust metal parts layer by layer.
- Materials: Stainless steel, titanium, aluminum, and other metal powders.
- Advantages: High strength, suitable for functional parts, complex geometries.
- Disadvantages: Expensive equipment and materials require extensive postprocessing, safety considerations due to metal powders.

6.6.7 Material jetting

- Principle: Material jetting involves depositing droplets of photopolymer material through a print head. UV light cures each layer as it is deposited.
- Materials: Photopolymer resins, waxes.
- Advantages: High resolution, multi-material and multi-color printing, smooth surface finish.
- Disadvantages: Expensive, limited material options, and postprocessing required.

6.6.8 Electron beam melting (EBM)

- Principle: EBM uses an electron beam to melt metal powder layer by layer in a vacuum environment, creating high-strength metal parts.
- Materials: Titanium, cobalt-chrome, and other metal powders.
- Advantages: High strength, suitable for aerospace and medical applications, reduced residual stress.

Process types	Brief Description	Related Technology	Companies	Materials
Powder Bed Fusion	Thermal energy selectively fuses regions of a powder bed	Electron beam melting (EBM), selective laser sintering (SLS), selective heat sintering (SHS), and direct metal laser sintering (DMLS)	EOS (Germany), 3D Systems(US), Arcam (Sweden)	Metals, Polymers
Directed Energy Deposition	Focused thermal energy is used to fuse materials by melting as the material is being deposited	Laser metal deposition (LMD)	Optomec (US), POM (US)	Metals
Material Extrusion	Material is selectively dispensed through a through Nozzle or orifice	Fused deposition modelling (FDM)	Stratasys (Israel), Bits from Bytes (UK)	Polymers
Vat Photo polymerization	Liquid photopolymer in a vat is selectively cured by light-activated polymerization	Stereo lithography(SLA), digital light processing (DLP)		Photopolymers
Binder Jetting	A liquid bonding agent is selectively deposited to join powder materials	Powder bed and inkjet head (PBIH), plaster-based 3D printing (PP)	3D Systems (US), Ex One (US)	Polymers, Foundry Sand, Metals
Material Jetting	Droplets of build material are selectively deposited	Multi-jet modelling (MJM)	Objet (Israel), 3DSystems (US)	Polymers, Waxes
Sheet Lamination	Sheets of material are bonded to form an object	Laminated object manufacturing(LOM), ultrasonic consolidation (UC)	Fabrisonic (US), Mcor (Ireland)	Paper, Metals

Figure 4.
Seven processes as described by ASTM F-42.

- Disadvantages: Expensive equipment, limited material options, vacuum requirement.

Each of these technologies offers unique advantages and is suitable for different applications (**Figure 4**).

7. Applications for maxillofacial surgery

7.1 Diagnostic applications

- Enhanced imaging for accurate diagnosis (**Figure 5**)
- Integration with medical imaging modalities (CT, MRI, etc.)
- Visualization of complex anatomical structures [14, 15].

Enhanced 3D imaging plays a critical role in maxillofacial surgery by providing detailed and accurate visualization of complex anatomical structures. This improves diagnostic accuracy and aids in precise treatment planning. Modalities like CBCT, USG, CT, and MRI can be used for obtaining better visualization.

7.2 Advanced technologies for 3D imaging

1. Volumetric rendering and visualization software
    - Function: Advanced software tools convert volumetric imaging data into detailed 3D visualizations, allowing for interactive exploration and manipulation of anatomical structures.
    - Examples: 3D Slicer, Mimics, and OsiriX.
    - Applications: Preoperative planning, virtual surgical simulations, and educational purposes.

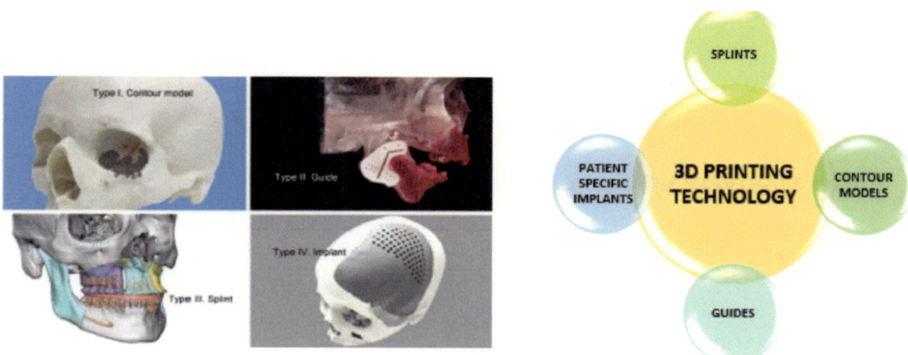

Figure 5.
Classification of applications of 3D printing technology in maxillofacial region.

2. 3D Printing and anatomical models

    - Function: 3D printing technology creates physical models of anatomical structures based on 3D imaging data. These models provide tactile feedback and enhance understanding of complex anatomies.

    - Applications: Surgical planning, custom implant design, and patient education.

3. Virtual Reality (VR) and augmented reality (AR)

    - Function: VR and AR technologies create immersive environments for visualizing and interacting with 3D imaging data. These technologies enhance spatial understanding and provide real-time guidance during surgical procedures.

    - Applications: Surgical training, intraoperative navigation, and patient consultation.

4. Artificial intelligence (AI) and machine learning

    - Function: AI algorithms analyze 3D imaging data to detect patterns, segment tissues, and assist in diagnosis. Machine learning models can predict surgical outcomes and suggest optimal treatment plans.

    - Applications: Automated diagnosis, personalized treatment planning, and enhanced image analysis.

7.3 Benefits of enhanced 3D imaging

1. Improved diagnostic accuracy

    - Enhanced 3D imaging provides detailed visualization of anatomical structures, leading to more accurate diagnoses and better-informed treatment decisions.

2. Precise treatment planning

    - Detailed 3D images allow for precise preoperative planning, reducing the risk of complications and improving surgical outcomes.

3. Enhanced surgical precision

    - Real-time 3D imaging and navigation technologies guide surgeons during procedures, enhancing precision and minimizing invasive techniques.

4. Patient-specific solutions

    - Custom anatomical models and implants based on 3D imaging data ensure personalized and optimal solutions for each patient.

Enhanced 3D imaging techniques and technologies are transforming maxillofacial surgery by providing accurate, detailed, and comprehensive visualizations that improve diagnostic and surgical outcomes. If you have any specific questions.

The integration of 3D printing with medical imaging modalities such as computed tomography (CT) and magnetic resonance imaging (MRI) has revolutionized personalized medicine and surgical planning.

7.4 Workflow integration

1. Data acquisition: Medical imaging modalities like CT and MRI are used to capture detailed images of a patient's anatomy. These images are stored in Digital Imaging and Communications in Medicine (DICOM) format, which is a standard for handling, storing, and transmitting medical imaging information (**Figure 6**) [2, 4, 5, 14, 16–18].

2. Image segmentation and processing: The acquired images are processed using specialized software to segment and isolate the anatomical structures of interest. This step involves identifying and separating different tissues, bones, and organs within the images.

3. 3D model creation: The segmented images are converted into 3D models using software tools such as Mimics, 3D Slicer, or OsiriX. These tools allow for the reconstruction of the patient's anatomy in a digital 3D format.

4. Design and customization: The 3D models are used to design and customize medical devices, implants, or surgical guides tailored to the patient's specific anatomy. This customization ensures a better fit and improved outcome.

5. 3D printing: The customized designs are sent to a 3D printer, which fabricates the physical objects layer by layer using materials such as plastics, metals, or biocom-

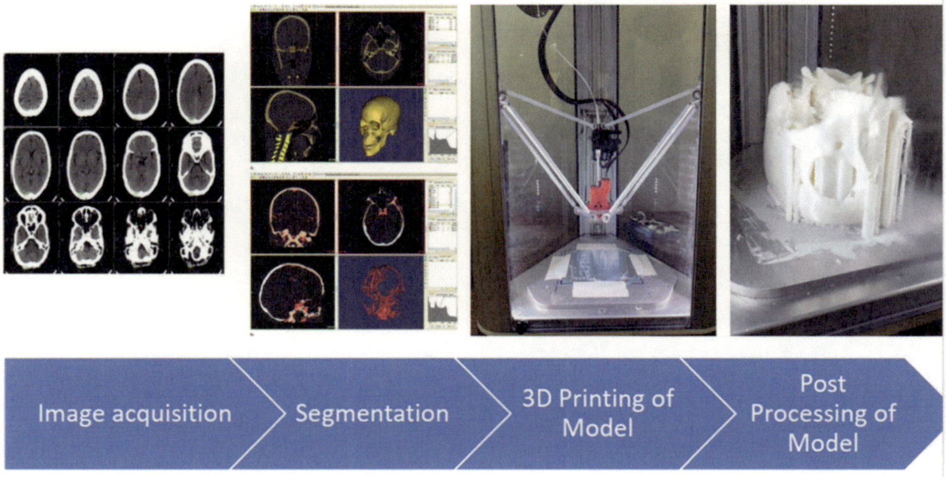

Figure 6.
Workflow of 3D printing a medical model.

patible resins. Common 3D printing technologies used include fused deposition modeling (FDM), stereolithography (SLA), and selective laser sintering (SLS)1.

6. Postprocessing: The printed objects may undergo postprocessing steps such as cleaning, curing, or surface finishing to achieve the desired properties and quality.

7.5 Applications and benefits

1. Surgical planning: 3D-printed models and surgical guides help surgeons plan complex procedures with greater precision, reducing surgical time and improving patient outcomes (**Figure** 7).

2. Custom implants: Patient-specific implants, such as cranial plates, dental implants, and joint replacements, are designed and manufactured to fit perfectly, enhancing biocompatibility and functionality.

3. Education and training: 3D-printed anatomical models are used for medical education and training, allowing students and professionals to practice procedures and understand complex anatomies better.

4. Prosthetics and orthotics: Customized prosthetics and orthotic devices are created to meet the unique needs of patients, improving comfort and functionality.

5. Research and development: 3D printing and medical imaging integration facilitate research in tissue engineering, drug delivery systems, and the development of new medical devices.

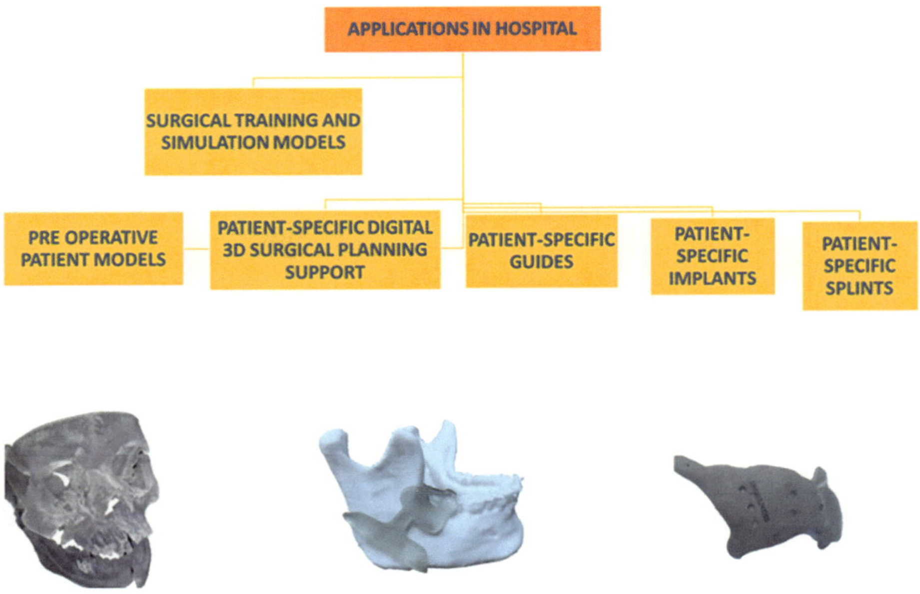

Figure 7.
Various applications of 3D printing in maxillofacial region.

7.6 Treatment planning

- Custom surgical guides and templates
- Simulation of surgical procedures
- Preoperative planning and risk assessment.

8. Surgical applications

8.1 Custom surgical guides and templates

i. Design and creation

ii. Principle: Custom surgical guides and templates are designed using advanced imaging techniques such as CT or MRI scans. These images are processed using computer-aided design (CAD) software to create a 3D model of the patient's anatomy. These 3D models are then utilized for surgical guide-making based on the bone's final position (**Figure 8**).

iii. Materials: Guides and templates are typically made from biocompatible materials like nylon, titanium, or resins suitable for 3D printing.

iv. Preoperative planning

v. Principle: Surgeons use the 3D models to simulate the surgical procedure, allowing them to plan the exact cuts, repositioning, and fixation required. These models provide haptic feedback to surgeons like the casts which are used in orthognathic. These, in turn, enable surgeons to visualize the anatomy three dimensionally and help in the incision planning and or bone movement more exactly. 3D models also play a vital role in patient education. This helps patients

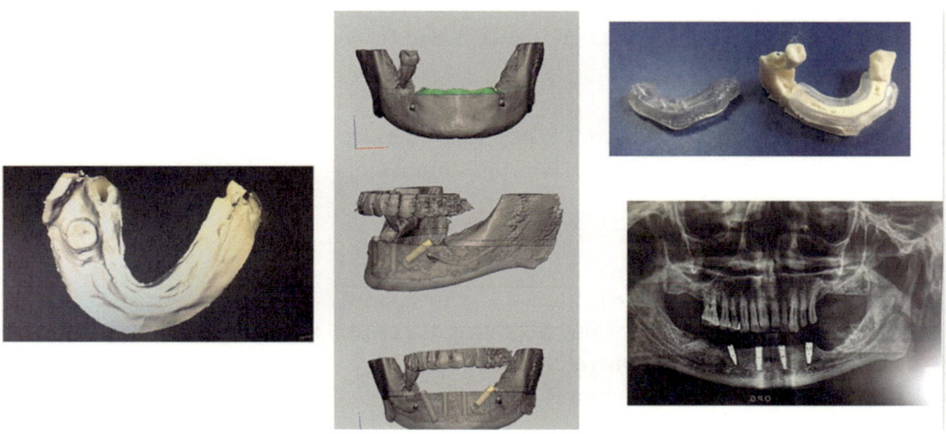

Figure 8.
Process of dental implant guide and alveoloplasty guide in an edentulous ridge using biocompatible material.

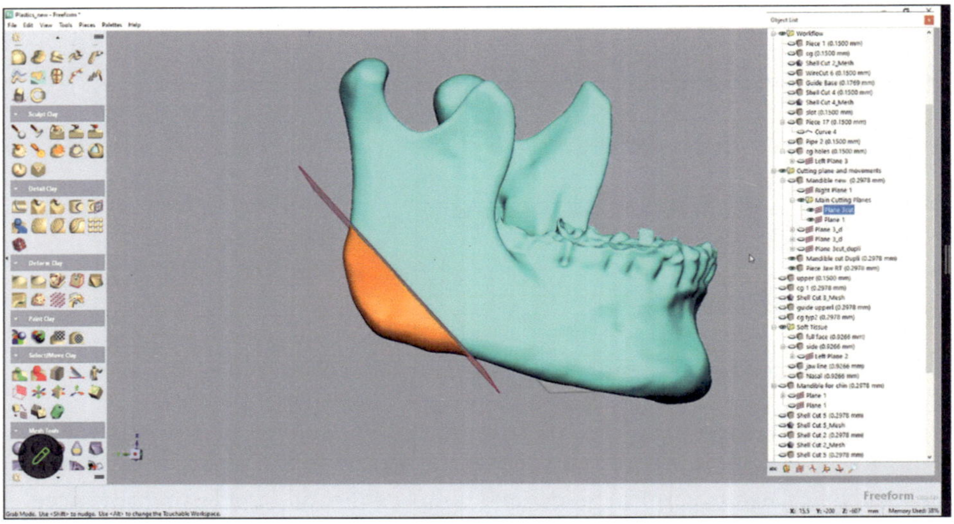

Figure 9.
Virtual surgical planning (VSP) for mandibular guides.

to visualize their treatment and outcome and be more vigilant of the postoperative care and responsibilities from the patient side. It thus improves patient perceptibility to the treatment and enhances the positive feedback, thereby resulting in early and enhanced recovery (**Figure 9**).

vi. Applications: Used in orthognathic surgery, craniofacial reconstruction, and implant placement.

vii. Intraoperative guidance

viii. Principle: During surgery, the custom guides and templates are used to ensure accurate execution of the preoperative plan. They help with precise bone cuts, alignment, and placement of implants. These precise cuts ensure the safety of important anatomical structures that lie in close proximity and thus provide execution of a clean surgical field. The screws in the guides also guide the position of the final implant and thus ensure the seamless procedure throughout.

ix. Applications: Enhances surgical precision, reduces the risk of errors, and minimizes the need for intraoperative adjustments.

x. Postoperative assessment

xi. Principle: After surgery, the guides and templates can be used to assess the accuracy of the procedure and make any necessary adjustments. This enables surgeons to do quality control, thereby creating a room for improvement and the future reduction of the errors if encountered.

xii. Applications: Ensures that the surgical outcomes align with the preoperative plan, improving patient satisfaction and recovery.

9. Benefits of 3D image processing & 3D printing in maxillofacial surgery

9.1 Improved accuracy and precision

- Reduction in surgical errors
- Enhanced anatomical understanding and visualization
- Better alignment and fit of implants.

9.2 Enhanced patient outcomes

- Reduced surgery time and shorter recovery periods
- Lower complication rates and improved healing
- Esthetic and functional improvements.

9.3 Cost-effectiveness

- Reduction in overall healthcare costs
- Efficient use of surgical resources
- Shortened hospital stays and fewer follow-up procedures.

10. Case studies

10.1 Case study 1

Dental rehabilitation using dental guide for surgical planning and placement of multiple implants (**Figure 10**)

- This case represents an edentulous jaw requiring dental rehabilitation with multiple implants.
- The placement of multiple implants can be planned on the surgical planning software. The implant guide can be prepared after the final positions of the implant are locked.
- As a result of virtual surgical planning (VSP) and dental guide, 6 implants can be placed at accurately planned positions in less time. This helps patients to be rehabilitated quickly in less time with better surgical accuracy and postoperative complications.

10.2 Case study 2

10.2.1 Maxillary reconstruction using guides for fibula

- This case represents a maxillary defect which requires rehabilitation with free fibula to accommodate teeth and allow the patient to eat food (**Figure 11**).

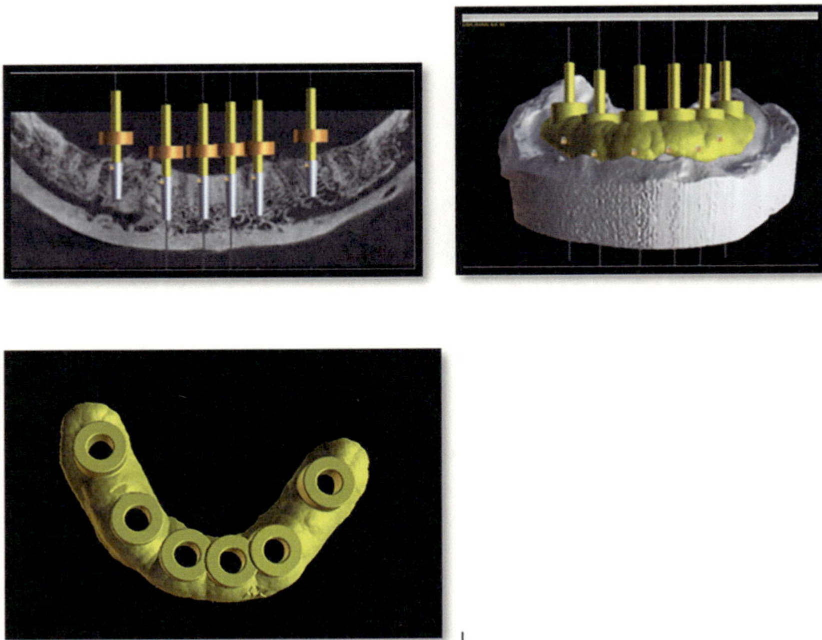

Figure 10.
Virtual planning of multiple implant positioning and dental guide fabrication.

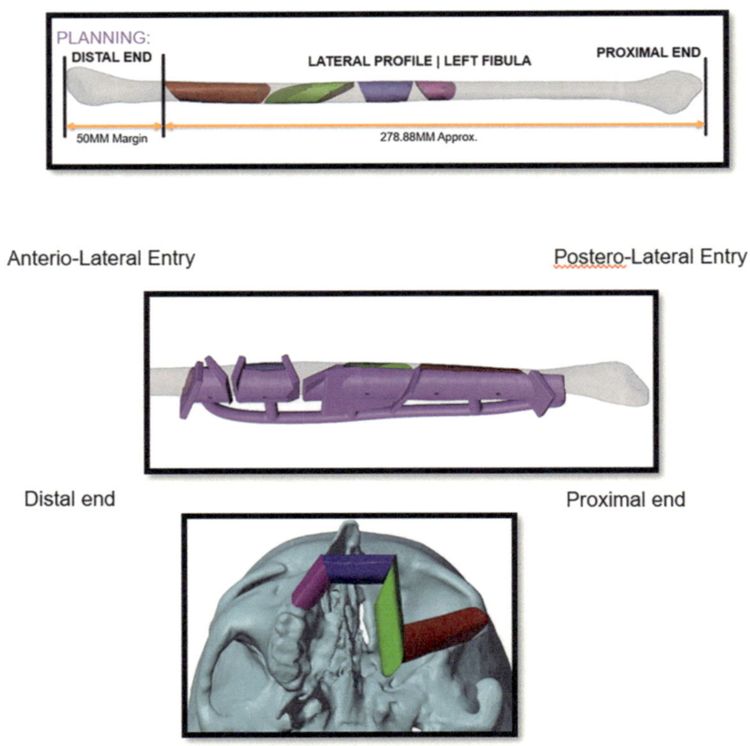

Figure 11.
Virtual surgical plan of harvesting the fibula to reconstruct maxilla.

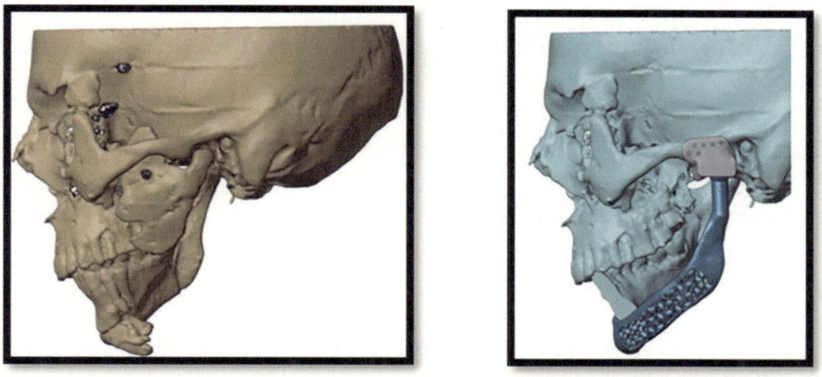

Figure 12.
Pre and post reconstruction of temporomandibular joint after gunshot injury defect in a patient.

- Utilization of 3D technologies in planning and execution, the surgical resection of fibula is planned with the surgeon, and a fibula guide is created to reconstruct maxilla during the surgery.

- The virtual surgical planning for harvesting fibula and accurately reconstructing the maxilla allows accurate surgical procedure with less complications and postoperative recovery.

10.3 Case study 3

10.3.1 Temporomandibular joint reconstruction

- This case represents a maxilla-mandibular defect along with temporomandibular joint reconstruction to rehabilitate the patient with lower jaw and joint (**Figure 12**).

- Virtual surgical planning to fabricate the left temporomandibular joint is done along with extension in mandible to recreate the natural position of jaw in the patient.

- The virtual surgical planning allows accurate positioning of the temporomandibular joint to facilitate mouth opening for the patient. Functional as well as esthetic outcome of the patient is satisfactory. The defect is reconstructed accurately to facilitate function and esthetics without much postoperative complications.

11. Future prospects and innovations

Innovative technologies like medical 3D printing, augmented, and virtual reality have been impacting human health in the past few years. Personalized medicine and patient-specific treatments hold a great future to provide state-of-the-art care for patients. The covid pandemic has proven that leveraging technology can help healthcare expand its capabilities and successfully serve the world population. Emerging technologies have the potential to enhance human performance to the extent of performing remote surgeries. Some of the areas which have the potential to bring about rapid development in the growth of science and technology include:

- Advances in 3D bioprinting and tissue engineering
- Integration with artificial intelligence and machine learning
- Development of hybrid imaging and printing systems

Some of the challenges in the newer developments which need more clarity and mitigation include

- Ethical and regulatory implications
- Technical limitations and areas for improvement
- Adoption barriers and potential solutions.

12. Conclusion

This chapter addresses the various tools, techniques, and benefits of using visualization and 3D image processing for complicated cases. This is followed by various examples of cases which are planned to use 3D printing. The chapter finally concludes addressing future prospects of emerging technologies in the present times.

Acknowledgements

I am thankful to All India Institute of Medical Sciences, New Delhi, our private practitioners along with the patients who trusted me to plan cases for them using 3D printing technology. We would like to acknowledge Indian Council of medical research (ICMR) for funding this chapter as per File no5/3/8/3/2022/MDMS.

Conflict of interest

The author declares no conflict of interest.

DOI: http://dx.doi.org/10.5772/intechopen.1009516

Author details

Ruchi Pathak Kaul[1,2]* and Sushma Sagar[2]

1 University College London, United Kingdom

2 All India Institute of Medical Sciences, New Delhi, India

*Address all correspondence to: r.kaul@ucl.ac.uk

References

[1] Synopsys, Inc. Simpleware Medical: Clinical Applications and Point-of-Care 3D Printing [Internet]. Sunnyvale (CA): Synopsys; 2024 [cited 2025 Feb 01]. Available from: https://www.synopsys.com/simpleware/clinical-applications.html

[2] Kaul RP, Parthasarthy J. Fundamentals of 3D Printing Technology for Medical and Dental Professionals (Illustrated). Available from: https://www.amazon.in/Fundamentals-Printing-Technology-Professionals-Illustrated-ebook/dp/B093JLYLS5/ref=cm_cr_arp_d_pb_opt?ie=UTF8

[3] Kaul RP, Malviya A, Sagar S, Kumar S, Gupta A, Kumar A. An experimental study conducted on material properties used in a FDM printer for medical models. Fortune Journal of Health Sciences. 2024;**7**:767-778

[4] Dutta A, Singh M, Kumar K, Navarro AR, Santiago R, Kaul RP, et al. Accuracy of 3D printed spine models for pre-surgical planning of complex adolescent idiopathic scoliosis (AIS) in spinal surgeries: A case series. Annals of 3D Printed Medicine. 2023;**11**:100-117

[5] Kaul RP, Sagar S. Personalization of surgery with 3D printing technology: A new frontier. The Indian Journal of Medical Research. 2020;**152**(Supplement):254-255. DOI: 10.4103/ijmr.IJMR_2338_19

[6] Paul GM, Rezaienia A, Wen P, Condoor S, Parkar N, King W, et al. Medical Applications for 3D Printing: Recent Developments Missouri Medicine. 2018;**115**(1):75

[7] Martelli N, Serrano C, van den Brink H, Pineau J, Prognon P, Borget I, et al. Advantages and disadvantages of 3-dimensional printing in surgery: A systematic review. Surgery. Jun 2016;**159**(6):1485-1498. DOI: 10.1016/j.surg.2015.12.017. Epub 2016 Jan 30

[8] Lee C, Ventola. Medical applications of 3D printing: Current uses and projected uses. P&T. 2014;**39**(10):704-711

[9] Chepelev et al. Radiological Society of North America (RSNA) 3D printing special interest group (SIG): Guidelines for medical 3D printing and appropriateness for clinical scenarios. 3D Printing in Medicine. 2018;**4**:11

[10] Parthasarathy J. 3D modelling, custom implants, and its future perspectives in craniofacial surgery. Annals of Maxillofacial Surgery. 2014;**4**(1):9-18

[11] Bauermeister AJ, Zuriarrain A, Newman MI. Three-dimensional printing in plastic and reconstructive surgery: A systematic review. Annals of Plastic Surgery. Nov 2016;**77**(5):569-576

[12] Witowski J, Sitkowski M, Zuzak T, Coles-Black J, Chuen J, Major P, et al. From ideas to long-term studies: 3D printing clinical trials review. International Journal of Computer Assisted Radiology and Surgery. 2018;**13**:1473-1478

[13] Huang MF, Alfi D, Alfi J, Huang AT. The use of patient-specific implants in oral and maxillofacial surgery. Oral and Maxillofacial Surgery Clinics of North America. 2019;**31**:593-600

[14] Hua J, Aziz S, Shum JW. Virtual surgical planning in oral and maxillofacial surgery. Oral and Maxillofacial Surgery Clinics of North America. 2019;**31**:519-530

[15] Tack P, Victor J, Gemmel P, Annemans L. 3D-printing techniques in a medical setting: A systematic literature review. Biomedical Engineering Online. 2016;**15**:115

[16] Matias M, Zenha H, Costa H. Custom-made implants for Craniomaxillofacial reconstructive surgery. Craniomaxillofac Trauma Reconstruction. 2017;**10**:89-98

[17] Marinho ROM, Freire-Maia B. Management of fractures of the zygomaticomaxillary complex. Oral and Maxillofacial Surgery Clinics of North America. 2013;**25**:617-636

[18] Ehrenfeld M, Manson PN, Prein J. Principles of internal fixation of the craniomaxillofacial skeleton trauma and orthognathic surgery. Midfacial Fractures. 2012;**3**:181-256